Applied Anatomy for the FRCA

Applied Anatomy for the FRCA

Edited by
Bobby Krishnachetty and Abdul Syed

Associate Editor
Harriet Scott

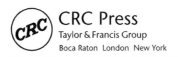

CRC Press
Taylor & Francis Group
Boca Raton London New York

CRC Press is an imprint of the
Taylor & Francis Group, an **informa** business

First edition published 2021
by CRC Press
6000 Broken Sound Parkway NW, Suite 300, Boca Raton, FL 33487-2742

and by CRC Press
2 Park Square, Milton Park, Abingdon, Oxon, OX14 4RN

ISBN: 978-0-367-07620-7 (pbk)
ISBN: 978-0-367-25492-6 (hbk)
ISBN: 978-0-429-02166-4 (ebk)

Typeset in RotisSerif
by Deanta Global Publishing Services, Chennai, India

Contents

Foreword

There is continued debate about how anatomy is best taught at the undergraduate level, but almost universal agreement that the subject's place in curricula has eroded dramatically in the last few decades. The inevitable consequence is young doctors who lack fundamental knowledge and exposure to anatomy upon graduating. Although there are some specialties that will not notice the deficiency, doctors wishing to train in anaesthesia, intensive care and pain medicine may feel themselves at a distinct disadvantage. Practice in these specialties requires anatomical knowledge to be applied almost daily and it is therefore right for FRCA exam candidates to continue to be rigorously tested for proficiency in this area. Herein lies the rationale for this book.

The challenge for any good textbook is to find the right balance between giving sufficient and too much information, having the correct ratio of text to illustration and to be interesting enough to be readable at the end of a busy clinical shift. The text is straightforward and is livened up by illustrations that are hand-drawn and digitally drawn images directed by the authors. This book has also been written by working clinicians who not only regularly put their own understanding of anatomy to the test in their clinical roles, but have taught the subject to postgraduate trainees over many years and have successfully prepared candidates for the FRCA examinations. This gives it a strong foundation of clinical and academic relevance.

I am confident that trainees will find this book a useful resource to help prepare for the FRCA exams, but clinical educators will also turn to it to refresh their own memory of difficult-to-recall areas of anatomy when they come to teach it. This book will hopefully provide a valuable addition to the trainee's library and will ultimately achieve its stated aim – to help deliver success in the FRCA examinations.

Prof. John Kinnear
Honorary Consultant in Critical Care Medicine
Head of ARU School of Medicine
Head of Zambia MMed Anaesthesia Training Programme

Contributors

Editors
Bobby Krishnachetty
Southend University Hospital
Southend, UK

Abdul Syed
Southend University Hospital
Southend, UK

List of Contributors
Lisa Elam
Barts and The London School of Anaesthesia
London, UK

Mark Gotecha
East of England School of Anaesthesia
Cambridge, UK

Gopal Govindarajan
Queen's Hospital
Romford, UK

Hannah Hines
Barts and The London School of Anaesthesia
London, UK

Anokha Oomman Joseph
North Middlesex Hospital
London, UK

Janso Padickakudi Joseph
Southend University Hospital
Southend, UK

Snehal Ramnath Kumbhare
Southend University Hospital
Southend, UK

Jignesh Khilan Kumar Patel
North Central Thames School of Anaesthesia
London, UK

Jagdish Sokhi
Imperial School of Anaesthesia
London, UK

Associate Editor
Harriet Scott
Barts and The London School of Anaesthesia
London, UK

Teena Thomas
Southend University Hospital
Southend, UK

Simon Trundle
Royal London Hospital
London, UK

Sarra Wang
Barts and The London School of Anaesthesia
London, UK

Artists
Ashitha Sahana Abdul
Chelmsford County High School
Chelmsford, UK

Elizabeth Filips
King's College London
London, UK

Bobby Krishnachetty
Southend University Hospital
Southend, UK

Billy Leung
Royal Berkshire Hospital
Reading, UK

Rino Maeda
Southend University Hospital
Southend, UK

Nandagudi S Niranjan
Broomfield Hospital
Chelmsford, UK

Amrit Roopra
Barts and The London School of Anaesthesia
London, UK

Our thanks to **Dr Manohary Selvakumaran** and **Dr Eric Makmur** of Southend University Hospital for the ultrasound images.

Introduction

Anatomy knowledge is a requirement for both the primary and final components of the FRCA. During medical training, acquiring this knowledge is not standard but follows a variety of teaching methods such as dissections, prosections and anatomage leading to varied levels of background interest and awareness.

Anatomy and the Anaesthetic Exam

Considerable knowledge in anatomy is an important curriculum requirement in current anaesthetic training leading up to certificate of completion of training (CCT). Albeit being an essential curriculum and exam requirement, it is rarely taught during anaesthetic training but is incorporated with regional anaesthetic procedures. The trainees are heavily judged on relevant anatomical topics in both parts of the fellowship examination, and lack of sufficient knowledge would lead to a failure in the exam. Questions related to anatomy appear in

- Primary FRCA – as multiple true/false questions and the objective structured clinical examination (MTFs and OSCEs), e.g. laryngeal nerve damage, fetal circulation and ultrasound guided nerve blocks
- Final FRCA – as short answer questions and the new constructed response questions (SAQs and CRQs), e.g. fetal circulation, pain pathway, labour analgesia and the dreaded vagus nerve!

The recent changes in the final FRCA structured oral examinations (SOE) has shed more light on anatomy and its clinical application. Despite this, anatomy is an area which is famously detested and feared by trainees. Hence, there is no doubt that revision for the exam should include dedicated time for anatomy.

Content and Layout

This book intends to cover the anatomy curriculum tailored to anaesthetists including answers to past exam questions. The book is divided into sections pertaining to anatomical regions (head and neck, thorax, abdomen, spine, upper and lower limbs). The topics of importance to anaesthetists in each section is presented under 'structures', 'circulation' and 'nervous system' (with relevance to regional anaesthesia). We believe this will make revising easy and targeted. It is important to note that this is not just an anatomy reference book but includes a wide range of questions of clinical relevance that are asked in the exam. This, in our opinion, is a big selling point for the book.

Contributors

The contributors are consultants and trainees within the East of England and the North East London school of anaesthesia. They are handpicked for their enthusiasm as educators and their continued interest in providing faculty support to the primary and final FRCA exam revision courses. Each topic is extensively researched and referenced, yet presented in a simple format for maximum retention.

Artists

We are very lucky to have found our artists who have produced amazing drawings. They range from an aspiring medical student to a retired cosmetic surgeon, who have produced hand-drawn and digitally illustrated images. The images are in colour which are not only aesthetically pleasing, but also easy to reciprocate.

Conclusion

It is needless to say that anatomy forms an important element in the anaesthetic exams. This book aims to provide sufficient knowledge to trainee anaesthetists preparing for the primary and final fellowship exams and other practising anaesthetists. The topics covered are derived from the curriculum and the subject matter includes the most up-to-date version of past exam questions. We have put a lot of thought into the content, diagrams and overall layout of this book, considering common gaps in knowledge and struggles encountered by trainees. We sincerely hope we have done justice to an extensive and difficult topic such as anatomy by writing this book which will supplement revision for FRCA as well as serve as a reference point for anatomy knowledge throughout your training.

What it is not: It is neither a standalone anatomy textbook nor a regional anaesthesia handbook.

For the anatomy haters: Basic knowledge is essential, but it is always attached to clinical relevance... So it is not all that boring!

Happy reading!

HEAD AND NECK

Structures

- Scalp and base of skull
- Brain
- Pituitary gland
- Eye and optic tract
- Nose
- Sagittal section of head and neck
- Cross section at C6
- Larynx with grades at laryngoscopy
- Triangles of neck

Circulation

- Arterial supply of head and neck
- Great veins of head and neck

Nervous System

- Cranial nerves – II, V, VII and X
- Scalp blocks
- Eye blocks
  - Sub-Tenon's block
  - Retrobulbar block
  - Peribulbar block
- Laryngeal nerve blocks
- Cervical plexus block

Structures

- Scalp and base of skull
- Brain
- Pituitary gland
- Eye and optic tract
- Nose
- Sagittal section of head and neck
- Cross section at C6
- Larynx with grades at laryngoscopy
- Triangles of neck

Scalp and Base of Skull

What are the layers of the scalp covering the skull (Figure 1.1)?

Use the SCALP mnemonic

- Skin with hair follicles and sebaceous glands
- Connective tissue with neurovasculature of the scalp
- Aponeurosis (galea aponeurotica)
- Loose areolar connective tissue which serves as a plane of access in neurosurgery. It is also called the 'danger zone of the scalp' as infection from scalp can reach the meninges through emissary veins.
- Periosteum

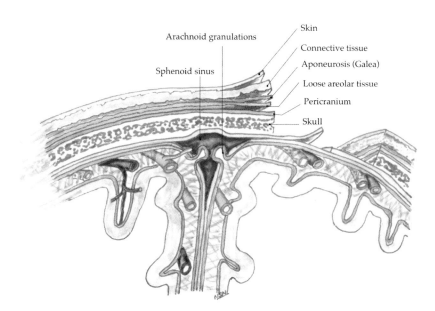

Figure 1.1   Layers of scalp.

Which bones make up the skull?

The skull is made up of eight bones which are interconnected by sutures which are immovable fibrous joints.

- One each of the frontal, sphenoid, occipital and ethmoid bones
- Two of the parietal and temporal bones

Briefly describe the structures that pass through the various foramina in the base of the skull.

Out of the different foramina, there are a few which are easy to remember: foramen caecum in front of the crista galli, cribriform plate, superior orbital fissure, foramen magnum, stylomastoid foramen, hypoglossal canal on either side of the foramen magnum.

The other foramina can be remembered as

OROS LAJ – in order of their appearance as shown in the figures (Figures 1.2 and 1.3).

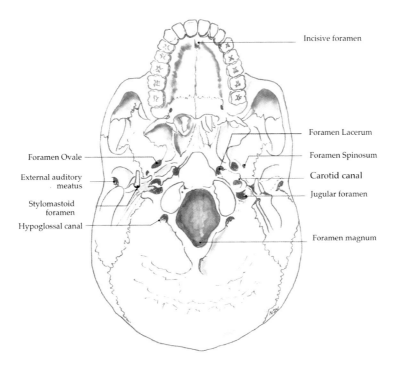

Figure 1.2   Base of skull – inferior surface.

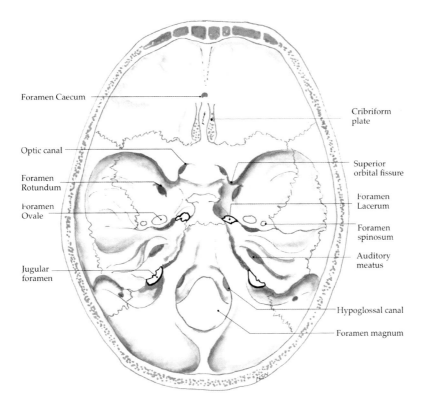

Figure 1.3   Base of skull – inner surface.

The base of the skull with its foramina and contents is shown in Table 1.1.

Table 1.1   Major Cranial Foramina and the Structures Passing Through

Foramen	Contents
Foramen caecum	Emissary vein from nose to superior sagittal sinus
Cribriform plate	Olfactory nerve Anterior ethmoidal nerve
Superior orbital fissure (Live Frankly To See Absolutely No InSult)	Lacrimal nerve (branch of ophthalmic nerve) Frontal nerve (branch of ophthalmic nerve) Trochlear nerve Superior branch of oculomotor nerve Abducens nerve Nasociliary nerve (branch of ophthalmic nerve) Inferior branch of oculomotor nerve Superior and inferior ophthalmic vein
Optic canal	Optic nerve Ophthalmic artery
Foramen rotundum	Maxillary nerve (V_2)
Foramen ovale (O-MALE)	Mandibular nerve (V_3) Accessory meningeal nerve Lesser petrosal nerve Emissary vein
Foramen spinosum (S-MEN)	Middle meningeal artery and vein Emissary vein Nervus spinosus
Foramen lacerum (L-GEMI)	Meningeal branch of ascending pharyngeal artery Emissary vein Traversed partially by Internal carotid artery Greater petrosal nerve
Auditory meatus	Facial nerve Vestibulocochlear nerve Labyrinthine vessels
Jugular foramen	Inferior petrosal sinus/sigmoid sinus Glossopharyngeal nerve Vagus nerve Accesory nerve Occipital artery
Carotid canal	Internal carotid artery with venous and sympathetic plexus

(Continued)

Table 1.1 (Continued)   Major Cranial Foramina and the Structures Passing Through

Foramen	Contents
Hypoglossal canal	Hypoglossal nerve Meningeal branch of hypoglossal nerve Emissary vein
Stylomastoid foramen	Facial nerve Posterior auricular artery
Foramen magnum	Medulla oblongata Meninges Spinal accessory nerves Spinal arteries Dural veins

For completeness, the foramina through which the cranial nerves exit the skull are summarised in Table 1.2.

Table 1.2   Foramina Through which the Cranial Nerves Exit the Brain

Cranial nerve	Foramina
I – olfactory	Cribriform plate of ethmoid
II – optic	Optic canal of sphenoid
III – oculomotor	Superior orbital fissure
IV – trochlear	Superior orbital fissure
V – trigeminal	V_1 – ophthalmic – superior orbital fissure V_2 – maxillary – foramen rotundum V_3 – mandibular – foramen ovale
VI – abducens	Superior orbital fissure
VII – facial	Internal auditory meatus $\longrightarrow$ facial canal $\longrightarrow$ stylomastoid foramen
VIII – vestibulocochlear	Internal auditory meatus
IX – glossopharyngeal	Jugular foramen
X – vagus	Jugular foramen
XI – accessory	Enters by the foramen magnum, exits by the jugular foramen
XII – hypoglossal	Hypoglossal canal

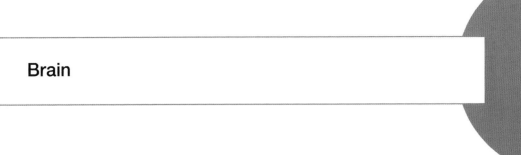

Brain

What is the normal cerebral blood flow to the grey and white matter? What is the overall cerebral blood flow to the brain? What percentage is this of cardiac output?

The normal cerebral blood flow to grey matter is 70 ml/100 g/min and to white matter is 20 ml/100 g/min. The overall cerebral blood flow to the brain is 50 ml/100 g/min.

The percentage of cardiac output is approximately 14% (700 ml/min).

Describe the meningeal layers that surround the brain and the spinal cord.

The brain and spinal cord are surrounded by three layers of membranes called the meninges. A tough outer layer (dura mater), a delicate middle layer (arachnoid mater) and an inner layer firmly attached to the surface of the brain (pia mater).

Describe the arterial supply to the dura mater.

The arterial supply to the dura mater consists of

- Anterior meningeal arteries which are branches of the ethmoidal artery
- Middle and accessory meningeal arteries arising from the maxillary artery
- Posterior meningeal artery which is a branch of the ascending pharyngeal artery
- Meningeal branches from the occipital artery and vertebral artery

What is the innervation of the dura mater?

The dura mater is supplied by the meningeal branches of all three divisions of the trigeminal nerve (V_1, V_2 and V_3) and the first, second and third cervical nerves.

Pituitary Gland

The pituitary gland is located in the *sella turcica* of the sphenoid bone at the base of the skull. The roof is formed by an incomplete fold of dura, the *diaphragma sella*, which is traversed by the pituitary stalk and optic chiasm. The fossa is limited posteriorly by the clivus of the sphenoid and inferiorly and anteriorly by the sphenoidal air sinuses. The lateral walls are in close relation to the cavernous sinus, internal carotid artery, CN III, IV, V1, V2 and VI (Figures 1.4 and 1.5).

The pituitary gland weighs 500–900 mg and is divided into the anterior and posterior glands. The two parts of the pituitary gland function as separate endocrine organs with different cell populations and functionality.

The *anterior pituitary gland (adenohypophysis)* is an evagination of the ectodermal Rathke's pouch. The anterior lobe is further divided into the par distalis, pars tuberalis and par intermedia.

The *posterior pituitary (neurohypophysis)* is divided into the pars nervosa and the infundibulum. Developmentally the posterior pituitary arises from the forebrain and is an extension of the hypothalamus.

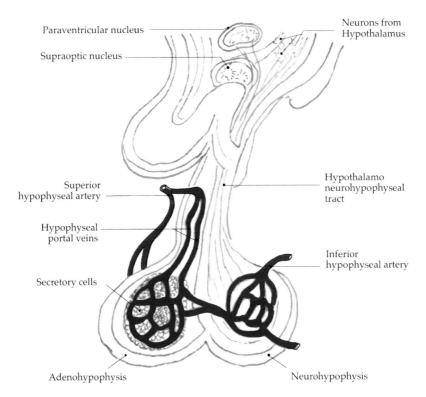

Figure 1.4   Pituitary gland – structure.

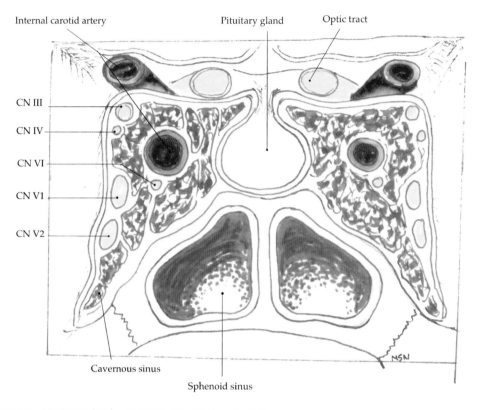

Figure 1.5   Pituitary gland – anatomical position and relations.

Arterial supply

- Superior and inferior hypophyseal arteries, which are branches of the internal carotid artery. They form a capillary network with the hypothalamo-hypophyseal portal system. The primary capillary network lies at the pituitary stalk, where the hypothalamic hormones are released. This capillary bed is drained by a set of long portal veins that give rise to the second capillary bed in the anterior pituitary. The veins originating in the neurohypophyseal capillary plexus give rise to the short portal veins that will also contribute to the adenohypophyseal capillary plexus and connect the two circulatory systems.
- This hypothalamo-hypophyseal portal system creates a communication between the endocrine and neural cells providing an easy short loop feedback between the two sets of cells.

Venous drainage

- Venous drainage from the gland is into the cavernous sinus and then onto the petrosal sinus and finally into the jugular vein.

What is a portal circulation and what are the other examples in the body?

A portal circulation begins and ends in capillaries. Arterial capillaries normally end up forming a vein that enters the right side of the heart. In a portal circulation, the primary capillary network drains into a vein known as a portal vein. This then branches to form a second set of capillaries before draining into the venous system. Other examples of a portal circulation are the hepatic portal, placental, renal, ovarian and testicular circulations.

Which hormones are released by the pituitary?

- Anterior pituitary – growth hormone (GH), adrenocorticotrophic hormone (ACTH), thyroid stimulating hormone (TSH), follicle stimulating hormone (FSH), luteinising hormone (LH) and prolactin
- Posterior pituitary – antidiuretic hormone (ADH) and oxytocin

What are the types of pituitary tumours? What are their clinical manifestations?

Pituitary tumours are classified by size into

Microadenomas

- <10 mm in diameter, most commonly occurring pituitary adenomas
- Clinical effects are mainly due to hormonal hyper-secretion
- The commonest pituitary hormone secreted by these tumours is prolactin (35%), followed by GH (20%) and ACTH (7%)

Macroadenomas

- >10 mm in size
- Non-secretory tumours
- Clinical effects are usually due to mass and pressure effects leading to visual disturbances, increased intracranial pressure and hypopituitarism due to destruction of pituitary tissue.

Hyperprolactinaemia – due to increased prolactin secretion

- Male – impotence, reduced facial hair and galactorrhoea
- Female – weight gain, menstrual disturbance, infertility and galactorrhoea

Acromegaly – due to increased GH, after epiphyseal closures

- Musculoskeletal features – prognathism, prominent supraorbital ridges, increased skull size, large hands and feet
- Soft tissues – macroglossia, enlarged nose, thickening of the laryngeal and pharyngeal soft tissues, laryngeal stenosis, hoarse voice due to recurrent laryngeal nerve palsy
- Heart – myocardial hypertrophy, interstitial fibrosis and cardiomegaly leads to ischaemic heart disease and left ventricular dysfunction
- Miscellaneous – sleep apnoea, hypertension and diabetes mellitus secondary to the anti-insulin effect of growth hormone

Cushing's disease – due to increased ACTH

- Central weight gain and obesity, moon face, extra fat around neck ('buffalo hump'), hirsutism, thin skin, abdominal striae, easy bruising, poor wound healing
- Proximal myopathy, fatigue, depression
- Hypertension and hyperglycaemia

What are the anaesthetic concerns for a patient undergoing surgery for acromegaly?

Anaesthetic concerns can be classified into

Neurosurgical anaesthesia and its complications

- Haemodynamic instability
- Maintenance of cerebral oxygenation
- Prevention of perioperative complications such as venous air embolism in the sitting position
- Rapid emergence to facilitate neurological assessment
- Adequate postoperative analgesia and antiemesis

Acromegaly and its implications

- Airway – the clinical features of acromegaly lead to an increased risk of a difficult ventilation and intubation. An awake fibreoptic intubation may be necessary.
- Respiratory – coarsening of features leading to upper airway obstruction leads to an obstructive picture on spirometry. Also, obstructive sleep apnoea can increase the risk of difficulties with ventilation and intubation and sensitivity to opioids.
- Cardiovascular – myocardial hypertrophy, interstitial fibrosis, hypertension and cardiomegaly lead to ischaemic heart disease and left ventricular dysfunction.
- Neurological – compression of surrounding structures leading to visual disturbances, increased ICP and cavernous sinus thrombosis.
- Endocrine – impaired glucose tolerance and diabetes mellitus complicates more than 25% of acromegalic patients hence the need for careful glucose monitoring and management.

Which electrolyte is most commonly affected after pituitary surgery?

After pituitary surgery the most commonly affected electrolyte is sodium. This can be due to diabetes insipidus (DI) due to decreased secretion of ADH. Inappropriate water loss leads to hypernatraemia and increased serum osmolality in the context of large volumes of dilute urine. Treatment aims at replacement of water and ADH. Intranasal or intravenous desmopressin (Deamino D Arginine Vasopressin, DDAVP) has been the mainstay of treatment.

The criteria for diagnosis of DI include

- Increased urine volume >3 L/day
- Increased serum sodium >145 mmol/L
- Increased serum osmolality >300 mOsm/kg
- Decreased urine osmolality <300 mOsm/kg
- Decreased urine specific gravity <1.005

Bibliography

Griffiths, S., & Perks, A. (2010). The hypothalamic pituitary axis Part 2: Anaesthesia for pituitary surgery. *Anaesthesia Tutorial of the Week, 189.*

Krishnachetty, B., & Sethi, D. S. (2015). *The Final FRCA Structured Oral Examination: A Complete Guide.* CRC Press: Boca Raton, FL.

Eye

What makes up the bony structure of the orbit?

The bony structure of the orbit can be described as follows

- General shape
  - Pyramidal
  - Apex points towards the optic canal
- Boundaries
  - Roof – frontal bone
  - Floor – zygoma, maxilla
  - Medial wall – sphenoid, maxilla, ethmoid, lacrimal bone
  - Lateral wall – zygoma, sphenoid

Can you name the important foramina contained within the orbit, and the structures passing through each?

There are a total of nine foramina or fissures within the orbit. The most important are shown in Figure 1.6.

- Optic foramen
  - Optic nerve, ophthalmic artery
- Superior orbital fissure (*see also Scalp and Base of Skull*)
  - Oculomotor, trochlear, abducens nerves, ophthalmic division (V1) of trigeminal nerve
  - Superior and inferior ophthalmic veins
- Inferior orbital fissure
  - Infra-orbital nerve (branch from maxillary division (V2) of trigeminal nerve) and vessels

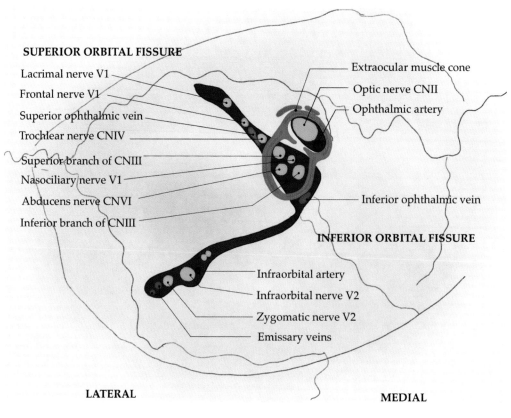

SUPERIOR ORBITAL FISSURE
Lacrimal nerve V1
Frontal nerve V1
Superior ophthalmic vein
Trochlear nerve CNIV
Superior branch of CNIII
Nasociliary nerve V1
Abducens nerve CNVI
Inferior branch of CNIII

Extraocular muscle cone
Optic nerve CNII
Ophthalmic artery

Inferior ophthalmic vein

INFERIOR ORBITAL FISSURE

Infraorbital artery
Infraorbital nerve V2
Zygomatic nerve V2
Emissary veins

LATERAL

MEDIAL

Figure 1.6   Superior and inferior orbital fissures and structures passing through.

What is the general structure of the eyeball?

- Axial length approximately 25 mm in diameter
- Three layers
  - Outer layer – sclera (posterior and opaque) and cornea (anterior and transparent) form the fibrous outer layer. Sclera receives attachments to the extraocular muscles, and is perforated posteriorly by the optic nerve.
  - Middle layer – choroid, ciliary body and iris form the vascular middle layer. Choroid lines the inside of the sclera, and is continuous with the iris anteriorly and is perforated by the optic nerve posteriorly.
  - Inner layer – retina forms the innermost layer within the posterior chamber and comprises of neural tissue.
- Two segments
  - Anterior segment
    - (further divided into anterior and posterior chambers; anterior chamber extends from cornea to iris and posterior chamber from iris to lens)
    - One sixth of the eyeball
    - Contains transparent watery fluid called aqueous humour

○ Posterior segment
   ◆ Five-sixths of the eyeball
   ◆ Contains transparent, gelatinous mass called vitreous body

What are the constituents of aqueous humour?

Aqueous humour is a clear gelatinous fluid contained within the anterior and posterior chambers of the eye supplying nutrients to the avascular cornea and lens and maintaining the intraocular pressure.

The fluid has similar composition to plasma but with less protein and glucose and more lactic acid and ascorbic acid.

It is produced predominantly by active secretion mechanisms (80%) with the Na^+/K^+ ATPase enzyme creating an osmotic passage of water into the posterior chamber. The other method of production of aqueous humour is through ultrafiltration of the plasma (20%).

The rate of production is approximately 2.5 μL/min, its total volume being 250 μL.

Can you describe the anatomy of the production and drainage of the aqueous humour?

It is produced by the *ciliary processes of the ciliary body* and is secreted into the posterior chamber. It then flows between the iris and lens and into the anterior chamber through the pupil. Most exits the anterior chamber via the trabecular meshwork at the iridocorneal angle into the *canal of Schlemm*. The canal of Schlemm is a scleral venous sinus which drains into the anterior ciliary veins (then into the superior ophthalmic vein and the cavernous sinus), with some exiting via the uveoscleral route being absorbed through the ciliary muscle into the sclera (Figure 1.7).

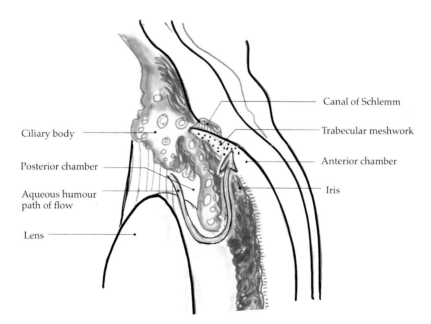

Figure 1.7   Drainage of aqueous humour.

How does pupil size affect drainage of the aqueous humour?

Pupillary dilatation narrows the iridocorneal angle and reduces the rate of drainage.

What are the determinants of intraocular pressure (IOP)?

The normal IOP is 10–25 mmHg.

Internal factors (due to the volume of the globe contents)

- Arterial blood pressure – blood flow to the eye is autoregulated, therefore a fall in blood pressure will decrease IOP. Significant increases in arterial blood pressure outside of the range of autoregulation will therefore increase IOP.
- Venous blood pressure – coughing, straining, vomiting and the Valsalva manoeuvre will increase venous congestion therefore increasing IOP. Head-up positioning of the patient will decrease venous congestion and IOP.
- Partial pressures – partial pressures of oxygen (PaO_2) and carbon dioxide ($PaCO_2$) affect blood vessel tone and therefore IOP. The effect is the same as the factors which affect cerebral blood flow.
- Aqueous humour production and drainage – can affect IOP, such as in glaucoma
- Vitreous humour volume – haemorrhage in the vitreous can increase IOP
- Presence of a foreign body – sulphur hexafluoride bubble or tumour

External factors (extraocular compression)

- Extraocular muscle tone – can increase IOP (such as is caused by a depolarising muscle relaxant) and therefore cause a decrease in IOP when paralysed
- Extrinsic compression – due to an improperly applied facemask, prone positioning or expanding orbital haematoma due to regional block complication can increase IOP
- Drugs – can both increase and decrease IOP depending on their mechanism of action (listed below)

How can drugs affect intraocular pressure?

- Induction agents: all anaesthetic induction agents and inhalational agents apart from ketamine reduce IOP. Etomidate can cause myoclonus and should probably be avoided. The fall in IOP is independent of their effect on blood pressure, central venous pressure and extraocular muscle tone. It is more likely to be as a result of direct action on central control mechanisms.
- Opioids: have no direct action on IOP but will attenuate elevated pressure caused by intubation and can increase IOP due to respiratory depression and increased $PaCO_2$.
- Muscle relaxants: suxamethonium causes a small transient rise in IOP (5–10 mmHg for 5–10 minutes due to prolonged contraction of the extraocular muscles), whilst non-depolarising muscle relaxants produce no change or even a fall in IOP.
- Mannitol can be given (0.5 mg/kg IV) as an osmotic diuretic which works by removing fluid from the vitreous chamber. Acetazolamide is a carbonic anhydrase inhibitor (500 mg IV) which acts by decreasing aqueous humour production by the ciliary body.

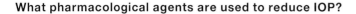

What pharmacological agents are used to reduce IOP?

Reducing aqueous humour production
- Beta blockers such as timolol reduce aqueous humour production through adenylate cyclase inhibition.

Increasing the drainage of aqueous humour
- Prostaglandin analogues such as latanoprost work by increasing the outflow of aqueous humour via the uveoscleral route.
- Cholinergic medications such as pilocarpine, and anticholinesterase inhibitors such as neostigmine contract the ciliary body and increase drainage through the trabecular network.

Both mechanisms
- Sympathomimetics such as ephedrine reduce aqueous humour production and increase drainage through ciliary body vasoconstriction and adenylate cyclase inhibition.
- Alpha 2 agonists such as brimonidine work by decreasing aqueous humour production and increasing uveoscleral outflow.

What is SF_6? What are the implications of its use for anaesthetists?

Sulphur hexafluoride is an inert, highly insoluble gas used by ophthalmic surgeons to provide tamponade for retinal surgery.

Nitrous oxide should not be used in patients where SF_6 has been used in their surgery (visual loss up to 6 weeks after the procedure due to nitrous oxide use has been reported). Exposure to nitrous oxide when SF_6 is present can lead to diffusion of nitrous oxide into the bubble faster than inert insoluble gases leave thereby increasing IOP.

How would you anaesthetise an unstarved patient requiring urgent surgery for a penetrating eye injury?

Concerns

- Unstarved patient – risk of aspiration and hence the need for rapid sequence induction
- Urgent surgery – no time to wait for a starved status
- Penetrating eye injury – avoid increased IOP for the fear of expulsion of eye contents
- Depolarising muscle relaxants aiding rapid sequence (to avoid aspiration) risks the rise of IOP

This was a problem in the pre-rocuronium (and sugammadex) era, where adjuncts were given to reduce the IOP rise with the use of suxamethonium.

Current practice: in an unstarved patient, a modified RSI induction would be indicated to minimise aspiration risk. Rocuronium at a dose of 1– 1.2 mg/kg would be preferred to suxamethonium due to non-depolarising muscle relaxants having minimal effect on IOP. A smooth induction using an appropriate induction agent (propofol) and volatile agent for maintenance (sevoflurane), with a short acting opioid should be used to attenuate the elevation in pressure due to intubation (remifentanil or alfentanil). Ventilation to control PaO_2 and $PaCO_2$ to reduce the risk of an increase in IOP due to derangements in these parameters. A head-up position should be maintained if possible during intubation and surgery to help with venous drainage. A plan for smooth extubation should be in place such as using remifentanil to minimise the risk of coughing. Prevention of nausea and vomiting by giving appropriate antiemetics during the surgery is vital to smooth emergence and recovery post eye surgery.

Explain the pathways involved in the pupillary light reflexes. *See also* Chapter 7.

- Afferent pathway: light is sensed by the optic nerve which is transmitted via the optic tract to the pretectal nucleus of the high midbrain. This signal is then transmitted to the Edinger-Westphal nucleus (of CN III).
- Efferent pathway starts via parasympathetic fibres which run from the Edinger-Westphal nucleus in the oculomotor nerve (CN III), synapsing in the ciliary ganglion. From here post ganglionic short ciliary nerves leave the ciliary ganglion and innervate the iris sphincter which causes pupil constriction.

Contraction of the pupillary muscles to dilate the pupil is triggered via sympathetic impulses along the short and long ciliary nerves originating in the superior cervical ganglion. These axons run along the internal carotid artery.

Sagittal Section of Neck

The candidates are shown an image of the sagittal section of the head and neck pertaining to the airway and asked to point out the structures of importance.

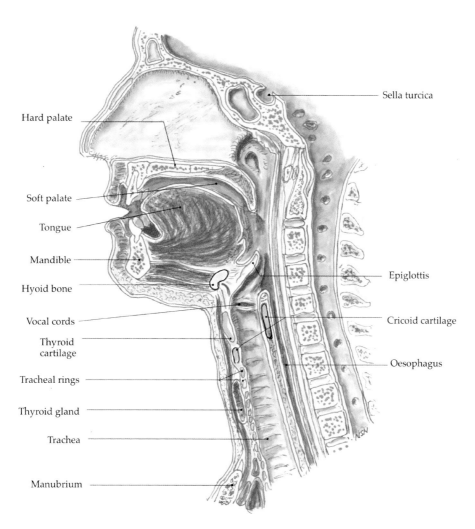

Figure 1.8   Sagittal section of the head and neck.

Make yourself familiar with Figure 1.8 and the structures.

1. Tongue
2. Hard palate
3. Soft palate
4. Hyoid bone (C3)
5. Thyroid cartilage (C4–C5)
6. Cricoid cartilage (C6)
7. Thyroid gland
8. Epiglottis
9. Vocal cords
10. C6 vertebral body

Nose

The nose is made of bones and cartilage and features the external cartilaginous nose, nares and nasal cavity. The nasal cavity is divided into right and left by the septum which comprises the ethmoid bone, vomer and septal cartilage.

The lateral wall of the nose has three nasal conchae (superior, middle and inferior) forming turbinates (horizontal bones with fibrovascular tissue) and four openings

- Sphenoethmoid recess – opening for the sphenoidal sinus
- Superior nasal meatus – opening for the posterior ethmoidal sinuses
- Middle nasal meatus – opening for the frontal sinus, maxillary, middle and anterior ethmoidal sinuses
- Inferior nasal meatus – opening for the naso-lacrimal duct

Arterial supply

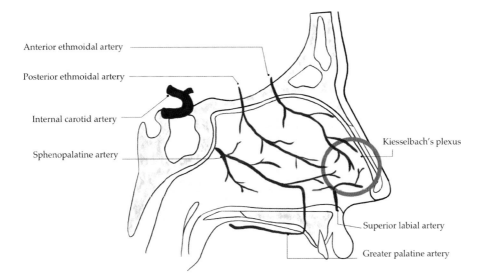

Figure 1.9   Nasal septum – arterial supply.

The overall arterial supply of the nose is by branches of internal and external carotid arteries.

External nose – branches of facial, ophthalmic and maxillary arteries

Lateral nasal wall – sphenopalatine, anterior and posterior ethmoid arteries

Nasal septum – sphenopalatine, anterior and posterior ethmoid arteries and superior labial and the greater palatine arteries. Little's area or Kiesselbach's plexus is situated in the antero-inferior part of nasal septum just above the vestibule and marks the confluence of different supplies (Figure 1.9).

Venous drainage

Submucous venous plexus draining into the cavernous sinus.

Nerve supply

In short, the nose is supplied by the first two branches of the trigeminal nerve (Figures 1.10 and 1.11)

- Sensory
  - External nose – infratrochlear, infraorbital and nasociliary nerve
  - Nasal cavity – palatine nerves from pterygopalatine (or sphenopalatine) ganglion and anterior ethmoidal nerve
- Special sensory (smell) carried via olfactory nerves
- Motor innervation to the nasal muscles is via the facial nerve

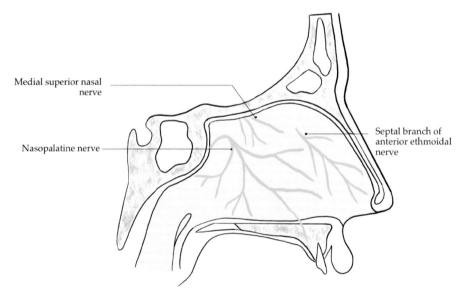

Figure 1.10   Nasal septum – nerve supply.

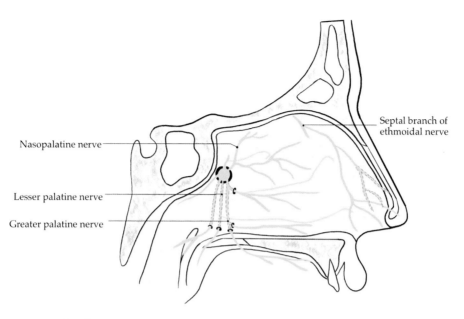

Figure 1.11   Lateral wall of nose – nerve supply.

When would you cannulate the nose?
- Provide oxygen via nasal specula
- Insertion of nasopharyngeal airway
- Nasotracheal intubation
- Insertion of nasogastric tubes or temperature probes

What are the indications and contraindications for the nasal route for intubation?

Indications

- Surgical access
- Angioedema of the tongue
- Mechanical obstructions to mouth opening from mandibular fixation
- Trismus
- Intraoral mass lesions
- Fixed neck contracture or severe degenerative cervical spine disease

Absolute contraindications

- Suspected epiglottitis
- Midface instability
- Severe coagulopathy
- Base of skull fracture
- Impending respiratory arrest

What is the 'danger area' of the face?

The lower part of external nose and the upper lip is called the dangerous area of the face as an infection in this region may spread to cavernous sinus through the inferior ophthalmic vein via the valveless anterior facial vein.

How would you topicalise the nose for awake fibreoptic intubation?

The nasal cavity is innervated by the *greater and lesser palatine nerves and the anterior ethmoidal nerve.*

Local anaesthetic can be given by spray or the use of atomiser, placement of swabs soaked with local anaesthetic, by inhalation via nebuliser or by performing nerve blocks of the palatine and anterior ethmoidal nerve.

These nerves can be blocked by taking a cotton-tipped applicator soaked in local anaesthetic and passing it along the upper border of the middle turbinate to the posterior wall of the nasopharynx, where it is left for 5–10 minutes.

Tongue

The tongue is a boneless, muscular organ which facilitates swallowing, speech and sensation of taste.

Muscles of the tongue

- Intrinsic – change the shape and size of the tongue
- Extrinsic – attached to the adjacent structures, e.g. hyoglossus, styloglossus, palataglossus

Blood supply

- Lingual artery (a branch of the external carotid artery) and tonsillar artery (a branch of the facial artery)

Venous drainage

- Lingual vein

Nerve supply

- Anterior 2/3
  - Sensory – lingual nerve (Trigeminal V3)
  - Special sensory – facial nerve
- Posterior 1/3
  - Sensory – glossopharyngeal nerve
  - Special sensory – glossopharyngeal nerve
- Motor
  - All muscles except palatoglossus – hypoglossal nerve
  - Palatoglossus – vagus nerve

Pharynx

The pharynx is a tubular structure that lies posterior to the nasal cavity, oral cavity and larynx with muscles that help with swallowing and speaking. Arterial supply is via branches of external carotid artery and drainage into internal jugular vein. The sensory and motor supply of the pharynx is from the trigeminal (maxillary branch), glossopharyngeal and the vagus nerves.

Larynx

In the Primary FRCA OSCE, an image may be provided either of the sagittal section of the neck or the laryngeal complex with cartilages and muscles and the candidate is required to name specific structures followed by issues with nerve injury. This question is generally answered badly, and the overall opinion is that the image provided is quite difficult to decipher. The candidate might also be asked to perform surgical cricothyroidotomy in a manikin.

In the Final FRCA SOE, a more detailed knowledge of the anatomy with its clinical application is required for a satisfactory pass.

Clinical application topics

- Cricothyroid puncture or surgical airway
- Anaesthesia of the larynx for awake fibreoptic intubation
- Nerve palsies
- Laryngeal injuries
- Post thyroidectomy airway emergency

The larynx is the organ of phonation and an important structure for anaesthetists in many clinical contexts.

The larynx extends from C3 (hyoid bone) to C6 (cricoid cartilage), at which level the trachea originates. It consists of three paired and three unpaired (single) cartilages and hyoid is the only bone in the pharyngo-laryngeal complex.

Unpaired/single cartilages

- Epiglottis (leaf-shaped)
- Thyroid (shield-like)
- Cricoid (signet ring-like)

Paired cartilages

- Arytenoid (pyramidal)
- Cuneiform (cylindrical)
- Corniculate (triangular)

A knowledge of the names of the cartilages and their relative positions will help name the structure attached to them. For example, the structure that connects the thyroid and the cricoid cartilages could only be the cricothyroid ligament (membrane) or cricothyroid muscle. The ligament is more central connecting the inferior border of the thyroid and the superior surface of the cricoid. Whereas the muscle is more lateral attaching to the inferior horn of the thyroid cartilage to the cricoid cartilage.

Epiglottis: the epiglottis is leaf-shaped and connected to the hyoid bone by the hyo-epiglottic ligament. The vallecula is the pouch between the epiglottis and the base of the tongue where the tip of the laryngoscope is placed during direct laryngoscopy in adults.

Thyroid cartilage: the thyroid cartilage is in the shape of a shield and gives the anterior laryngeal prominence. It is quadrangular with superior and inferior cornu which articulate with the hyoid and cricoid respectively through specific ligaments.

Cricoid cartilage: the cricoid cartilage is positioned below the thyroid cartilage with the thinner portion attaching to the thyroid cartilage via the avascular cricothyroid membrane. The broader part is posterior and houses the arytenoid cartilage on the top.

Arytenoid, cuneiform and corniculate cartilages: these cartilages are present at the back of the larynx between the thyroid and the cricoid cartilages. They connect to the epiglottis by the aryepiglottic folds which are further strengthened by the cuneiform and corniculate cartilages which are found embedded in these folds (Figure 1.12).

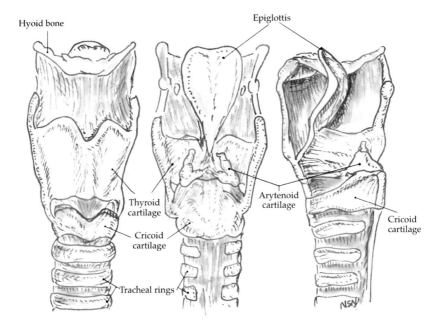

Figure 1.12   Cartilages of the larynx.

Vocal cords

The vocal cords are formed by the thickening of the upper edge of cricothyroid membrane connecting to the arytenoid cartilage posteriorly. The white colour of the cords is because of the absence of the submucosal covering.

Muscles

Extrinsic muscles – move the larynx as a whole

- Elevators – suprahyoid muscles (stylohyoid, geniohyoid, mylohyoid, thyrohyoid and stylopharyngeus)
- Depressors – infrahyoid muscles (omohyoid, sternothyroid, sternohyoid and thyrohyoid)

Intrinsic muscles – control the vocal cords and the glottic opening (Figure 1.13)

The intrinsic muscles connect between cartilages as listed below (T, thyroid; C, cricoid; A, arytenoid) (Table 1.3).

Table 1.3   Muscles of the Larynx

	T – C	Cricothyroid
	T – A	Thyroarytenoid
	T – A	Vocalis
	C – A	Cricoarytenoid – lateral
	C – A	Cricoarytenoid – medial
	A – A	Transverse arytenoid

Cricothyroid muscle – the **only TENSOR** of the cord.

Posterior cricoarytenoid muscle – the **only ABDUCTOR** of the cord.

All other intrinsic muscles are responsible for relaxation and adduction of the cords.

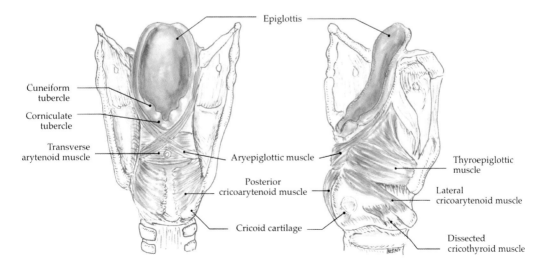

Figure 1.13   Muscles of the larynx.

Arterial supply

Superior and inferior laryngeal arteries which arise from the superior and inferior thyroid arteries which in turn are branches of the external carotid artery.

Venous drainage

Superior and inferior laryngeal veins drain into the superior and inferior thyroid veins which in turn empty into the internal jugular veins and left brachiocephalic veins, respectively.

Lymphatic drainage

Deep cervical and upper tracheal lymph nodes drain the upper and lower half, respectively.

Nerve supply

The sensory and motor supply of the larynx is by the vagus via the superior and recurrent laryngeal nerves.

Superior laryngeal nerve (SLN)

The SLN originates from the inferior ganglion (C1 level) of the vagus nerve and descends posterior to the carotid artery towards the larynx. At the level of greater horn of hyoid bone, it divides into external and internal branches. The internal branch (iSLN) provides sensory innervation of mucous membrane of the larynx above the level of vocal cords including base of the tongue and epiglottis. The external branch (eSLN) provides motor supply to cricothyroid muscle.

The iSLN can be injured during surgical interventions of the anterior neck such as carotid endarterectomy and after cervical spine injury.

The eSLN is in close proximity to the superior thyroid vascular pedicle at the superior pole of the thyroid and there is a risk of injury during thyroid surgery.

Recurrent laryngeal nerve (RLN)

The right RLN is a branch of right vagus nerve and it loops the right subclavian artery and runs parallel to the tracheoesophageal groove.

The left RLN originates from the left vagus nerve as it crosses the aortic arch and it loops the arch and descends parallel to the tracheoesophageal groove. The longer course of the left RLN makes it more prone to injury than the right RLN.

In the neck, both nerves accompany the inferior thyroid pedicle and it is at high risk of injury during thyroid surgery (Figure 1.14 and Table 1.4).

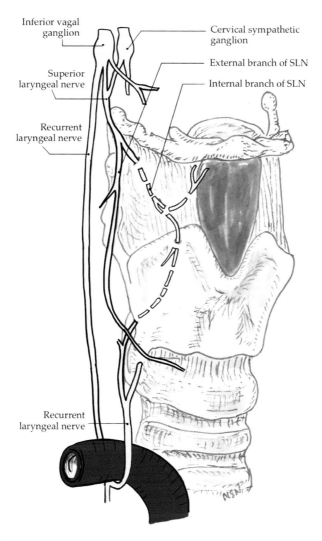

Figure 1.14   Nerves of the larynx.

Table 1.4   Innervation of the Larynx

	SLN	RLN
Sensory	Base of tongue, epiglottis, larynx above the level of vocal cords (iSLN)	Larynx below the level of vocal cords
Motor	Cricothyroid muscle only (eSLN)	All other intrinsic muscles

What are the causes of laryngeal nerve palsy?

Damage to vagus, SLN or RLN can be due to

- Trauma
- Iatrogenic causes, secondary to
  - Surgical – thyroid, lung, heart or cervical spine surgery
  - Anaesthetic – prolonged intubation, nerve blocks
- Neoplastic – lung malignancy and metastatic lesions
- Infective – viral
- Miscellaneous
  - Cardiovocal syndrome (Ortner's syndrome) – hoarseness due to a left recurrent laryngeal nerve palsy caused by cardiovascular pathology
  - Neurological syndromes – various neurological syndromes are named secondary to the level of lesion of vagus nerve; Wallenberg – lateral medulla, Vernet's – jugular foramen

What happens when the vagus nerve is damaged at the base of skull (with respect to laryngeal innervation)?

High vagal lesions cause complete unilateral vagal paralysis affecting both SLN and RLN.

Sensory

- Unilateral loss of the sensation of larynx

Motor

- Loss of abductors and adductors – ipsilateral cords in the paramedian (cadaveric) position
- Dysphagia from unilateral palatal weakness
- Palatal droop on the ipsilateral side and deviation of the uvula to the contralateral side

When the injury is unilateral, the loss of function can be temporary and less pronounced as opposed to bilateral damage (Tables 1.5 and 1.6).

Table 1.5   Summary of SLN (Superior Laryngeal Nerve) Damage

	Unilateral SLN	Bilateral SLN
Modality		
Sensory	Unilateral sensory loss above the cord	Bilateral sensory loss above the cords
Motor	Unilateral cricothyroid palsy	Bilateral cricothyroid palsy
Function		
Voice	Temporary hoarse voice	Hoarse voice
Risk of aspiration	Unlikely	Likely
Airway obstruction	No	No

Table 1.6   Summary of Bilateral RLN (Recurrent Laryngeal Nerve) Damage

	Partial RLN damage*	Complete RLN damage*
Modality		
Sensory	Sensory loss below the cords	Sensory loss below the cords
Motor	Paralysis of abductors (posterior cricoarytenoid) – cords in closed position	Paralysis of all intrinsic muscles (except cricothyroid) – cords in open position
Function		
Voice	Hoarseness, dysphonia	Dysphonia
Risk of aspiration	Unlikely	Yes
Airway obstruction	Yes	No

The RLN carries the abductor and adductor fibres and hence its injury results in damage to both. Varying degrees of damage result in involvement of abductors more than the adductors according to Semon and Rosenbach. Semon's law is based on the assumption that *the nerve fibres supplying the abductors lie in the periphery of the recurrent laryngeal nerve and any progressive lesion involves these fibres first as they are more susceptible to pressure before involving the deeper adductor fibres.*

In summary, bilateral partial RLN damage (0.2% after thyroidectomy) causes complete acute airway obstruction whilst in bilateral complete damage (1–2%) the cords are open and increases the aspiration risk.

So if RLN palsy is unavoidable choose a complete injury!

How can you prevent laryngeal nerve damage during surgical procedures?

- Preoperative laryngoscopy to rule out preoperative nerve involvement
- Good surgical conduct – complete dissection and exploration of RLN during surgery
- Awareness of anatomical variations
- Continuous RLN monitoring may be useful in certain cases

What are the causes of airway complications post thyroidectomy?

Airway complications are more prevalent in the recovery period compared to during induction and intubation.

General causes

- Laryngospasm
- Foreign body
- Obesity/obstructive sleep apnoea syndrome
- Inadequate reversal of neuromuscular blocking drug

Specific to thyroidectomy

- Haematoma (1–2%)

  The commonest cause for acute airway obstruction in the first 24 hours. Definitive therapy is surgical evacuation of haematoma. If re-intubation is necessary consideration should be given to awake fibreoptic intubation due to airway distortion.

- Laryngeal oedema (0.1%)
- Bilateral RLN palsy or paresis (<2%)
- Hypoparathyroidism/hypocalcaemia (3–5%)

  The commonest cause of airway compromise after 24 hours, hypocalcaemia usually manifests 24–48 hours post surgery as tingling in lips followed by laryngeal stridor and airway obstruction, carpopedal spasm, tetany, laryngospasm, seizures, QT prolongation and cardiac arrest. It is usually managed with intravenous calcium gluconate and CPAP for associated airway compromise.

- Tracheomalacia

  Rare and considered historical as it is nearly obsolete in modern day thyroidectomies. Confounding factors could be long standing goitre with retrosternal extension and presence of tracheal compression.

How can the cricothyroid membrane be used for oxygenation in an emergency?
- Cricothyroid cannula and jet ventilation
- Surgical cricothyroidotomy and ventilation
- Seldinger mini-tracheostomy

NAP4 suggests that cricothyroid cannulation has a higher failure rate than surgical cricothyroidotomy in an emergency. The scalpel-bougie-cricothyroidotomy technique or the 'three-step' technique is considered as the most efficient and reliable method of obtaining emergency front of neck access (FONA) in 'can't intubate can't oxygenate' situations.

Other possible questions…

1. Describe the technique of front of neck access (FONA) or demonstrate in a manikin in OSCE.
2. How would you anaesthetise the airway for an awake fibreoptic intubation?

Bibliography

Batuwitage, B., & Charters, P. (2017). Postoperative management of the difficult airway. *BJA Education, 7*(17), 235–241.

Burdett, E., & Mitchell, V. (2011). Anatomy of the larynx, trachea and bronchi. *Anaesthesia & Intensive Care Medicine, 12*(8), 335–339.

Erman, A. B., Kejner, A. E., Hogikyan, N. D., & Feldman, E. L. (2009, February). Disorders of cranial nerves IX and X. *Seminars in Neurology 29*(01), 85–92.

Grades at Laryngoscopy

Cormack-Lehane classification describes laryngeal view at direct laryngoscopy (Figure 1.15).

- Grade 1: full view of glottis
- Grade 2a: partial view of glottis
- Grade 2b: only posterior extremity of glottis seen or only arytenoid cartilages
- Grade 3: only epiglottis seen, none of glottis seen
- Grade 4: neither glottis nor epiglottis seen

Intubation is likely to be difficult with a Grade 2b view or worse.

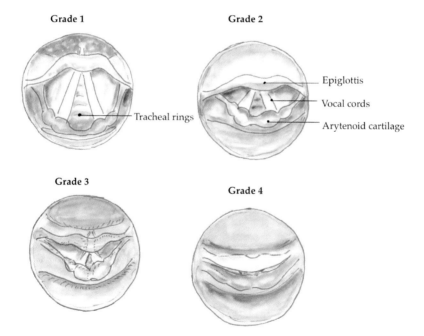

Figure 1.15   Grades at laryngoscopy.

Bibliography

Krage, R., Van Rijn, C., Van Groeningen, D., Loer, S. A., Schwarte, L. A., et al. (2010). Cormack–Lehane classification revisited. *British Journal of Anaesthesia, 105*(2), 220–227.

Cross Section of Neck at C6 Level

Figure 1.16 shows the structures at the level of cross section at C6 or C7 vertebra.

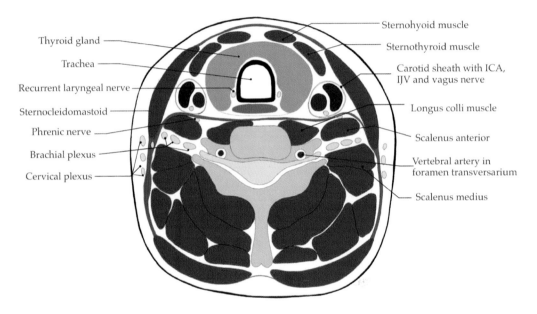

Figure 1.16   Cross section of neck at C6 level.

Easily identifiable structures

- Skin and subcutaneous tissue
- Platysma, sternohyoid and sternothyroid muscles
- Thyroid gland, trachea, oesophagus
- Carotid sheath with contents (common carotid artery medially, IJV laterally and the vagus nerve)
- C6 or C7 vertebra

The structures laid out in Table 1.7 might not be easy now, but you will certainly be able to identify them after reading this topic!

Table 1.7   Important Structures in the Neck at the Level of C6

Muscles
Sternocleidomastoid Scalene muscles Longus colli
Nerves
Recurrent laryngeal nerve Phrenic nerve Brachial plexus (or C6 nerve root) Sympathetic trunk Superficial cervical plexus
Vessels
Vertebral artery and vein
Fascial planes of deep cervical fascia
Investing layer Pretracheal layer Prevertebral layer

Muscles

- Sternocleidomastoid – large muscle bulk lateral and anterior to the carotid sheath, comprising of a sternal head (manubrium of sternum to superior nuchal line of occiput) and a clavicular head (medial one third of clavicle to mastoid process) and innervated by accessory nerve and branches from the anterior rami of C2–C3.

- Scalene muscles – a group of three paired muscles (anterior scalene, middle scalene, posterior scalene) that originate on the transverse processes of the C2–C7 vertebrae and insert on the first and second ribs, and innervated by the anterior rami of C4–C6.

- Longus colli muscle – 'long muscle of the neck', posterior to the oesophagus, running along the anterior surface of the vertebrae between the atlas and T3 vertebra, and innervated by the anterior rami of C2–C6.

Nerves

- Recurrent laryngeal nerve – in the tracheo oesophageal groove laterally
- Phrenic nerve – posterior to the carotid sheath and in front of scalenus anterior
- Brachial plexus (or C6 nerve root) – nerves between anterior and middle scalene muscles
- Sympathetic trunk – medial to the carotid sheath just in front of the longus colli muscle and transverse process
- Superficial cervical plexus – the nerve point of the neck, also known as Erb's point, where the four superficial branches of the cervical plexus nerves surface at the lateral border of sternocleidomastoid (namely, the greater auricular nerve, lesser occipital nerve, transverse cervical nerve and supraclavicular nerve)

Vessels

- Vertebral artery and vein – in the foramen transversarium of the transverse process

Fascial layers

- The deep cervical fascia is deep to the platysma. It is organised into several layers and named according to its position and the structures it surrounds.
- Investing layer – outermost of the deep fascial layers and surrounds all structures in the neck
- Pretracheal layer – in the anterior part of the neck enclosing the trachea, oesophagus, thyroid gland and the infrahyoid muscles (sternohyoid medially, sternothyroid in the middle and omohyoid laterally)
- Prevertebral layer – surrounds the vertebral column and muscles associated with it (scalene, prevertebral and back muscles). It envelops the brachial plexus at its exit in the neck and also forms the carotid sheath and communicates with the mediastinum, forming a likely path for extravasated blood from vascular puncture.

Clinical importance of the fascial planes

Loose areolar tissue and connective tissue fill the area between the layers and form potential spaces. The retropharyngeal space is the largest and a clinically relevant interfascial space between the posterior part of pretracheal fascia and the prevertebral fascia. It extends from the base of the skull down to the superior mediastinum. By compartmentalising the neck, it can contain infection and prevent spread. But perforations of the prevertebral fascia due to infection can lead to retropharyngeal abscess. Similarly, air from a ruptured trachea or oesophagus (pneumomediastinum) may pass superiorly in the neck.

Areas of interest to anaesthetists include the following.

- Cricoid cartilage – signet ring shaped, with the narrow portion at the front. It slopes posteriorly and lies just above the arytenoid cartilages. This is the level at which force is applied to the oesophagus against the C6 vertebral body to reduce risk of aspiration of gastric contents whilst performing rapid sequence intubation.
- Carotid sheath – a fascial sheath running from the base of the skull to the root of the neck which contains the carotid artery, internal jugular vein and vagus nerve. This is the level of IJV cannulation which also marks the midpoint of the lateral border of sternocleidomastoid muscle.
- Scalene muscles and brachial plexus – the anterior scalene originates from C3–C6 and inserts onto the first rib. The phrenic nerve runs on the anterior surface of the muscle and the subclavian vein lies anterior to it.
- Superficial cervical plexus – originates from the anterior rami of C2–C4, and sometimes C1. It emerges from the lateral border of sternocleidomastoid at the level of C6 (Erb's point).
- Sympathetic trunk/chain – the cervical chain ganglia lie between the prevertebral fascia and carotid sheath. The middle cervical ganglion lies at the level of the C6 vertebral body. The needle entry point for stellate ganglion block is at this level.

Triangles of Neck

The front and side of the neck is divided by the sternocleidomastoid muscle into anterior and posterior triangles. These are further divided into other triangles by the muscles present in this area. Below is the summary of all triangles with boundaries and contents and their clinical importance to anaesthetists (Tables 1.8, 1.9, 1.10, 1.11, 1.12, 1.13, 1.14 and 1.15; Figure 1.17).

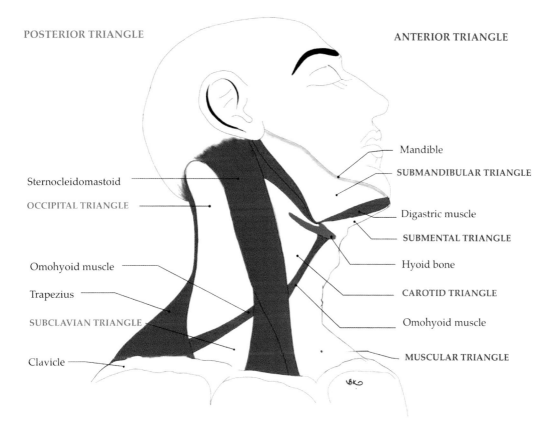

Figure 1.17   Triangles of neck.

Table 1.8   Anterior Triangle – Boundaries, Contents and Clinical Importance

Anterior triangle	
Boundaries Superior – base of mandible Posterior – sternocleidomastoid muscle Anterior – median line of neck	Contents Muscular triangle, carotid triangle, submandibular triangle, submental triangle
Importance: landmarks for tracheostomy, cricothyrodotomy, carotid sinus massage and internal jugular vein cannulation	

Table 1.9   Muscular Triangle – Boundaries, Contents and Clinical Importance

Muscular triangle	

Boundaries
Superior – hyoid bone
Medial – midline of the neck
Supero-laterally – omohyoid muscle
Infero-laterally – sternocleidomastoid muscle
	Contents
	Muscles – thyrohyoid, sternothyroid,
	  sternohyoid
	Vessels – superior and inferior thyroid artery,
	  anterior jugular veins
	Viscera – thyroid and parathyroid gland,
	  larynx, trachea, oesophagus

Importance: landmarks for tracheostomy, cricothyrodotomy	

Table 1.10   Carotid Triangle – Boundaries, Contents and Clinical Importance

Carotid triangle	
Boundaries Superior – digastric muscle Lateral – sternocleidomastoid muscle Inferior – omohyoid muscle	Contents Arteries – common, external and internal carotid artery Veins – internal jugular vein Nerves – vagus, hypoglossal, sympathetic trunk

Importance: the vessels are superficial in the triangle and hence there is easy access for internal
  jugular vein cannulation, carotid artery dopplers, stellate ganglion block, carotid sinus massage
  and vagal manoeuvres.	

Table 1.11   Submandibular Triangle – Boundaries, Contents and Clinical Importance

Submandibular triangle	
Boundaries Superior – body of mandible Anterior – anterior belly of digastric Posterior – posterior belly of digastric	Contents Viscera – submandibular and parotid gland Vessels – facial and lingual artery Nerves – hypoglossal nerve
Importance: nil specific for anaesthetists	

Table 1.12   Submental Triangle – Boundaries, Contents and Clinical Importance

Submental triangle	
Boundaries Inferior – hyoid bone Medial – midline of the neck Lateral – anterior belly of the digastric	Contents Submental lymph nodes and tributaries of the anterior jugular vein
Importance: nil specific for anaesthetists	

Table 1.13   Posterior Triangle – Boundaries, Contents and Clinical Importance

Posterior triangle	
Boundaries Anterior – sternocleidomastoid Posterior – trapezius Inferior – clavicle	Contents Occipital triangle, supraclavicular triangle
Importance: frequent site for regional anaesthesia and for acute and chronic pain procedures. It holds the entire brachial plexus from roots to divisions, the cervical plexus and subclavian artery.	

Table 1.14   Occipital Triangle – Boundaries, Contents and Clinical Importance

Occipital triangle	
Boundaries Anterior – sternocleidomastoid Posterior – trapezius Inferior – omohyoid	Contents Vessels – external jugular vein Nerves – accessory nerve, phrenic nerve, supraclavicular nerves, cervical plexus, uppermost part of brachial plexus
Importance: cervical plexus and interscalene block	

Table 1.15   Supraclavicular Triangle – Boundaries, Contents and Clinical Importance

Supraclavicular/subclavian triangle	
Boundaries Anterior – sternocleidomastoid Superior – inferior belly of omohyoid Inferior – clavicle	Contents Vessels – subclavian artery Nerves – supraclavicular nerves, trunks of brachial plexus
Importance: brachial plexus block, supraclavicular approach to subclavian venous cannulation	

Circulation

- Arterial supply of head and neck
- Great veins of head and neck

Cerebral Circulation

Talk me through the blood supply to the Circle of Willis starting from the aortic arch.

The Circle of Willis lies in the interpeduncular fossa at the base of the brain, alongside the origins of many of the cranial nerves and represents the cerebral circulation. Anteriorly it is bordered by the optic chiasm and posteriorly by the pons. The arterial supply of the brain arises from the internal carotid arteries (70%) and the vertebrobasilar system (30%) (Figure 1.18).

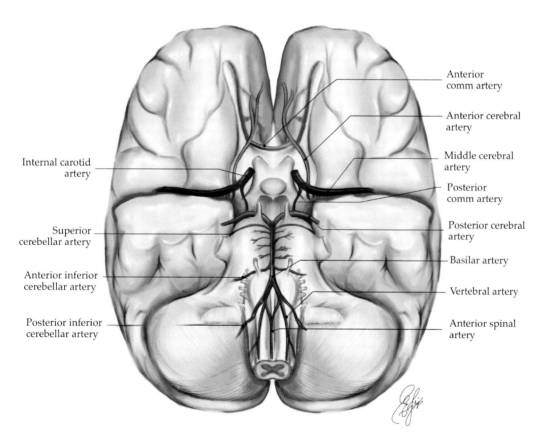

Figure 1.18   Arterial supply of brain – Circle of Willis.

Carotid system

- Origin

  The right common carotid artery arises from a bifurcation of the brachiocephalic trunk (the right subclavian artery is the other branch).

  The left common carotid artery branches directly from the arch of aorta.

  The left and right common carotid arteries ascend up the neck, lateral to the trachea and the oesophagus. They do not give off any branches in the neck.

- Course

At the level of the superior margin of the thyroid cartilage (C4), the carotid arteries split into the external and internal carotid arteries. The internal carotid arteries do not supply any structures in the neck, entering the cranial cavity via the carotid canal in the petrous part of the temporal bone.

Vertebrobasilar system

- Origin

  The right and left vertebral arteries arise from the subclavian arteries, medial to the anterior scalene muscle.

- Course

  The vertebral arteries then ascend up the posterior side of the neck, through the foramen transversarium in the transverse processes of the cervical vertebrae. They enter the cranial cavity via the foramen magnum, and converge and give rise to the basilar arteries, which supply the brain. The vertebral arteries supply no branches to the neck, or extracranial structures.

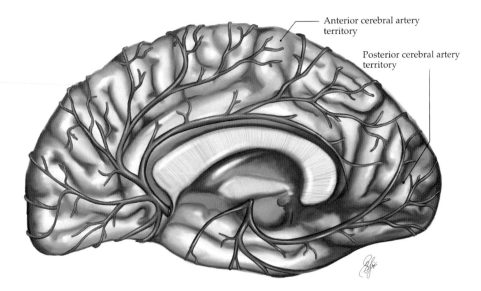

Anterior cerebral artery territory

Posterior cerebral artery territory

Figure 1.19   Arterial supply – medial surface of brain.

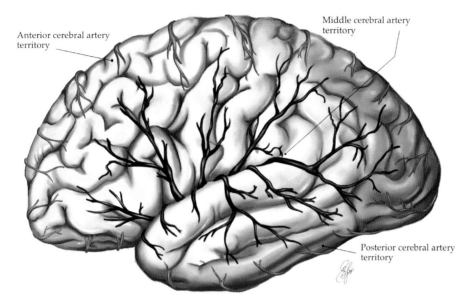

Figure 1.20   Arterial supply – lateral surface of brain.

What territories are supplied by the anterior, middle and posterior cerebral arteries (ACA, MCA and PCA)? What are the features of disruption of blood supply of one of these branches? (Figures 1.19 and 1.20)

Table 1.16   Cerebral Artery Territory and Features of Ischaemia

Vessel	Region	Clinical features in involvement
ACA	Middle of the frontal lobe	• Loss of higher function • Contralateral weakness legs > arms
MCA	Remainder of the frontal, temporal and parietal lobes	• Contralateral weakness – face > arms > legs • Visual field loss – homonymous hemianopia • Non-dominant hemisphere – visual and spatial neglect • Dominant hemisphere – aphasia, agraphia, acalculia
PCA	Occipital lobe and part of the cerebellum	• Contralateral homonymous hemianopia • Thalamic involvement – loss of pain/temperature • Cerebellar features • Cortical blindness

What about the venous drainage?

The cerebrum, cerebellum and brainstem are drained by numerous veins, which empty into the dural venous sinuses which lie between the periosteal and meningeal layers of the dura mater. They are best thought of as collecting pools of blood, which drain the central nervous system, the face and the scalp. All dural venous sinuses ultimately drain into the internal jugular vein.

There are 11 venous sinuses in total. Veins draining the brain parenchyma may be divided into superficial and deep veins. The superficial veins primarily drain the cerebral cortex, whereas the deep veins drain the deep structures within the hemispheres. These veins do not typically follow the arterial supply and there is significant variation in anatomy between different subjects.

- Superficial venous system: cortical veins drain eventually into the sagittal sinuses
- Deep venous system: drain into the transverse, straight and sigmoid sinuses

How do you classify acute stroke?

Stroke is not usually classified by isolated territory, but by clinical features according to the Oxford Bamford Classification (2006).

The components observed are

- Unilateral motor deficit
- Homonymous hemianopia
- Disruption of higher cerebral function (dominant hemisphere – aphasia/dysphasia or non-dominant hemisphere – neglect)

Depending on how many of these features are present, four possible syndromes are possible.

1. Total anterior circulation infarct (TACI): 10–20% strokes – worst prognosis
2. Partial anterior circulation infarct (PACI): 30–40% strokes
3. Posterior circulation infarct (POCI): 20–30% strokes
4. Lacunar infarct: 20–30% pure motor, pure sensory, ataxic hemiparesis

What are watershed infarcts?

Watershed infarcts are ischaemic lesions that are characteristically present at the junction of two main arterial territories accounting for 10% of strokes. They can be due to systemic hypotension with or without decreased cardiac output.

A 65-year-old female is admitted with thunderclap headache, vomiting and neck stiffness.

What is your differential diagnosis?
- Subarachnoid haemorrhage (SAH) is most likely. 80% of SAH is caused by a rupture of berry (saccular) aneurysms, with arteriovenous malformations accounting for 10%.
- Other intracranial haemorrhage/thrombosis (e.g. cerebral venous sinus thrombosis)
- Infection – meningitis
- Primary headache/headache syndromes – migraines, cluster headaches, etc.
- Hypertensive crisis
- Carotid artery dissection

What are the common sites for aneurysms?

Aneurysms commonly occur at the sites of bifurcations, around the Circle of Willis.

- 40% at anterior communicating artery and ACA
- 30% at MCA branches

- 20% at MCA origin
- 5% within the posterior communicating artery

What are the causes of cerebral vascular aneurysms?

These can be classified into

- Modifiable – hypertension, hypercholesterolaemia, smoking and substance abuse (e.g. cocaine, alcohol)
- Non-modifiable – genetic conditions (e.g. some forms of polycystic kidney disease, Ehler Danlos type 4) and a positive family history of SAH
- Others include trauma, mycotic aneurysms and AV malformations

How will you proceed if the patient has a SAH and the radiologists want to take her to the neuroradiology suite to insert an endovascular coil?

Initial management should focus on cardiorespiratory stabilisation to maintain cerebral perfusion and minimise the risk of re-bleeding and secondary brain injury. It is achieved by securing the airway, controlling ventilation and careful arterial pressure management.

- PaO_2 of 13 kPa
- Normocapnia (4.5–5.0 kPa)
- Blood pressure to maintain cerebral perfusion pressure and avoid big swings in blood pressure
- Treat pain and seizures, avoid hyperthermia

What are your concerns with anaesthetising the patient in the neuroradiology suite?

General considerations

- Transfer and management of critically ill patient
- Poor access to the patient
- Remote site anaesthesia
- Potential for hypothermia with long procedures
- Radiation exposure

Equipment considerations

- Sufficient slack in tubing of lines and airways to allow safe movement of patient
- May need to deliberately induce hypo-/hypertension
- Need for invasive monitoring
- Need for urinary catheter – significant volume of flush and contrast media

Specific considerations

- Monitoring of anticoagulation required to prevent thromboembolic events
- Specialised neuroanaesthetic technique with neuroprotection
- Smooth and rapid emergence from GA to facilitate early neurological assessment

What are the complications of SAH?

Neurological complications

- Re-bleed
- Hydrocephalus
- Seizures
- Cerebral vasospasm – see explanation below
- Delayed cerebral ischaemia (DCI)

Systemic complications

- Cardiovascular – brain injury results in a massive catecholamine release with increased sympathetic outflow and dysfunction of the autonomic nervous system. This results in a hyperdynamic circulation with increased myocardial oxygen demand and workload leading to transient myocardial ischaemia and failure.
- Pulmonary – 80% of patients may have impaired oxygenation due to aspiration pneumonitis, neurogenic or cardiogenic pulmonary oedema, pneumonia, acute lung injury or ARDS.
- Metabolic – hyperglycaemia is a marker of the severity of SAH and is associated with a worse outcome. However, tight glycaemic control may be detrimental because of the risk of hypoglycaemia.
- Electrolytes – hyponatraemia may be due to administration of excessive hypotonic fluids, cerebral salt wasting syndrome, or the syndrome of inappropriate antidiuretic hormone secretion (SIADH).

What is delayed cerebral ischaemia?

Neurological deterioration related to ischaemia that persists >1 hour and has no other cause (e.g. hydrocephalus, seizures, etc.). Examples of neurological deterioration include reduced GCS, changes to speech and focal motor deficits.

The aetiology of DCI is unclear but most likely multifactorial in origin, including impaired auto regulation, impaired vessel relaxation or excess reactivity and irritation of arteries by haemoglobin and local mediators.

Explain vasospasm in the context of SAH?

Vasospasm is arterial narrowing demonstrated on imaging, including doppler or digital cerebral angiography (gold standard) that may or may not produce clinical features. Over 60% of patients will develop DCI/vasospasm during days 4 to 10 post SAH.

Diagnosis is by a combination of clinical suspicion and investigations.

Investigations

- Transcranial doppler – non-invasive
- CT angiography – 90% specificity
- Digital subtraction angiography – gold standard, invasive
- CT perfusion – gives regional brain tissue perfusion

Management

- Nimodipine – dihydropyridine calcium channel antagonist – blocks Ca^{2+} in L-type channels. The mechanism of action is not completely understood although there is grade 1 evidence for its use (Cochrane review, 2007). A dose of 60 mg qds for 3 weeks from diagnosis reduces the risks of vasospasm.

- Triple H therapy – hypertension, hypervolaemia, haemodilution, to increase cerebral blood flow and oxygen delivery. A systematic review in 2010 has discredited its use, although hypertension is an important factor. Haemodilution is no longer practised and euvolaemia is the ideal fluid balance post SAH, but this can be difficult with patients developing neurogenic pulmonary oedema and disorders of sodium homeostasis.

- Magnesium – is neuroprotective and has vasodilatory properties. The IMASH trial (magnesium sulphate in aneurysmal subarachnoid haemorrhage, 2010) showed no benefit in treating DCI. Current guidance is to maintain magnesium levels within the normal range.

- Statins – attenuate the production of reactive oxygen species in brain injury and diminish the inflammatory reaction by modulating the cytokine response. Current evidence for the use of statins in the treatment of SAH and prevention of DCI and vasospasm is equivocal.

Other possible questions...

1. When do we consider monitoring cerebral perfusion?

Bibliography

Dankbaar, J. W., Slooter, A. J., Rinkel, G. J., & vander Schaaf, I. C. (2010). Effect of different components of triple-H therapy on cerebral perfusion in patients with aneurysmal subarachnoid haemorrhage: A systematic review. *Critical Care, 14*(1), R23.

Luoma, A., & Reddy, U. (2012). Acute management of aneurysmal subarachnoid haemorrhage. *Continuing Education in Anaesthesia, Critical Care & Pain, 13*(2), 52–58.

Raithatha, A., Pratt, G., & Rash, A. (2013). Developments in the management of acute ischaemic stroke: Implications for anaesthetic and critical care management. *Continuing Education in Anaesthesia, Critical Care & Pain, 13*(3), 80–86.

Venous Drainage of the Brain

The brain parenchyma is drained by a set of superficial and deep veins, which drain into the dural (i.e. contained within the dura mater) venous sinuses in the subarachnoid space (Figures 1.21 and 1.22).

Unpaired sinuses

- Superior sagittal sinus, which sits between the cerebral hemispheres in the superior border of the cerebral falx, drains eventually into the right internal jugular vein.
- Inferior sagittal sinus, which sits between the cerebral hemispheres in the inferior border of the cerebral falx, drains eventually into the left internal jugular vein.
- Straight sinus, a continuation of the inferior sagittal sinus after it receives the great cerebral vein of Galen

The 'confluence of sinuses' is the area which receives the superior sagittal sinus and the straight sinus.

Paired sinuses

- Cavernous sinus drains via the superior and inferior petrosal sinuses
- Transverse sinus, which drains into the
- Sigmoid sinus which becomes the
- Internal jugular vein at the jugular foramen

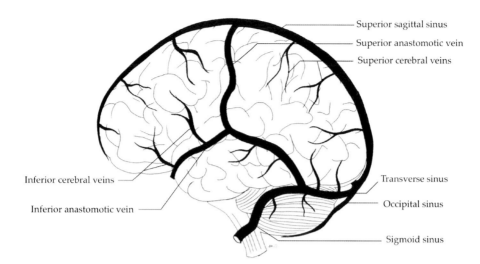

Superior sagittal sinus
Superior anastomotic vein
Superior cerebral veins

Inferior cerebral veins
Inferior anastomotic vein

Transverse sinus
Occipital sinus
Sigmoid sinus

Figure 1.21   Venous drainage – lateral surface of brain.

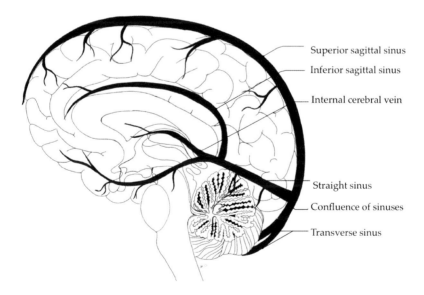

Superior sagittal sinus
Inferior sagittal sinus
Internal cerebral vein

Straight sinus
Confluence of sinuses
Transverse sinus

Figure 1.22   Venous drainage – medial surface of brain.

Figure 1.23 is a representation of the venous drainage in an easy to understand view.

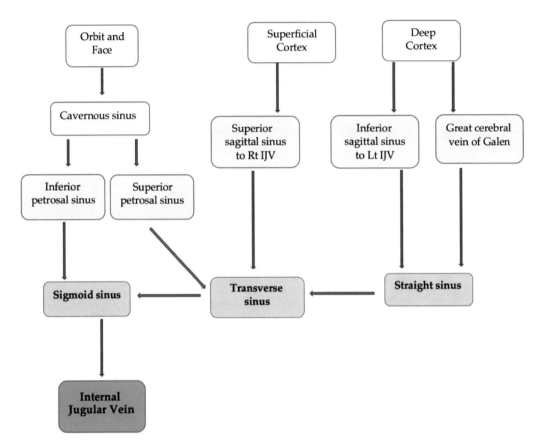

Figure 1.23   Schematic representation of venous drainage of the brain.

What do you know about cerebral venous thrombosis and in particular cavernous sinus thrombosis?

Cerebral venous thrombosis is an umbrella term to describe clot formation in any of the cerebral venous sinuses. It causes venous infarction and can present acutely like a stroke and depending on the site of thrombosis, focal neurology may be present. Most commonly, it occurs due to infection of the frontal sinuses and is accompanied by fever. Other aetiologies include surgery, trauma, clotting disorders, pregnancy and use of oral contraceptive pill.

Cavernous sinus thrombosis is a type of cerebral venous thrombosis, in which the blood clot is located in the cavernous sinus. The most common precipitating factor is infection of the nose, sinuses, teeth or eyes that spreads directly to the cavernous sinus.

Great Veins of the Neck

Internal jugular vein

The internal jugular vein (IJV) is the main conduit of venous drainage of the head and neck and starts at the base of skull as the sigmoid sinus exits through the jugular foramen. The left internal jugular vein receives blood from the inferior sagittal sinus and the larger right IJV from the superior sagittal sinus. The internal jugular vein receives the pharyngeal, facial, lingual and thyroid branches in the upper part of the neck and terminates by combining with the subclavian vein to form the brachiocephalic vein. The longer, left brachiocephalic vein crosses over to the right side and combines with the right brachiocephalic vein, forming the superior vena cava, ultimately draining into the right atrium (Figure 1.24).

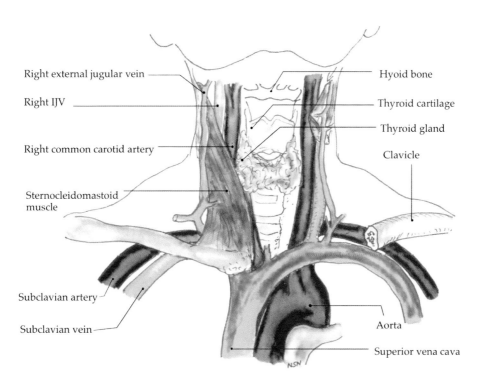

Figure 1.24   Great veins of neck.

Course

The surface marking of the IJV is from the point between the mastoid process and the angle of the mandible to the sternoclavicular joint.

Then it descends posterior to the sternocleidomastoid muscle and behind the sternal end of the clavicle. At its inferior end, both IJVs tend to shift to the right. On the right side this means the IJV is lateral to the common carotid artery and on the left side it overlaps the left common carotid artery, although there is much inter-person variability.

Relations

- *Posterior*

  Muscles – rectus capitis, levator scapulae, scalenus anterior and medius

  Nerves – cervical plexus, phrenic nerve

  Vessels – thyrocervical trunk, first part of vertebral and subclavian arteries

  Lymphatics – thoracic duct on the left side and lymphatic duct on the right side
- *Anterolateral*

  The IJV is crossed by two muscles, two arteries, two nerves and one vein

  Muscles – posterior belly of digastric and superior belly of omohyoid

  Arteries – posterior auricular artery, occipital artery

  Nerves – spinal accessory nerve, inferior root of ansa cervicalis
- *Medial*

  Internal carotid artery and 9th, 10th, 11th and 12th cranial nerves in the upper part and common carotid artery and vagus nerve in the lower part (within the carotid sheath)

Figure 1.25 is an image of the carotid sheath on ultrasound. How can you identify the structures within the sheath?

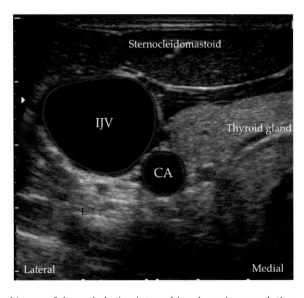

Figure 1.25   Ultrasound image of the neck during internal jugular vein cannulation.

Ultrasound image of IJV

Real-time ultrasound imaging of the internal jugular vein is performed during central line placement. Ultrasound guidance is used to reduce the risk of carotid artery injury and cannulation, pneumothorax and damage to other surrounding structures. A high-frequency vascular probe (e.g. 7.5 MHz) produces high-quality images. A slight head-down position is used to increase venous filling of the vessel, thereby increasing its diameter and facilitating cannulation. This position also minimises the risk of air embolism.

Ultrasound imaging reveals two sonolucent circles. The carotid artery is smaller in diameter and medial to the internal jugular vein. The internal jugular vein is compressible and non-pulsatile.

What anatomical abnormalities of this vein can make cannulation hazardous or impossible?

The two most common anatomical abnormalities of the internal jugular vein are duplication and fenestration. Duplication results from distal branching of the IJV, resulting in two branches draining separately into the subclavian vein. Fenestration is when there is branching, and distal re-unification.

Subclavian vein

The subclavian vein is a large, central vein that starts at the outer border of the first rib, as a continuation of the axillary vein and also receives the external jugular vein. It courses behind the clavicle and combines with the internal jugular vein at the medial border of the anterior scalene muscle to form the brachiocephalic vein at the venous angle. The venous angle receives the thoracic duct on the left and the right lymphatic duct on the right.

Course

The surface marking of the subclavian vein is along the course of the clavicle, though it arches upward behind the clavicle and then slopes down to meet the internal jugular vein behind the sternoclavicular joint.

It stays anterior to the subclavian artery, from which it is separated by the anterior scalene muscle.

Relations

- Anterior – clavicle
- Posterior – subclavian artery, anterior scalene muscle, first rib
- Inferior – pleura

What are the indications for central venous access?
- Access for infusions or interventions
  - Irritant drugs (e.g. vasopressors, chemotherapy)
  - Total parental nutrition
  - Renal replacement therapy

- Transvenous pacing
- Monitoring
  - Central venous pressure
  - Serial blood sampling
  - Pulmonary artery floatation catheter

What are the alternatives to internal jugular or subclavian central venous access?

Femoral access can be gained as an alternative to internal jugular or subclavian central venous access. This is particularly useful in an emergency resuscitative scenario, where access to the head, neck and chest are required for concomitant intubation or chest compressions. Femoral lines have higher rates of bacterial colonisation and possibly catheter-related infections than IJV or subclavian lines.

What are the alternatives for longer-term central venous access?

Peripherally inserted central lines (PICC) can be used for medium-term access. These are lines inserted into a peripheral vein and fed up into the central venous system. Other options for long-term access include tunnelled lines (e.g. surgically inserted Hickman line) or implanted devices (e.g. surgically inserted port).

Outline the risks associated with central venous cannulation and how they can be minimised.

Table 1.17   Complications of Central Venous Cannulation and Methods to Minimise Them

Risk	Consequence	Methods to minimise risk
Carotid injury/ cannulation	Arterial injury, stroke	Real-time ultrasound
Haemorrhage/ haematoma	Haemorrhage/haematoma	Appropriate catheter size, limiting attempts at cannulation
Air embolism	Air embolism	Head-down tilt, careful aspiration and flushing of lines
Injury to adjacent structures	Pneumothorax, haemothorax, chylothorax	Knowledge of anatomy, correct technique
Catheter-related infection	Sepsis	Aseptic technique and catheter maintenance (see Epic3)
Catheter misplacement	Arrhythmia	Confirmation of position: clinical, ultrasound visualisation, pressure transducer, blood gas analysis, chest x-ray

What do you understand by catheter-related blood stream infection (CRBSI)? What are the steps to minimise it?

CRBSI or catheter-related sepsis is defined as the presence of bacteraemia originating from an intravascular catheter. This could not only be from peripheral or central intravenous catheters but also from intra-arterial cannulae. The catheters are embedded with plasma proteins soon after insertion and form a nidus for colonisation of organisms that migrate from the skin along the catheter track. The bacterial colonisation can be extraluminal or endoluminal. Once the threshold count of organisms is reached, this then triggers a systemic inflammatory response through to multiorgan failure.

The most common offending organisms are staphylococcus aureus, coagulase negative staphylococcus, enterococci and candida.

Epic3 2014: this study produced national evidence-based guidelines for preventing healthcare-associated infections (HCAI) in NHS hospitals in England. The relevant points in the guidelines summary for intravascular access devices are as follows

Catheter type

- Use a single-lumen catheter unless multiple ports are essential
- For total parenteral nutrition, a dedicated CVC or lumen should be used
- Consider the use of an antimicrobial impregnated catheter for high risk patients

Catheter insertion site

- Assess the risks for infection vs mechanical complications and patient comfort
- Use the subclavian route unless contraindicated
- Use peripherally inserted catheters as an alternative to central venous catheters

Antisepsis

- Skin – single-use application of 2% chlorhexidine gluconate in 70% isopropyl alcohol and allowing it to dry
- General – maximal barrier precautions
- Antimicrobial lock solutions or systemic antibiotics should not be used routinely for prevention of CRBSI

Post procedure care

- Dressing – sterile, transparent, semipermeable polyurethane dressing changed every 7 days, or sooner
- Consider the use of a chlorhexidine impregnated sponge dressing in adult patients to reduce catheter related bloodstream infection

Catheter maintenance

- Cleaning hub with 2% chlorhexidine gluconate in 70% isopropyl alcohol and allowing it to dry
- Daily review of need for access and to exclude signs of infection
- Removal of central venous catheter at earliest opportunity

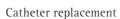

Catheter replacement

- Avoid guidewire-assisted catheter exchange for patients with CRBSI

Education

- Use quality improvement interventions to support the appropriate use and management of intravascular access devices
- Continuing professional education

Describe how you would perform cannulation of the internal jugular and the subclavian veins.

Table 1.18   Comparison of Techniques and Complications during Cannulation of Internal Jugular and Subclavian Vein

Preparation	
Informed consent, equipment (including ultrasound) Antisepsis – wash hands, sterile barrier precautions • Prepare skin with antiseptic (2% chlorhexidine) and sterile drape	
Internal jugular venous cannulation	**Subclavian venous cannulation**
Advantages • Superficial location and a straight course to the superior vena cava (on the right) • Avoidance of the subclavian 'pinch-off syndrome'	Advantages • Reduced risk of thrombosis and infectious complications • Better patient comfort
Landmarks	
Sedillot's triangle Medial – sternal head of the sternocleidomastoid muscle Lateral – clavicular head of the sternocleidomastoid Inferior – superior border of the medial third of the clavicle The IJV lies posterior to the apex of the triangle at a depth of approximately 1–1.5 cm	Space between the first rib and clavicle at the junction between the medial one third and lateral two-thirds of the clavicle
Position of patient and operator	
Patient position – head down with head turned to contralateral side Operator position – at the top of bed behind the patient's head	Patient position – head down with head turned to contralateral side Operator position – on the side of venous cannulation

(Continued)

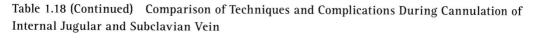

Table 1.18 (Continued) Comparison of Techniques and Complications During Cannulation of Internal Jugular and Subclavian Vein

Ultrasound guidance	
The internal jugular vein frequently lies anterolateral to the carotid artery but may also lie directly anterior to the artery, predisposing to arterial puncture which is hugely reduced by the use of ultrasound. Short axis view at or 1 cm above the apex of Sedillot's triangle demonstrates the carotid artery and internal jugular vein as two sonolucent circles. The artery is smaller, non-compressible and pulsatile and IJV is larger, compressible and collapsible. Long axis helps identify correct position of the guide wire and catheter in the vein.	The transducer is placed in the infraclavicular fossa in order to obtain a short axis view of the subclavian vein and artery. Then the vein is positioned centrally on the screen and the transducer is rotated retaining image of the vein, until a longitudinal view is obtained. This view enables visualisation of the axillary vein and distal subclavian vein, as well as the pleural lining below the vessel.

Technique	
Needle is angled 45° to the skin and the needle is advanced in a sagittal plane.	Needle is advanced parallel to the floor to avoid pneumothorax and directed to the sternal notch.

Seldinger technique: the vessel is accessed with a narrow-gauge needle through which a guidewire is advanced. ECG monitoring is used at this stage to rule out arrhythmias by preventing the wire from extending into intracardiac chambers. The needle is then removed, and the catheter inserted over the guidewire. The length of the catheter is determined by the height, sex of the patient and choice of the central vein. As a rough rule, in order to achieve correct positioning, Peres' formula can be used.

- Right IJV: height/10 (~12–13 cm in males and 11–12 cm in females)
- Left IJV: (height/10) + 4 cm (~13–14 cm in males and 12–13 cm in females)
- Right subclavian: (height/10) – 2 cm
- Left subclavian: (height/10) + 2 cm

Complications	
1. Carotid arterial puncture – risk reduced by avoiding medial angulation of needle & ultrasound use 2. Pneumothorax – risk reduced by staying high at Sedillot's triangle 3. Infection – this is more common with IJV compared to subclavian cannulations. The methods of prevention are described above.	1. Subclavian artery puncture – avoided by aiming the needle to the sternal notch 2. Pneumothorax – risk reduced by keeping needle parallel to the floor 3. Subclavian 'pinch-off syndrome' happens when the catheter is compressed between clavicle and first rib leading to obstruction, tearing, transection and catheter embolisation

(Continued)

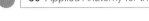

Table 1.18 (Continued)   Comparison of Techniques and Complications During Cannulation of Internal Jugular and Subclavian Vein

Post procedure confirmation
The optimal position of the catheter tip is found to be at the right atrio-caval junction as the blood flow at this junction is high thus preventing thrombosis. More proximal catheters can abut the wall of the vein and result in preventing injection/aspiration, pain on injection of irritant drugs, perforation of the vein, thrombosis and infection. More distally placed catheters have the risk of arrhythmias, haemothorax, damage of the tricuspid valve and atrial or ventricular wall. The surface landmark corresponding to this position is the angle of Louis or the manubrio-sternal angle.   *Confirmation of position*   • Ultrasound visualisation of needle insertion, guidewire and catheter placement   • Pressure transducer   • CXR   • Injection of agitated saline and observation of bubbles on bedside echo

What is the NICE guidance regarding the use of ultrasound in central venous catheterisation?

Ultrasound does not obviate the need for anatomic knowledge, so knowledge on anatomical landmarks remain necessary for orientation of the probe and the needle. Ultrasound use differentiates the internal jugular vein from the carotid artery, reduces the incidence of arterial puncture, guards against through-and-through puncture of the internal jugular vein and injury to nearby structures.

NICE recommends the use of 2-D ultrasound as the preferred method for insertion of internal jugular vein catheters in adults and in children in the elective setting. It should be 'considered in most clinical situations' both in the elective and emergency setting (NICE Technology Appraisal No 49, 2002).

- *Internal jugular vein*

  Results from seven RCTs suggested that real-time 2-D ultrasound guidance was associated with reduced risks of failed catheter placements, catheter placement complications and failure on the first catheter placement attempt and fewer attempts.

- *Subclavian vein*

  Only one RCT was identified that analysed the effect of 2-D ultrasound guidance. In comparison with the landmark method, 2-D ultrasound guidance was associated with reduced risks of catheter placement failure and catheter placement complications.

  But it is important to note that the operators in the trial were relatively inexperienced in both the landmark and 2-D ultrasound guided method.

- *Femoral vein*

  Compared with the landmark method, 2-D ultrasound guidance reduced the risk of failed catheter placement and the time to successful catheterisation, but the differences were not statistically significant.

Describe the blood supply and venous drainage of the tonsils.

The clinical application of this topic is the anaesthetic management of post tonsillectomy bleed.

Tonsils are highly vascularised lymphoid tissues situated in the tonsillar fossa of the pharynx (Figure 1.26).

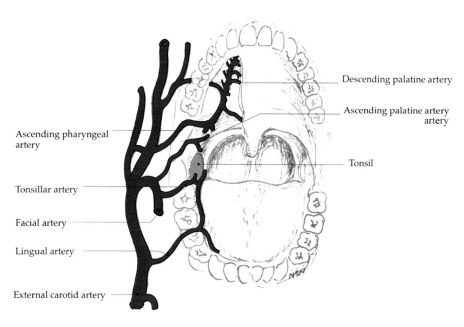

Descending palatine artery

Ascending palatine artery
artery

Tonsil

Ascending pharyngeal
artery

Tonsillar artery

Facial artery

Lingual artery

External carotid artery

Figure 1.26   Arterial supply – tonsils.

They receive blood from the external carotid artery and its branches

- Tonsillar artery and ascending palatine artery (branches of facial artery)
- Lesser palatine artery (from descending palatine, a branch of maxillary artery)
- Dorsal lingual artery (a branch of lingual artery)
- Ascending pharyngeal artery (a branch of external carotid artery)

Venous drainage is to the peritonsillar plexus, which drains into the lingual and pharyngeal veins and eventually into the internal jugular vein.

Bibliography

Bannon, M. P., Heller, S. F., & Rivera, M. (2011). Anatomic considerations for central venous cannulation. *Risk Management & Healthcare Policy, 4*, 27.

Fletcher, S. (2005). Catheter-related bloodstream infection. *Continuing Education in Anaesthesia, Critical Care & Pain, 5*(2), 49–51.

Loveday, H. P., Wilson, J., Pratt, R. J., Golsorkhi, M., Tingle, A., et al. (2014). epic3: National evidence-based guidelines for preventing healthcare-associated infections in NHS hospitals in England. *The Journal of Hospital Infection, 86*(Supplement 1), S1–S70.

National Institute for Clinical Excellence (2002). *Guidance on the Use of Ultrasound Locating Devices for Placing Central Venous Catheters.* London: NICE [NICE Technology Appraisal No 49.].

Rupp, S. M., Apfelbaum, J. L., Blitt, C., Caplan, R. A., Connis, R. T., et al. (2012). Practice guidelines for central venous access: A report by the American Society of Anesthesiologists Task Force on Central Venous Access. *Anesthesiology, 116*(3), 539.

Shrestha, G. S., Gurung, A., & Koirala, S. (2016). Comparison between long-and short-axis techniques for ultrasound-guided cannulation of internal jugular vein. *Annals of Cardiac Anaesthesia, 19*(2), 288.

Smith, R. N., & Nolan, J. P. (2013). Central venous catheters. *BMJ, 347*, f6570.

Nervous System

- Cranial nerves – II, V, VII and X
- Scalp blocks
- Eye Blocks
  - Sub-Tenon's block
  - Retro bulbar block
  - Peri bulbar block
- Laryngeal nerve blocks
- Cervical plexus block
- Stellate ganglion block – discussed in ANS

Cranial Nerves

When would you assess cranial nerves in a patient?

Anaesthetists might be involved with cranial nerve monitoring intraoperatively for specific ENT and neurosurgical procedures, in order to preserve function and avoid damage, or on the intensive care unit in brain stem death testing.

The facial nerve is also used to monitor depth and reversibility of neuromuscular blockade.

Which cranial nerves are commonly monitored perioperatively?

Commonly

- Facial nerve
  - Depth + reversibility of neuromuscular blockade
  - Surgery on parotid gland (most commonly parotidectomy)
  - Neurosurgery for acoustic neuroma

- Vagus nerve
  - Recurrent laryngeal nerve (branch of vagus) is monitored in surgery on the thyroid gland or the vocal cords.

Less commonly

- Glossopharyngeal nerve
  - Radical neck dissection
- Trigeminal nerve
  - Microvascular decompression for trigeminal neuralgia
- Accessory/hypoglossal nerves
  - Skull base surgery for glomus jugulare tumours (benign lesion in the jugular foramen)

What are the indications/pre-conditions for brainstem death testing?

The Academy of Medical Royal Colleges published a 42-page document in 2008 titled 'A Code of Practice for the Diagnosis and Confirmation of Death'. This document details the specific conditions necessary for the diagnosis and confirmation of brain stem death. In summary:

All of the following conditions must be fulfilled before a diagnosis of death can be made due to irreversible cessation of brainstem function.

- Aetiology of irreversible brain damage must be known
- Potentially reversible causes of coma must be excluded
- Potentially reversible causes of apnoea must be excluded – e.g. neuromuscular blocking drugs
- There should be no evidence that this state is due to depressant drugs – e.g. prolonged effects of analgesic, anaesthetic or benzodiazepine infusion, especially in the context of organ failure
- Primary hypothermia as the cause of unconsciousness must be excluded
  - Minimum T_{core} >34°C at time of testing
- Potentially reversible circulatory, metabolic and endocrine disturbances must be excluded as the cause for unconsciousness. The following must be observed
  - MAP >60 mmHg
  - P_aCO_2 <6.0 kPa
  - P_aO_2 >10 kPa
  - pH 7.35–7.45
  - Serum Na^+ 115–160 mmol/L
  - Serum K^+ >2 mmol/L
  - Serum PO_4^- & Mg^{2+} 0.5–3 mmol/L
  - Blood glucose 3–20 mmol/L
  - Hormone assays if suspicious of myxoedema, thyroid storm or Addisonian crisis

How would you test the vestibulo-ocular reflex?
- Sit patient up at 30° (unless contraindicated by an unstable spinal injury)
- Inspect external auditory meatus to ensure patency by visualising ear drums
- Inject 50 ml of ice-cold water slowly over 1 minute
- **Nystagmus is absent in brain stem death**

In ITU brain stem death testing, which cranial nerve reflexes are tested? And what are the afferent and efferent pathways for each?

Table 1.19   Cranial Nerves and Reflex Pathways Tested During Brainstem Death Test

Reflex	Afferent	Efferent	Response
Pupillary light reflex	II	III	Pupils remain fixed (no constriction) to bright light
Corneal reflex	V	VII	No blink to light touch of cotton wool to cornea
Response to facial pain	V	VII	No facial motor response to supra-/infra-orbital pain stimulus
Vestibulo-ocular reflex	VIII	III, IV, VI	No eye movement to ice cold water into auditory meatus
Gag reflex	IX	X	No gag when spatula inserted into back of pharynx
Cough reflex	X	X	No cough when larynx/trachea stimulated (bronchial catheter inserted to carina)

Which cranial nerves are not tested and why?

I, XI and XII are not tested as they are not involved in a reflex arc.

Optic Nerve

The optic nerve receives its inputs at the optic disc of the retina. It leaves the retina at its site of origin (optic disc) and follows an intraconal course (approximately 2.5 cm), exiting the orbit at the optic foramen superomedially to the ophthalmic artery to enter the middle cranial fossa. It passes medially to the internal carotid artery before reaching the optic chiasm, located above the sella turcica. The intracranial component of the nerve is 1.25 cm long. There is some decussation of fibres at the chiasm after which the nerve travels on its respective side to synapse in the lateral geniculate body within the thalamus. Fibres pass from here to the occipital cortex.

A small number of fibres bypass the lateral geniculate body to go to the superior colliculus. These fibres are associated with ocular and pupillary reflexes.

Which fibres of the optic nerve decussate?

Fibres from the medial side of the retina (associated with temporal vision) decussate at the optic chiasm and travel to the contralateral side of the cortex. Fibres from lateral half of retina travel ipsilaterally.

What visual disturbance might you expect with lesions at different levels?

Retina/optic nerve lesion

- Blindness associated with the side of the lesion

Lesions of optic tract and central pathways

- Homonymous defects

Lesion at optic chiasm (e.g. from pituitary tumour)

- Bitemporal hemianopia (loss of temporal vision in both eyes)

Trigeminal Nerve

The trigeminal nerve is the largest of the cranial nerves with one motor and three sensory nuclei (Figure 1.27).

- Motor nucleus – upper pons below the floor of fourth ventricle
- Sensory nuclei
  - Mesencephalic nucleus (proprioception) – midbrain
  - Principal sensory nucleus (touch) – upper pons
  - Nucleus of spinal tract (pain/temperature) – pons to spinal cord

Course

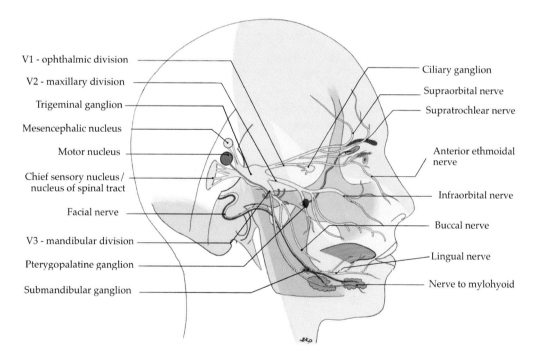

Figure 1.27 Trigeminal nerve – origin and course.

- Sensory fibres decussate, emerging at the upper pons as a large sensory and smaller motor root.
- Trigeminal ganglion (also known as Gasserian or semilunar ganglion) is a crescent-shaped swelling formed by the sensory fibres situated at the apex of the petrous temporal bone.

The ganglion is surrounded superiorly by the temporal lobe, medially by the internal carotid artery and cavernous sinus, and inferiorly lies the motor root.

- The motor fibres bypass the ganglion and join the mandibular division.

What is the sensory distribution and what are the important branches of the three main divisions?

- Ophthalmic (V1) – sensory only
  - Emerges via the supraorbital fissure to supply sensation to nose, forehead, eyelids, scalp and globe
  - Important branches include frontal, lacrimal and nasociliary nerves
- Maxillary (V2) – sensory only
  - Leaves the base of skull via the foramen rotundum and branches supply the pterygopalatine fossa, lower eyelid, cheek, upper lips, temple and teeth
  - Becomes the infraorbital nerve as it exits the infraorbital foramen
- Mandibular (V3) – sensory + motor
  - Exits via the foramen ovale
  - Sensory branches include auriculotemporal, buccal and lingual nerves
  - Motor branches include masseteric and lateral pterygoid nerves
  - Mixed (motor + sensory) branches include inferior dental nerve
  - Supplies ear, temple, jaw, lower lips and teeth

Apart from the trigeminal nerve, which other nerve supplies sensation to the face?

Greater auricular nerve from cervical plexus.

Do you know any local anaesthetic blocks for superficial facial surgery?

(See also Scalp Blocks)

- Infratrochlear (eyelids, nose and conjunctivae)
  - Blocked along medial orbit wall, 1 cm above inner canthus
- Supraorbital and supratrochlear (forehead)
  - Blocked a few millimetres above supraorbital ridge
- Infraorbital (lower eyelid and upper lip)
  - Blocked at infraorbital foramen, 1.5 cm below infraorbital margin in line with the pupil
- Mental (chin, lower lip)
  - Midpoint between upper and lower border of mandible, in line with pupil

What are the causes of trigeminal neuralgia?

- Demyelination – may be first presentation in patients with multiple sclerosis
- Compression – by abnormal blood vessel or space occupying lesion in posterior fossa
- Central – abnormal neurons in pons with spontaneous and uncontrollable firing
- Pontine infarct

What are the clinical features of trigeminal neuralgia?

- Severe, paroxysmal lancinating pain in the trigeminal distribution (usually mandibular/perioral)

- Often triggered by chewing or touching the face
  - Usually unilateral (bilateral in 3–5%)

What are the treatment options for trigeminal neuralgia?
- Pharmacological
  - Carbamazepine is first line. 100 mg BD, to maximum 1600 mg/day
  - Gabapentin, pregabalin and amitriptyline, for their use in neuropathic pain though evidence of efficacy in treating trigeminal neuralgia is not strong
  - Baclofen and lamotrigine can be used as add on therapy
  - IV phenytoin has been used in acute, intractable pain
- Surgical
  - Peripheral neurolysis of trigeminal nerve branches with LASER, alcohol injection or neurectomy
  - Trigeminal ganglion ablation by radiofrequency (thermal), chemical (phenol, alcohol) or mechanical (balloon compression) techniques (Figure 1.28)
  - Craniotomy for microvascular decompression
  - Gamma knife stereotactical radiosurgery
- Other
  - Psychological intervention – assess for signs of depression
  - Neuromodulation
  - Non-invasive repetitive transcranial magnetic stimulation of motor cortex

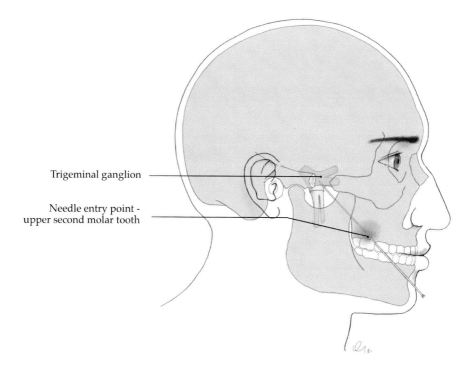

Figure 1.28   Trigeminal nerve block.

Facial Nerve

What is the course of the facial nerve?

- A large motor root and a smaller mixed sensory/visceral efferent root (nervous intermedius) emerge from the pontomedullary junction.
- They enter the internal auditory meatus, before passing through the facial canal and middle ear to reach the geniculate or facial ganglion.
- The nerve exits the skull via the stylomastoid foramen, before winding around styloid process and entering the parotid gland (Figure 1.29).

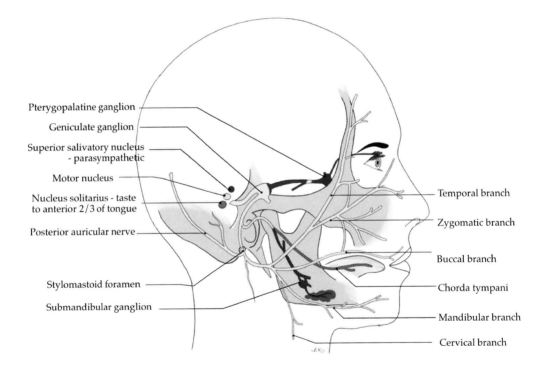

Figure 1.29   Facial nerve – origin and course.

What are the functions of the facial nerve?

- Motor – nerves of facial expression
- Sensory – taste to anterior two-thirds of the tongue and sensation from the external auditory meatus and tympanic membrane
- Parasympathetic – supply to the salivary, palatine and lacrimal glands

Which branches arise at the geniculate ganglion and what are their functions?

- Greater petrosal nerve – secretomotor to lacrimal gland
- Chorda tympani – taste to anterior two-thirds of tongue

What are the names of the motor branches which supply the muscles of facial expression?

Two Zulus Battered My Cat

- Temporal branch
- Zygomatic branch
- Buccal branch
- Mandibular branch
- Cervical branch

During which types of procedures might facial nerve monitoring be used?

- Parotidectomy
- Middle ear surgery (e.g. mastoidectomy)
- Posterior fossa surgery (e.g. acoustic neuroma or surgery at cerebello-pontine angle)

How is facial nerve monitoring done and what impact does it have upon anaesthesia?

Monitoring is done by

- EMG monitoring – spontaneous activity suggests that the surgeon is operating in close proximity to the nerve.
- Direct electrical stimulation – stimulation of the nerve and observation of the response to test integrity
- Train of four to assess depth of neuromuscular blockade

Anaesthetic plan

- Avoid neuromuscular blocking drugs.
- Remifentanil and propofol are often used as part of a TIVA technique to achieve desired intubating conditions and muscle relaxation.
- In surgery where SSEPs are monitored, avoid volatile. Muscle relaxants can be used so long as EMG/MEPs do not need to be monitored.

Vagus Nerve

The vagus nerve (CN X), is the longest, most complex and only asymmetrical cranial nerve. You will be expected to demonstrate a basic understanding of its course through the body, and knowledge of the main branches and where they arise.

Nuclei

- Nucleus ambiguous (motor)
- Nucleus tractus solitarius (sensory)
- Dorsal nucleus (parasympathetic)

Approximately ten rootlets arise symmetrically from the left and right sides of the medulla to form single left and right vagus nerves. These pass through the jugular foramen travelling within the dural sheath together with the accessory nerve.

The vagus nerve then descends within the carotid sheath, posterior to the internal carotid artery and the internal jugular vein. From the root of the neck, the paths of the right vagus nerve (RVN) and left vagus nerve (LVN) differ.

Left vagus nerve (LVN)

- Enters thorax between the left carotid and left subclavian arteries, travelling posterior to the left brachiocephalic vein
- Descends anterior to aortic arch, at which point the left recurrent laryngeal nerve is given off, which in turn crosses under the aortic arch and ascends in the tracheo-oesophageal groove
- The LVN further descends posterior to the lung root where it gives off the left pulmonary plexus.
- Two or more cords of the left pulmonary plexus unite with branches of right vagus nerve to form the oesophageal plexus.
- The anterior vagus nerve (now containing fibres from left and right) is formed from the oesophageal plexus. It passes through the diaphragm at T10 and enters the abdomen anterior to the oesophagus.
- In the abdomen, the LVN, or anterior vagus nerve, gives off gastric, pyloric and hepatic branches.

Right vagus nerve (RVN)

- The RVN gives off the right recurrent laryngeal nerve in the neck, at the level of the right subclavian artery.
- As it passes behind the right brachiocephalic vein, the RVN continues its descent into the thorax, in close proximity to the trachea.

- At the lung root, the right pulmonary plexus arises, from which fibres forming the oesophageal plexus unite with branches of the left vagus nerve to form the posterior vagus nerve.

- Like the anterior vagus nerve arising predominantly from the LVN, the posterior vagus nerve (arising predominantly from the right) enters the abdomen posterior to the oesophagus after piercing the diaphragm at T10.

- In the abdomen, the RVN, or posterior vagus nerve, also gives off branches to the stomach, however the bulk of the RVN will form the coeliac branch which forms the coeliac ganglion. This in turn supplies the intestines, kidneys and adrenals (Figure 1.30).

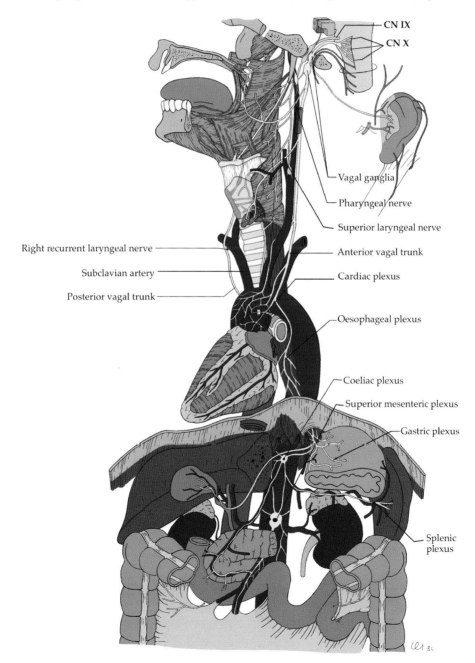

Figure 1.30   Vagus nerve.

What are the main branches of the vagus nerve arising in the head, neck, thorax and abdomen?

- Head
  - Auricular branch
- Neck
  - Pharyngeal nerve
  - Superior laryngeal nerve
  - Right recurrent laryngeal nerve
  - Superior cardiac plexus
- Thorax
  - Left recurrent laryngeal nerve
  - Inferior cardiac plexus
  - Pulmonary plexus
  - Oesophageal plexus
  - Anterior vagal trunk (LVN)
  - Posterior vagal trunk (RVN)
- Abdomen
  - Gastric
  - Hepatic
  - Intestinal
  - Coeliac plexus

What is the course of the recurrent laryngeal nerve?

The RLN supplies all intrinsic muscles of the larynx, except for cricothyroid muscle (supplied by the external branch of superior laryngeal nerve)

- Right RLN arises from the vagus at the level of the subclavian artery. It loops under this artery, before ascending in the tracheo-oesophageal groove up to the larynx.
- Left RLN comes off the vagus nerve at the level of the aortic arch. It loops under the arch, before similarly ascending in the tracheo-oesophageal groove up to the larynx.

Through which foramen does the vagus nerve exit the cranium?

The jugular foramen.

What are the clinical features of vagus nerve transection at the jugular foramen?

High vagal lesions are seen less commonly than low vagal lesions. The causes could be due to trauma, infection and neoplasm. Clinical features include

- Dysphonia or hoarse voice, due to vocal cord paralysis
- Bovine cough due to poor initial explosive impulse due to inability to close glottis fully and generate pressure
- Nasal speech
- Nasal regurgitation or abnormal swallowing with increased risk of aspiration

- Reduced bowel motility
- Loss of vagal reflexes (gag, cough, oculo-cardiac, carotid sinus pressure)

During which procedures is RLN monitoring often used?

Thyroidectomy and parathyroidectomy.

How might the RLN be injured or damaged?

- Neck
  - Thyroid or parathyroid surgery
  - Malignancy (thyroid, oesophagus)
- Chest
  - Cardiothoracic surgery
  - Aortic aneurysm
  - Trauma
  - Malignancy (lymphoma, lung, oesophagus)

Which clinical situations commonly produce vagal reflex bradycardia?

- Physiological
  - Pregnancy (IVC compression)
  - Baroreceptor reflex
    - Acute rise in BP (increased baroreceptor firing resulting in increased vagal activity)
  - Valsalva manoeuvre (phase 1)
- Surgical
  - Ophthalmic: oculocardiac reflex (squint surgery)
  - General: laparoscopic procedures (peritoneal distension), anal dilatation, traction to gall bladder, liver or bowel
  - Urological: bladder, urethral or testicular surgery
  - Gynaecological: cervical dilatation, uterine or ovarian traction
- Anaesthetic
  - Tilt table
  - Neuraxial block
  - Laryngospasm
  - Drugs: vasopressors, anticholinesterase

What are the important anaesthetic considerations for somebody undergoing a mastoidectomy?

Mastoidectomy is performed to remove diseased mastoid air cells, or abnormal growth of mastoid cells. Important anaesthetic considerations include

- LMA vs ETT. Either is acceptable, however the patient should ideally be mechanically ventilated. Remember the head is away from anaesthetic machine and tilted on a head ring. Access to the airway is difficult intraoperatively
- Avoid neuromuscular blocking drugs as facial nerve monitoring might be required

- Avoid nitrous oxide due to its high solubility in relation to nitrogen
  - Bloodless operating field in order to facilitate surgery
    - Head up
    - Avoid coughing
    - Hypotensive anaesthesia may be judiciously employed (remifentanil is very good at keeping heart rate constant and inducing hypotension)
  - Antiemetic: high incidence of PONV
  - Temperature regulation: long procedure so active warming methods (warm blankets/ forced warm air blanket, warmed fluids)
  - VTE Prophylaxis: TEDS/sequential compression devices

How would you assess the airway of a patient presenting for thyroidectomy?

- History
  - Enquire about positional breathlessness or noisy breathing
  - Enquire about dysphagia
  - Enquire about duration of goitre. Long standing goitre is associated with tracheomalacia.
- Examination looking for
  - Stridor
  - SVC obstruction (oedema, venous distension)
  - Neck examination, particularly looking at consistency and size of goitre
  - Airway examination, particularly looking at range of neck movement
- Investigations
  - Check if nasendoscopy has been performed
  - Imaging (CXR, CT neck) to look for retrosternal extension of goitre and tracheal deviation

How can the recurrent laryngeal nerve be monitored intraoperatively?

The recurrent laryngeal nerve can be monitored using a specialised endotracheal tube which contains surface electrodes that guide the placement of the tube between the cords. These electrodes enable EMG monitoring.

What implications does this have for anaesthesia?

The tracheal tube needs careful placement in order to work reliably. Intraoperative neuromuscular blocking drugs should be avoided.

What are the possible postoperative complications pertinent to the anaesthetist after thyroidectomy?

- Postoperative stridor
  - Haemorrhage/haematoma
  - Tracheomalacia
  - Bilateral recurrent laryngeal nerve palsies

- Other
  - Hypocalcaemia. This may present as neuromuscular excitability, tetany or perioral tinging. Facial twitching may be seen when tapping over the facial nerve at the parotid gland. ECG may demonstrate a prolonged QT interval.
  - Thyroid storm
  - Pneumothorax (if retro-sternal dissection)

How would you manage a patient with stridor post thyroidectomy?

This could rapidly deteriorate and become life threatening. It is important to call for senior anaesthetic and ENT help early.

- Give 100% oxygen.
- Remove clips to relieve compression from a haematoma. It may be necessary to do this at the bedside if the patient is in extremis and unable to wait to get to theatre.
- Nebulised adrenaline if stridor is due to oedema.
- Inform theatres and move to theatres if safe to do so.
- Prepare for urgent re-intubation with a selection of tube sizes available. Consider reinforced tube if due to tracheomalacia.
- Prepare for tracheostomy.
- If patient's condition allows, consider nasendoscopy to evaluate cord function.

Bibliography

Simpson, P., Bates, D., Bonner, S., Costeloe, K., Doyal, L., et al. (2008). *A Code of Practice for the Diagnosis and Confirmation of Death*. London Academy of Medical Royal Colleges.
Vasappa, C. K., Kapur, S., & Krovvidi, H. (2016). Trigeminal neuralgia. *BJA Education, 16*(10), 353–356.

Scalp Blocks

Blocking the nerves supplying the scalp had shown to blunt the reflex responses during surgery and also reduce the intra- and postoperative analgesic requirements.

Indications

- Neurosurgery – awake and routine craniotomies, stereotactic procedures, operations needing intraprocedural functional testing, etc.
- Surgery of the head and face – cleft lip and palate surgery, laceration repair, otoplasty, tympanoplasty, etc.
- Diagnostic and therapeutic management of chronic headache

Innervation of the scalp

The scalp is innervated by the following nerves and the area of supply by these nerves is depicted in the image (Figure 1.31).

1. Supraorbital and supratrochlear nerves from the ophthalmic division (V1) of the trigeminal nerve
2. Zygomaticotemporal nerve from the maxillary division (V2) of the trigeminal nerve
3. Auriculotemporal nerve from the mandibular division (V3) of the trigeminal nerve
4. Greater occipital nerve (C2)
5. Lesser occipital nerve (C2)
6. Greater auricular nerve (C2, C3)

The scalp can be anaesthetised by performing individual nerve blocks or by infiltration of local anaesthetic around the scalp. Use of ultrasound is highly recommended to avoid accidental vascular injection, injury to surrounding structures and to prevent local anaesthetic toxicity by limiting the total volume of local anaesthetic used.

Supraorbital and supratrochlear nerves (V1)

The frontal nerve is a branch of the ophthalmic nerve (V1) that divides into the terminal branches, supraorbital and supratrochlear nerves which can be blocked at one injection point.

Indications: frontal craniotomy, surgery on the eye and eyelid, nose and frontal sinus, and in providing analgesia in acute herpes zoster.

Procedure: the supraorbital foramen (at the junction of the medial one third and the lateral two-thirds of the orbital rim) is palpated and a 25G needle is inserted beneath the eyebrow and is directed medially and cranially. 1 ml of local anaesthetic is injected to block the supraorbital nerve. To block the supratrochlear nerve, the needle is redirected about 1 cm toward the midline and another ml injected after negative aspiration.

Specific complications: haematoma, intravascular injection and damage to the eye.

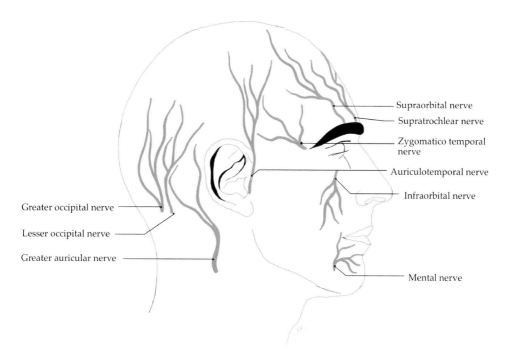

Figure 1.31   Face and scalp nerves.

Infraorbital (V2) nerve

(This is not a part of the 'scalp block' but it is included for completeness.)

The infraorbital nerve is the terminal branch of the maxillary nerve (V2) and surfaces the face through the infraorbital foramen where it is blocked.

Indications: cleft lip/palate repair, endoscopic sinus surgery, rhinoplasty and transsphenoidal hypophysectomy.

Procedure: the infraorbital foramen is identified just below the orbital rim 3 cm from the midline of the face. In the intraoral approach, a 25G needle is inserted into the buccal mucosa at the level of the first premolar and directed upward and outward and 1–2 ml of local anaesthetic is injected after negative aspiration.

Specific complications: haematoma, persistent paraesthesia and numbness of the upper lip, penetration of the foramen leading to damage of nerve and orbital contents.

Zygomaticotemporal nerve (V2)

The nerve lies in the temporal fossa and pierces the temporalis fascia 2.5 cm above the zygomatic arch.

Procedure: infiltration from the lateral edge of the supraorbital margin to the distal aspect of the zygomatic arch.

Specific complications: haematoma formation, increased systemic absorption due to high vascularity.

Auriculotemporal nerve (V3)

This nerve is a branch of the mandibular nerve (V3) and runs along with the superficial temporal artery.

Procedure: injection of local anaesthetic about 1 cm anterior to the ear, at the level of the tragus, avoiding the superficial temporal artery.

Specific complications: haematoma formation, increased systemic absorption due to high vascularity.

Greater and lesser occipital nerves (C2)

These nerves enter the back of the head along posterior border of the sternocleidomastoid muscle and run behind the ear (Figure 1.32).

Procedure: an imaginary line is drawn between the external occipital protuberance and mastoid process. The greater occipital nerve lies at the junction of the lateral and middle thirds on that line, and the lesser occipital nerve is between the middle and the medial thirds. A 25G needle is inserted medial to the occipital artery and 2–4 ml of local anaesthetic is infiltrated in a fan-like distribution to cover both nerves.

Specific complications: haematoma formation, increased systemic absorption due to high vascularity.

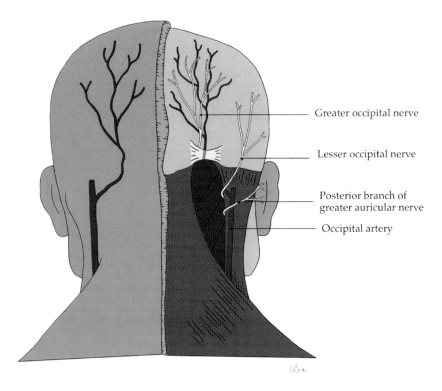

Greater occipital nerve

Lesser occipital nerve

Posterior branch of
greater auricular nerve

Occipital artery

Figure 1.32   Occipital nerve block.

Greater auricular nerve (C2, C3)

This nerve surfaces at the posterior margin of the sternocleidomastoid muscle at the level of the cricoid cartilage and ascends to the ear.

> Procedure: inject around 2 ml of the local anaesthetic about 1–2 cm posterior to the ear, at the level of the tragus.

> Specific complications: haematoma formation, increased systemic absorption due to high vascularity.

Table 1.20 Summary of Scalp Blocks

Nerve	Notes
Supraorbital/supratrochlear (V1)	
Indications	Frontal craniotomy, surgery on the eye and eyelid, nose and frontal sinus, and in providing analgesia in acute herpes zoster
Procedure	The supraorbital foramen (at the junction of the medial one third and the lateral two-thirds of the orbital rim) is palpated and a 25G needle is inserted beneath the eyebrow and is directed medially and cranially. 1 ml of local anaesthetic is injected to block the supraorbital nerve. To block the supratrochlear nerve, the needle is redirected about 1 cm toward the midline and another ml injected after negative aspiration. Specific complications: haematoma, intravascular injection and damage to the eye
Zygomaticotemporal nerve (V2)	Procedure: infiltration from the lateral edge of the supraorbital margin to the distal aspect of the zygomatic arch Specific complications: haematoma formation, increased systemic absorption due to high vascularity
Auriculotemporal nerve (V3)	Procedure: injection of local anaesthetic about 1 cm anterior to the ear, at the level of the tragus, avoiding the superficial temporal artery Specific complications: haematoma formation, increased systemic absorption due to high vascularity
Greater and lesser occipital nerves (C2)	Procedure: an imaginary line is drawn between the external occipital protuberance and mastoid process. Greater occipital nerve lies at the junction of the lateral and middle thirds on that line, and lesser occipital nerve is between the middle and the medial thirds. A 25G is inserted medial to the occipital artery and 2–4 ml of local anaesthetic is infiltrated in a fan-like distribution to cover both nerves. Specific complications: haematoma formation, increased systemic absorption due to high vascularity
Greater auricular nerve (C2, C3)	Procedure: inject around 2 ml of the local anaesthetic about 1–2 cm posterior to the ear, at the level of the tragus. Specific complications: haematoma formation, increased systemic absorption due to high vascularity

Bibliography

Burnand, C., & Sebastian, J. (2013). Anaesthesia for awake craniotomy. *Continuing Education in Anaesthesia, Critical Care & Pain, 14*(1), 6–11.

Guilfoyle, M. R., Helmy, A., Duane, D., & Hutchinson, P. J. (2013). Regional scalp block for postcraniotomy analgesia: A systematic review and meta-analysis. *Anesthesia & Analgesia, 116*(5), 1093–1102.

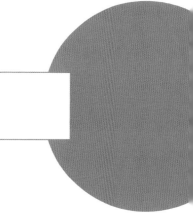

Eye Blocks

What is the nerve supply to the eyeball?

Sensory

- Optic nerve receives light input from the retina
- Ophthalmic (V1) branch of trigeminal nerve
  - Frontal nerve (conjunctiva and upper eyelid)
  - Nasociliary nerve (cornea, iris and ciliary muscle)
  - Lacrimal nerve (lacrimal gland)
- Maxillary (V2) branch of trigeminal nerve
  - Infraorbital nerve (lower eyelid)

Autonomic

- Sympathetic – pupillary dilatation
  - By long and short ciliary nerves via superior cervical ganglion
- Parasympathetic – pupillary constriction
  - By short postganglionic ciliary nerve via ciliary ganglion
  - Preganglionic supply via CN III

Motor ($3LR_6SO_4$)

- Lateral rectus (abduction) – abducens nerve (CN VI)
- Superior oblique (medial rotation, abduction and depression 'down and out') – trochlear nerve (CN IV)
- Inferior rectus (depression), medial rectus (adduction), inferior oblique (lateral rotation, abduction and elevation), superior rectus (elevation) – oculomotor nerve (CN III)

Which eye blocks might anaesthetists perform for eye surgery, and can you give a brief description of each?

All the nerves responsible for the sensory, motor and autonomic innervation of the eyeball transit through the intraconal space (except the trochlear nerve and branch of the facial nerve). Whatever the technique, the local anaesthetic injected must spread into the cone for a successful block. This explains why the retrobulbar block has a faster onset whilst in the peribulbar block the local anesthetic injected extraconally needs time to spread into the cone to produce the effect. This can be overcome by increasing the volume of local anaesthetic injected.

In sub-Tenon's block, local anaesthetic spreads into the episcleral space and the extraocular muscle sheaths with lower volumes and extends to the subconjunctival space and the optic nerve sheath with higher volumes.

A successful block will result in

- Ptosis
- Proptosis
- Akinesia
- Anaesthesia
- Mydriasis

Indications

Cataract surgery but is also effective in a variety of other eye surgeries, including vitreoretinal surgery, strabismus correction and trabeculectomy.

Drugs used

Local anaesthetic: 2% lignocaine and/or bupivacaine 0.5% depending on anaesthetic and surgical preference considering the potential length of operation.

Hyaluronidase: to increase the effectiveness of the block by enabling the spread of local anaesthetic through the tissues. Hyaluronidase can be used in a concentration of approximately 25–75 units/ml of local anaesthetic.

Adrenaline: used in a concentration of 1:100000 to decrease systemic absorption of the anaesthetic drug and provide a longer duration of action.

Sub-Tenon's block (episcleral injection) (Figure 1.33)

- Ask patient to look up and out.
- Apply topical local anaesthetic and antiseptic to lower fornix.
- Using special forceps (Moorfield's) to expose a thick fold of conjunctiva in the inferonasal quadrant, make a small 1–2 mm cut with round tip scissors (Westcott's).
- Slowly advance a blunt, 25 mm 19G sub-Tenon's cannula, following the curvature of the globe posteriorly.
- Confirm negative aspiration before injecting 2–5 ml of local anaesthetic solution depending on the surgical time.

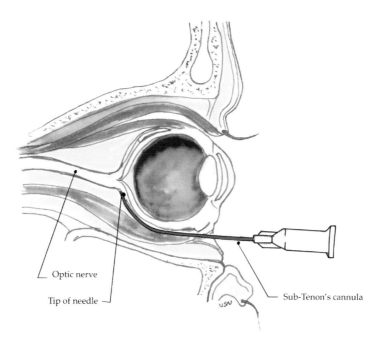

Figure 1.33 Sub-Tenon's block.

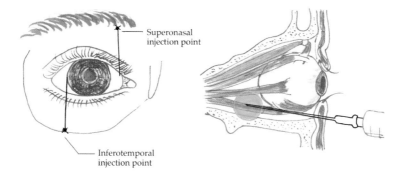

Figure 1.34 Peribulbar block.

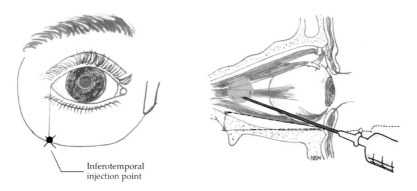

Figure 1.35 Retrobulbar block.

Peribulbar block (extraconal injection) (Figure 1.34)

- Ask patient to look straight ahead.
- Apply topical local anaesthetic and antiseptic.
- The point of injection is at the junction of the lateral one third and medial two-thirds of the eye. A 25G 16 mm needle is inserted through the conjunctiva or percutaneously with bevel facing up and advanced aiming at an inferotemporal angle parallel to the floor of the orbit. The needle tip should remain extraconal and should not be advanced further than the posterior border of the globe.
- Inject 6–12 ml of local anaesthetic after confirming negative aspiration.
- Apply pressure to the eye to promote spread.

Retrobulbar block (intraconal injection) (Figure 1.35)

- Ask patient to look straight ahead.
- Apply topical local anaesthetic and antiseptic.
- A 24 mm 25G needle is inserted at the same insertion point as above either through the conjunctival fold or percutaneously through the lower eyelid. The needle is advanced parallel to floor of orbit. At about 10–15 mm, it is redirected medially and upwards to enter the muscle cone and inject 3–5 ml local anaesthetic after negative aspiration.
- Apply pressure to the eye to promote spread.

What are the possible complications from performing eye blocks?

Table 1.21   Block-Specific Complications of Eye Blocks

Retrobulbar block
Puncture of globe
Haemorrhage due to arterial puncture (venous puncture is less severe)
Oculocardiac reflex due to haemorrhage
Central retinal artery occlusion due to haemorrhage
Subarachnoid or intradural injection (injection into optic sheath)
Optic nerve injury
Peribulbar block
Globe perforation
Transient blindness
Periorbital ecchymoses
Brainstem anaesthesia due to injection of local anaesthetic into optic sheath
Spread of local anaesthetic to contralateral eye
Sub-Tenon's block
Chemosis
Subconjunctival haemorrhage
Scleral perforation

Bibliography

Local Anaesthesia for Intraocular Surgery. (2012). London: The Royal College of Anaesthetists and the Royal College of Ophthalmologists.

Parness, G., & Underhill, S. (2005). Regional anaesthesia for intraocular surgery. *Continuing Education in Anaesthesia, Critical Care & Pain, 5*(3), 93–97.

Ripart, J., Lefrant, J. Y., de La Coussaye, J. E., Prat-Pradal, D., Vivien, B., et al. (2001). Peribulbar versus Retrobulbar Anesthesia for ophthalmic Surgery. An Anatomical Comparison of Extraconal and Intraconal Injections. *Anesthesiology: The Journal of the American Society of Anesthesiologists, 94*(1), 56–62.

Rodgers, H., & Craven, R. (2014). Local anaesthesia for ocular surgery. *Anaesthesia & Intensive Care Medicine, 15*(1), 34–36.

Laryngeal Nerve Blocks

What are the indications for awake fibreoptic intubation (AFOI)? How would you anaesthetise a patient for an AFOI?

Indications

Awake intubation is indicated when there is known/suspected difficulty with mask ventilation and/or tracheal intubation. In the case of easy mask ventilation but isolated difficulty with tracheal intubation, an asleep technique may be appropriate. The role of AFOI in a partially obstructed airway (critical airway) is debatable. Another indication is to avoid iatrogenic injury, e.g. a patient with an unstable C-spine.

Predictors of difficult direct laryngoscopy and mask ventilation

- Difficult tracheal intubation
  - Previous difficult intubation
  - Infections – dental abscess, Ludwig's angina
  - Tumours – tongue base, larynx, thyroid
  - Iatrogenic – radiotherapy to mouth/neck, previous airway or cervical spine surgery
  - Trauma – unstable cervical spine fracture, facial fracture, airway burns
  - Arthritis – rheumatoid arthritis, ankylosing spondylitis
  - Congenital – Pierre–Robin, Treacher Collins, Goldenhar's syndrome
- Difficult mask ventilation
  - Previous difficult mask ventilation
  - Obesity, obstructive sleep apnoea/snoring

Technique of AFOI

As those of you who have done AFOI in practice are aware, preparation is key. The act of passing the endotracheal tube into the trachea forms a very small part of the procedure.

- History, examination and consent

  Ensure there are no contraindications, explain the procedure to the patient and gain consent. Explanation is crucial and a patient who understands what the procedure entails will be far more compliant.

- Oral or nasal route

  Although nasal route is better tolerated by the patient and has an easier line of access to the larynx compared to the oral route, this should be guided by the type of surgery and presence of other abnormalities precluding the choice of one over the other. A split nasopharyngeal airway or specialised oropharyngeal airway (Berman or Ovassapian) can aid in the process of guiding the scope into the laryngeal inlet.

- Pre-requisites

Full AAGBI monitoring, a flushed intravenous line and emergency drugs and a clear plan B!

- Assign roles – one anaesthetist for drugs and one for airway and experienced operating department practitioner and a runner

- Preoxygenation

There are various different ways to achieve adequate preoxygenation using nasal specs, face mask or transnasal humidified rapid-insufflation ventilatory exchange (THRIVE).

- Use of adjuvants

Antisialagogues – glycopyrrolate (4 mcg/kg) to reduce secretions.

Vasoconstrictors – ephedrine 0.5%, phenylephrine 0.5–1%, xylometazoline 0.05% can be used to achieve vasoconstriction and prevent bleeding during the procedure. Co-phenylcaine (combination of 5% lignocaine and 0.5% phenylephrine) is available which is commonly used.

- Sedation

Propofol and/or remifentanil target controlled infusion, fentanyl in 25 mcg aliquots or midazolam 1–2 mg can be used as per individual practice to achieve safe sedation for anxiolysis and patient comfort. Avoid sedation in patients with difficult airway where oversedation leads to unresponsiveness and complete airway obstruction.

- Calculating the total dose of lignocaine

Calculate the total dose according to body weight and use within limits. The British Thoracic Society guidelines for flexible bronchoscopy state the safe maximum dose of lignocaine as 8 mg/kg as opposed to the standard 4 mg/kg.

Note

For topical spray – limit is 8 mg/kg

For regional blocks – limit is 4 mg/kg

Innervation of the airway

- Techniques of achieving airway anaesthesia

Anaesthesia can be achieved either by topical anaesthesia (topical sprays, gargles or nebulisation of local anaesthetic) or discrete nerve blocks. The following are the various methods used to topicalise and block the nerves in the airway. Individual practice differs depending on experience and institutional preference.

Table 1.22   Innervation of Airway

Nose
Ethmoidal nerve (CN 1) – anterior 1/3 of the nasal septum and the nares Maxillary nerve (CN 5) – remaining part of the septum, the nasal cavity and the turbinates via the sphenopalatine ganglion situated posterior to the middle turbinate
Oropharynx
Lingual nerve (CN 5) – anterior 2/3 of tongue Glossopharyngeal nerve (CN 9) – posterior 1/3 of tongue, uvula, tonsils, vallecula, anterior surface of the epiglottis, pharynx
Larynx
Internal branch of superior laryngeal nerve (CN 10) – posterior surface of epiglottis, larynx above the vocal cords Recurrent laryngeal nerve (CN 10) – larynx below the cords

Topical anaesthesia

Table 1.23   Techniques of Topical Anaesthesia of the Airway

Nose
• 2–3 sprays of co-phenylcaine per nostril (one spray = 5 mg lignocaine) • Nasopharyngeal airway smothered with instillagel • Nebulisation with 5 ml of 2–4% lignocaine over 15–20 min • Moffett's solution – 2 ml of 10% cocaine, 1 ml of 1:1000 adrenaline, 2 ml of sodium bicarbonate and 5 ml of sodium chloride. Use of commercial or improvised mucosal atomising device (MAD) helps with a wider spread.
Oropharynx
• Gargling of 5 ml of 2% instillagel (and spit out) • Two sprays of 1% lignocaine to each tonsillar pillar • Benzocaine lozenges
Larynx

• 'Spray as you go' (SAYG) using epidural catheter in the fibreoptic scope port
  ○ 1–2 ml 2% lignocaine at the level of epiglottis
  ○ 1–2 ml 2% lignocaine at the level of cords
  ○ 1–2 ml 2% lignocaine at the level of trachea

Airway nerve blocks

Table 1.24   Nerve Blocks to Anaesthetise the Airway

Nose – ethmoidal and maxillary nerve
• Lignocaine soaked swabs to the nasal cavity
Oropharynx – glossopharyngeal nerve
• Lignocaine spray or soaked swabs in the tonsillar fossa • Injection of 2 ml 1–2% lignocaine to the palatopharyngeal fold (intraoral)
Larynx – vagus nerve
Internal branch of superior laryngeal nerve lies underneath the thyrohyoid membrane inferior to the greater cornu of the hyoid. • Injection of 2 ml of 2% lignocaine bilaterally after walking off the greater cornu inferiorly and piercing the thyrohyoid membrane will effectively block the larynx above the level of cords (or) • Placement of pledgets soaked in 2% lignocaine on either side of the root of the tongue in piriform fossa
Recurrent laryngeal nerve is better blocked by the transtracheal/cricothyroid puncture. • 22G cannula with a 10 ml syringe containing 5 ml of 2–4% lignocaine is passed through the cricothyroid membrane. After aspirating air and confirming tracheal placement the drug is injected at end-expiration. The inspiration and coughing that follows disperses the lignocaine in the trachea and below.

- Technique
  - Lubricate the scope and railroad appropriately sized endotracheal tube over it. Either standing in front of the patient or behind the head, orientate yourself, your scope and your screen.
  - Advance scope through naso and oropharynx, visualising landmarks as you go. Once the larynx is visualised, anaesthetise using SAYG, advance scope until carina is visible.
  - Advance endotracheal tube ensuring carina is visible still. Withdraw scope whilst holding tube.
  - Confirm tube placement: $EtCO_2$, chest rise, auscultation.
  - Induce general anaesthesia as planned.
  - Document.

Bibliography

Leslie, D., & Stacey, M. (2014). Awake intubation. *Continuing Education in Anaesthesia, Critical Care & Pain, 15*(2), 64–67.

Cervical Plexus

The cervical plexus is of relevance to the anaesthetist as it can be blocked for a variety of superficial procedures to the neck, clavicle, thyroid and most commonly for anaesthetists, for carotid endarterectomy procedures where it confers the advantage of being able to perform surgery in an awake patient.

Can you describe the anatomy of the cervical plexus?

The cervical plexus is formed from the ventral rami of C1–C4 which pass along the transverse process of their respective vertebrae, before receiving grey rami communicantes from the superior cervical ganglion. As they pass behind the vertebral artery and reach the end of the transverse process, they split into ascending and descending branches, before forming nerve loops which form the cervical plexus.

There are four major branches arising from the cervical plexus

1. Superficial cervical plexus (sensory)
2. Deep cervical plexus (motor)
3. Phrenic nerve (discussed in detail a little later)
4. Communicating branches (communicate with hypoglossal, accessory and vagus nerves and sympathetic nervous system via superior cervical ganglion)

Superficial cervical plexus (sensory)

The nerves supplying the lateral aspect of the neck arise from the anterior primary rami of C2, C3 and C4. C1 is motor and has no sensory supply to skin.

The nerves emerge at the posterior border of sternocleidomastoid at approximately the midpoint between mastoid and sternum, also called Erb's point (Figure 1.36 and Table 1.25).

Table 1.25 Branches and Area of Innervation of the Superficial Cervical Plexus

Branch	Sensory supply to skin covering
Lesser occipital nerve (C2)	Upper + posterior ear
Greater auricular nerve (C2, C3)	Lower third ear + angle of mandible
Transverse cervical nerve (C2, C3)	Chin to suprasternal notch
Supraclavicular nerve (C3, C4)	Lower neck, clavicle and upper chest

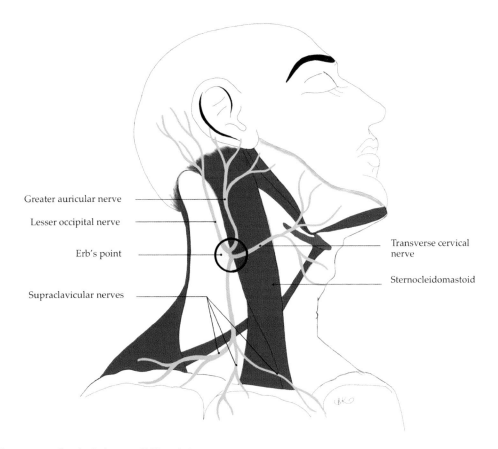

Greater auricular nerve

Lesser occipital nerve

Erb's point

Supraclavicular nerves

Transverse cervical nerve

Sternocleidomastoid

Figure 1.36   Cervical plexus – Erb's point.

Deep cervical plexus (motor)

The deep cervical plexus is entirely motor (C1–C4), supplying the anterior vertebral and neck muscles, including scalenus medius, sternocleidomastoid, levator scapulae, rhomboids, trapezius and infrahyoid (omohyoid, sternohyoid, sternothyroid, thyrohyoid) muscles.

Can you briefly describe a regional technique for performing carotid endarterectomy under local anaesthesia?

Superficial and deep cervical plexus blocks can be performed to provide regional anaesthesia for carotid endarterectomy.

- Consent for risks and benefits
- Prepare equipment, monitoring, IV access and emergency drugs
- Position patient
  - Supine or semi recumbent
  - Head extended and turned away from side to be blocked

- Identify landmarks
  - Draw line between mastoid process and Chassaignac's tubercle (transverse process of C6), along posterior border of the sternocleidomastoid muscle
  - Deep plexus block: mark transverse processes of C2–C6 along this line with C2 located 2 cm below (caudad to) the mastoid process, and then 2 cm between each subsequent transverse process
  - Superficial plexus block: choose the midpoint of this line, normally marked by the external jugular vein crossing the muscle at this point
- Aseptic precautions
- LA infiltration to skin at C2, C3, C4 levels (for deep plexus block) and midpoint (for superficial plexus block)
- 1.5-inch, 25G needle with flexible tubing (pre-prime to avoid injecting dead space air)
- Deep plexus block: in turn at each of C2, C3, C4, slowly insert and advance the needle to contact the transverse process (1–2 cm in most patients). Withdraw the needle by 1–2 mm, then confirm negative aspiration before injecting 5 ml of 0.25% bupivacaine at each level.
- Superficial plexus block: at the midpoint of the line, which will be the midpoint of the posterior border of the sternocleidomastoid muscle, insert the needle to inject 10–15 ml of 0.25% bupivacaine subcutaneously between skin and muscle, fanning out 2–3 cm in all directions from the needle insertion point to ensure block of all four sensory nerves.

What are the specific complications of a deep and superficial cervical plexus block?

- Phrenic nerve block
- Intrathecal or epidural injection
- Vertebral artery injection
- Cervical sympathetic block (manifesting as Horner's syndrome)
- Brachial plexus block
- Recurrent laryngeal nerve block

How do you monitor cerebral perfusion during surgery?

In the awake patient, neurological function can be monitored directly by asking patients to perform simple tasks intraoperatively. Other methods include

Stump pressure

- Sited distal to clamp, measures perfusion pressure around the Circle of Willis
- Non-sensitive measure of cerebral ischaemia
- Does not identify emboli

Transcranial doppler

- Doppler probe is placed on the petrous temporal bone
- Measures blood flow through the middle cerebral artery
- Detects flow and emboli
- Operator dependent

EEG

- EEG is affected by cerebral ischaemia but not emboli
- Difficult to interpret as GA can affect signal

Somatosensory evoked potentials

- More sensitive compared to EEG
- Cannot detect emboli

Near infrared spectroscopy

- Measures arterial, venous and capillary oxygenation thereby producing a regional cerebral oxygenation value.

List the advantages and disadvantages of performing a carotid endarterectomy under regional (RA) and general anaesthesia (GA).

Table 1.26   GA vs RA in Carotid Endarterectomy

	Advantages	Disadvantages
GA	Patient is still Potential for neuroprotection Controlled ventilation and CO_2 Attenuated stress response	Lack of neurological monitoring Intraoperative hypotension Postoperative hypertension Increased rate of shunt use Delayed recovery from GA may mask neurological complications
RA	Direct, real time neurological monitoring Cerebral autoregulation preserved Avoids risks of GA and airway intervention Decreased shunt rate Allows arterial closure at normal arterial pressure thereby potentially decreasing risk of postoperative haematoma	Risks/complications associated with performing cervical plexus block Stress/pain increasing risk of myocardial ischaemia Restricted access to airway during surgery Requires a cooperative patient who is able to tolerate being supine Risk of converting to GA intraoperatively

Do you know any studies comparing general vs regional anaesthesia for this procedure?

GALA trial

- Randomised multicentre trial 2001–2007
- 3500 subjects
- Postoperative evaluations made by stroke physicians/neurologists that were blinded to mode of anaesthesia at 1 month
- No major differences in outcomes between two groups

What are the features of local anaesthetic toxicity and how would you manage it?

The Association of Anaesthetists (formerly AAGBI) have produced a two-sided guideline for the management of this life-threatening complication associated with local anaesthetic use

A summary of the AAGBI Safety Guideline 'Management of Severe Local Anaesthetic Toxicity' is provided below.

Recognition

- Signs of toxicity include confusion, agitation or loss of consciousness, with or without seizure activity
- Cardiovascular collapse in the form of tachyarrythmias, bradyarrythmias or asystole
- LA toxicity can manifest a while after initial injection

Immediate management

- Stop injecting LA, call for help, manage airway with 100% oxygen and establish IV access
- Hyperventilation may be of benefit in the presence of metabolic acidosis
- Control seizures (benzodiazepines, propofol or thiopental)
- If possible, draw blood for analysis, but do not delay definitive treatment

Treatment

- Provide ALS and manage arrhythmias as indicated by the patient's condition
- In circulatory arrest, give 20% lipid emulsion IV, 1.5 ml/kg bolus, followed by infusion at 15 ml/kg/hr. The initial bolus dose can be repeated after 5 minutes and then once more after a further 5 minutes, if cardiovascular stability is not restored. The infusion can be doubled to 30 ml/kg/hr. Do not give any more than three boluses
- Maximum cumulative dose of intralipid = 12 ml/kg
- CPR should continue for at least an hour, as this is how long it can take to see any recovery
- Do not use lidocaine for arrhythmia control

Follow up

- Post resuscitation care in ITU
- Exclude pancreatitis with daily amylase and lipase for at least two days
- Report to www.npsa.nhs.uk, and if intralipid is used then also to www.lipidregistry.org

What are the maximum doses of commonly used local anaesthetics?

Table 1.27   Maximum Recommended Doses of Commonly
Used Local Anaesthetic Agents

	Max. dose without adrenaline (mg/kg)	Max. dose with adrenaline (mg/kg)
Lidocaine	3	7
Bupivacaine	2	2
Ropivacaine	3	3
Prilocaine	6	–
Cocaine	1.5	

A carotid endarterectomy is being performed under a superficial cervical plexus block. A few minutes after clamping the carotid artery, the patient becomes unresponsive to verbal command.

How would you manage this situation?

Immediately inform the surgeon who will place a shunt. Recovery following shunt placement should be rapid, but if there remains a neurological deficit, or slow recovery, then convert to GA.

Whilst the shunt is being placed, prepare to convert to GA, give supplementary oxygen and increase blood pressure to increase CPP via the contralateral blood supply to the Circle of Willis.

How would you manage a patient with post CEA bleeding?

Postoperatively, the patient should be managed in a high dependency unit. The formation of haematoma following carotid endarterectomy poses a threat to the airway. Patients might present with stridor and difficulty breathing.

In the event of haematoma formation, the priorities in management would be

- Call senior anaesthetist and vascular surgeon urgently whilst resuscitating in an A–E fashion
- Prepare to take to theatre for re-exploration
- If patient is unstable and it is not safe to move to theatre, releasing wound clips in recovery or HDU to release the haematoma will help
- Anticipate difficult airway

THORAX

2

Structures

- Apertures in the neck
- Tracheobronchial tree
- Lung
  - Fissures
  - Bronchopulmonary segments
  - Root of lung
- Pleura
- Mediastinum
- Heart
- Diaphragm
- Rib

Circulation

- Lung
- Heart

Nervous System

- Phrenic nerve
- Intercostal nerve block
- Thoracic wall blocks – pectoralis and serratus anterior blocks

Structures

- Apertures in the neck
- Tracheobronchial tree
- Lung
  - Fissures
  - Bronchopulmonary segments
  - Root of lung
- Pleura
- Mediastinum
- Heart
- Diaphragm
- Rib

Apertures in the Neck

Superior thoracic aperture

The superior thoracic aperture '(otherwise called thoracic inlet or outlet)' lies in an oblique transverse plane and connects the thoracic cavity with the root of the neck. Its anteroposterior diameter is 4.5–6 cm and the transverse diameter is 9–11 cm.

Boundaries

- Anterior – superior border of manubrium sterni
- Posterior – anterior border of the T1 vertebral body
- Lateral – medial border of first rib

The superior thoracic aperture lies in an oblique transverse plane (45°) as the first rib slopes downwards and forwards from its posterior end to anterior end. Because of this angle, the apex of the lung and pleura project upward into the neck (Figure 2.1).

What is Sibson's fascia and what are its functions?

It is a dense fascial sheet otherwise known as the suprapleural membrane, which covers the dome of the pleura. The apex of Sibson's fascia is connected to the C7 transverse process and its base is connected to the inner border of first rib and its costal cartilage.

Its functions are to

- Shield the underlying cervical pleura and the lung apex beneath it
- Resist the intrathoracic pressure being transmitted to the neck during respiration

Coming back to the thoracic inlet, name the structures going through It?

Only important structures are listed (Figure 2.2).

Midline and paramedian structures

- Sternothyroid muscles
- Trachea
- Oesophagus
- Thoracic duct
- Recurrent laryngeal nerve

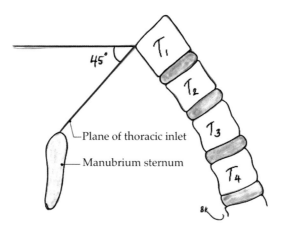

Figure 2.1 Thoracic inlet.

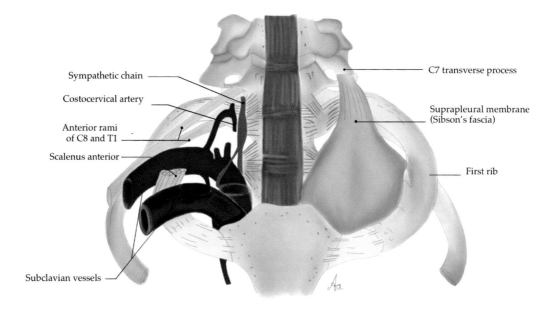

Figure 2.2 Thoracic inlet – structures and relations.

Lateral structures

- Apices of lung and pleurae
- Sympathetic trunks
- Brachiocephalic/subclavian veins
- Vagi and phrenic nerves
- Brachiocephalic artery on the right
- Common carotid and subclavian arteries on the left

What is its clinical significance?

Thoracic inlet (or outlet) syndrome (TOS) occurs when the above structures get compressed by the scalene muscles, an abnormal rib or by trauma.

- Neurogenic TOS – compression of the brachial plexus between the first rib and the scalene muscles. The clinical features include numbness, tingling, wasting and pain along distribution of compressed nerve. The symptoms get worse when the arm is raised overhead.

- Venous TOS – compression of the subclavian vein between the clavicle and the first rib causing a thrombus. This is characterised by a sudden swollen and discoloured arm requiring thrombolysis and surgical decompression.

- Arterial TOS – compression of the subclavian artery by an anomalous first rib. There could be ischaemic symptoms in the upper limb necessitating urgent surgery.

Inferior thoracic aperture

The inferior thoracic aperture is larger and more oblique than the thoracic inlet and connects the thorax with the abdomen.

Boundaries

- Posterior – T12 vertebral body
- Posterolateral – 11th and 12th ribs
- Anterolateral – costal cartilages of 7th to 10th ribs
- Anterior – xiphisternum

Contents

The diaphragm occupies this opening and separates the thoracic and abdominal cavities. So, the structures exiting the inferior outlet are those passing through the diaphragmatic foramina (T8, T10, T12 and other smaller foramina).

Cross Section at T4 Level

Figure 2.3 depicts the cross section at the level of T4

- Beginning and termination of the arch of the aorta
- The mediastinum is divided into superior and inferior mediastinum via a line connecting T4 and the manubriosternal angle (angle of Louis).

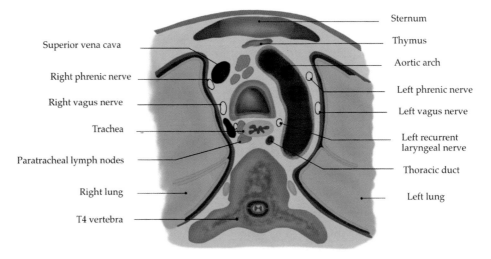

Figure 2.3   Cross section of thorax at T4 level.

Structures present at the level of T4

From anterior to posterior

- Thymus
- Superior vena cava
- Arch of aorta
- Left and right phrenic nerve
- Left and right vagus nerve
- Trachea
- Left and right recurrent laryngeal nerve

- Oesophagus
- Thoracic duct
- Sympathetic trunk

Clinical importance of T4 level

- Level of nipples or manubriosternal angle
- Lower border of trachea (carina) at expiration
- SVC opening into right atrium – landmark for checking IJV central line
- T4 is the accepted upper limit of block to cold for caesarean section under regional anaesthesia
- Position of deep cardiac plexus
- Left recurrent laryngeal nerve loops around aortic arch

Tracheobronchial Tree

Trachea

The trachea which measures 10–12 cm in length and 2–2.5 cm in width is a semi-cylindrical chondromembranous structure with a flattened posterior aspect. It is comprised of 15–20 cartilages which are incomplete posteriorly, where the oesophagus and trachea share a fibroelastic membrane. It originates at the level of the cricoid cartilage (C6) and terminates by bifurcating into right and left main bronchi at the carina (T4 on expiration and T6 on full inspiration).

Blood supply – inferior thyroid artery and veins
Nerve supply – recurrent laryngeal nerve and sympathetic fibres from middle cervical ganglion
Lymphatic drainage – deep cervical, pretracheal and paratracheal lymph nodes

Relations of the trachea

In the neck – trachea lies in the midline
<ul><li>Anterior: skin, fascia, isthmus of thyroid over 2–4 tracheal rings, sternothyroid and sternohyoid muscles, jugular arch and thyroidea ima artery (if present)</li><li>Posterior: oesophagus, recurrent laryngeal nerve in groove between trachea and oesophagus and vertebral bodies</li><li>Lateral: thyroid gland, carotid sheath, lung and pleura and great vessels</li></ul>
In the thorax – trachea deviates slightly to the right due to the arch of aorta
<ul><li>Anterior – inferior thyroid veins, the remains of the thymus, brachiocephalic and left common carotid arteries and aortic arch</li><li>Posterior – oesophagus and left recurrent laryngeal nerve</li><li>Lateral – right: mediastinal pleura, azygous vein and the right vagus nerve</li><li>Lateral – left: mediastinal pleura, left common carotid and subclavian arteries, the aortic arch and the left vagus nerve</li></ul>

Discuss how the trachea can be damaged. Describe the mechanisms of injury.

This answer can be broken down in several ways, however the most straightforward option would be to present internal vs external mechanisms of injury.

- Internal injury
  - Inhalation of foreign body

- Aspiration of caustic substances including GI contents
- Smoke inhalation (burns)
- Internal thoracic injury causing rupture/tear
- External injury
  - Trauma (blunt or penetrating)
  - Compression (strangulation, hanging, haemorrhage in neck compartment)
  - Iatrogenic injury (central venous line insertion, tracheostomy, neck/thyroid surgery, cervical spine surgery), hyperextension causing rupture

What is the difference between penetrating and blunt injuries to the trachea?

Penetrating injury – either by sharp instruments or gunshot wound. Usually occur in the cervical region and are associated with involvement of nearby structures such as oesophagus, heart, spinal cord, major vessels and nerves.

Blunt injury – can be due to direct trauma or hyperextension of the neck from motor vehicle accidents. They are associated with extensive injuries to the face, head, chest and abdomen. The mechanism of injury could be due to

- Sudden anteroposterior compression leading to disruption of lung at carina
- High airway pressure due to compression of chest against a closed glottis causing tracheobronchial rupture
- Rapid deceleration injury causing shearing at the fixation sites such as carina and cricoid cartilage
- Clothesline injury – compression of trachea between cervical vertebrae (seen in hanging injury)

What are the clinical features of tracheal injury?

The clinical features result from airway injury per se or from associated injuries such as oesophageal injury, haemopneumothorax, major vascular injury, recurrent laryngeal nerve and spinal cord injury.

Signs and symptoms include pain, dyspnoea, drooling, stridor, hissing of air, voice alteration, surgical emphysema (subcutaneous or mediastinal), bleeding, haemoptysis and pneumothorax.

How would you manage tracheal injury? Is it safe to intubate and ventilate?

- ABCDE approach – tracheal injury falls under A!
- Do NOT forget major haemorrhage control in trauma, i.e. if the carotid artery is bleeding out, compression before intubation is a sensible option.
- And always have a plan B!

Airway management is tailored to the type of injury, the nature and extent of airway compromise and haemodynamic and oxygenation status.

Small (<2 cm) mucosal injuries with no associated injuries in patients who are able to breathe spontaneously may be treated conservatively. It is important to identify the point of injury before deciding on airway management. For example, if the injury is proximal to the cricothyroid membrane, a tracheostomy may become plan A. If, however, the injury is distal to the cricothyroid membrane, isolation and one lung ventilation may be necessary.

- Blunt tracheal or laryngeal trauma

  Clinically blunt injuries are identified by the presence of hoarseness, cough, stridor and associated carotid vascular injury. The presence of subcutaneous emphysema suggests the possibility of airway disruption. Intubation is better performed in the operating theatre with bronchoscopy and cricoid pressure is generally avoided in laryngeal trauma.

- Penetrating airway trauma

  Direct laryngoscopy with rapid sequence induction or primary surgical airway would be the preferred and successful technique in the management of penetrating neck trauma. Associated great vessel disruption should be recognised/considered and embracing supine or Trendelenburg position can reduce the risk of an air embolism. Again cricoid pressure and positive pressure bag ventilation is avoided until airway is secured. Awake fibreoptic intubation may not be ideal because of the presence of airway oedema, bleeding and secretions or the patient might be obtunded.

You are called to see a 62-year-old male with a history of foreign body inhalation following a dental appointment. He appears comfortable, has mild stridor, normal oxygen saturations and his chest is clear on auscultation. The ENT surgeon is available and would like to perform a rigid bronchoscopy to remove the object.

How would you proceed to anaesthetise this patient?

Foreign body aspiration is a common cause of accidental morbidity and mortality in children under the age of 5 years. In adults, the major causes of foreign body inhalation are altered mental status (sedative use, alcohol, trauma), advanced age (>70 years) and impaired cough reflex (stroke, epilepsy, Parkinson's disease).

The symptoms depend on size, type and shape of the foreign body, duration and location of airway obstruction and patients could be asymptomatic. In children with cough and stridor with no clear history, alternate diagnosis of croup, acute epiglottitis and acute tracheitis should be excluded.

- Signs and symptoms of upper airway obstruction – cough, choking, cyanosis, desaturation, stridor and tachypnoea
- Signs and symptoms of lower airway obstruction – respiratory distress, tachypnoea, wheeze and absent breath sounds on the affected side

Organic objects such as peanuts or other food material can elicit an inflammatory process and causes oedema and chemical pneumonitis. Some foreign bodies can get lodged in distal smaller airways and create a 'ball valve' effect where in air trapping and distal atelectasis happens.

Complications of airway foreign body

- Asphyxia and death
- Pneumonia, bronchiectasis and atelectasis
- Bronchial stricture and inflammatory polyps

How would you proceed to anaesthetise this patient?

- Preassessment and investigations

  Rapid yet careful assessment with particular attention to history and airway signs. If the patient is asymptomatic and stable, a chest radiography may be helpful in localising the foreign body although most objects in children are not radio opaque. Chest CT scans can aid further in the diagnosis especially in delayed presentation or patients with chronic respiratory symptoms and reduce the number of unwarranted bronchoscopies.

- Premedication and fasting

  Anticholinergics are used to decrease airway secretions and reduce vagal tone (bradycardia) during bronchoscopy. Dose in children: atropine 20 mcg/kg or glycopyrrolate 4 mcg/kg.

  If the patient is stable with no or minimal distal airway obstruction, optimal fasting times are followed to decrease the risk of aspiration of gastric contents because the airway cannot be fully protected during the procedure.

- Choice of anaesthetic induction

  Intravenous access and monitoring as per AAGBI guidelines are instituted. It should be borne in mind that $EtCO_2$ monitoring may be inaccurate during the procedure due to leakage of gases around the bronchoscope. Appropriate personnel (senior anaesthetist, skilled anaesthetic assistant and an ENT surgeon) and good communication between all members of staff is vital. Induction of anaesthesia by the inhalation or intravenous route are both described in the literature and depends on personal preference and the experience of the anaesthetist. Whatever the choice of induction may be, spontaneous ventilation must be maintained until it is certain that the patient can still be ventilated post induction. Forced bagging may risk loss of the airway due to fragmentation or dislodgement of the foreign body and may also increase the chance of hyperinflation, pneumothorax and aspiration of gastric contents.

  After induction, administration of topical local anaesthetic (1% lignocaine to maximum of 4 mg/kg) to the airway is favourable as it obtunds the airway reflexes and results in a smooth bronchoscopy.

- Spontaneous or mechanical ventilation (Table 2.1)

  Studies have failed to show the superiority of either mode of ventilation and the outcomes are almost universally good. Breathing circuits can be connected to the sidearm of the rigid bronchoscopes for ventilation.

  Jet ventilation is another known method of oxygenation during the procedure and anaesthesia is maintained with intravenous agents.

- Procedure

  Rigid bronchoscopy is the gold standard, but flexible scopes can be used in children or in diagnostic procedures. Instruments available for foreign body extraction include forceps, snares, baskets, suction catheters, fogarty balloons, magnet catheters and cryotherapy probes.

  After the removal of the inhaled foreign body, in the absence of complications, mask ventilation can be applied until adequate spontaneous ventilation is reached.

- Postoperative period

  Patients are monitored for stridor and airway obstruction due to oedema or procedural complications such as pneumothorax and pneumomediastinum.

  If stridor occurs or worsens, nebulised adrenaline 1:1000 and/or intravenous dexamethasone for 24 hours is recommended.

  Regular physiotherapy and antibiotics should be prescribed if secondary infection is suspected.

Table 2.1   Comparison of Modes of Ventilation in Patients with Foreign Body Inhalation

Spontaneous ventilation	Mechanical ventilation
Advantages 1. Less risk of dislodgement of foreign body 2. Continuous ventilation throughout procedure 3. Aids in rapid assessment of airway adequacy post retrieval	Advantages 1. Use of muscle relaxant to aid instrumentation 2. Use of balanced anaesthesia with multiple drugs decreases effects on cardiac output
Disadvantages 1. Increased depth of anaesthesia needed for the procedure can cause cardiovascular and respiratory depression. 2. Increased resistance to ventilation during the use of the telescope worsens hypoventilation.	Disadvantages 1. Manual ventilation can dislodge the foreign object more distally requiring difficult retrieval and can convert the proximal partial obstruction to complete obstruction. 2. Increased chance of ball valve effect

If the same patient had presented in extremis with stridor, choking sensation and deteriorating oxygen saturations, how would this change your management?

In witnessed choking, where the patient is conscious, they should be encouraged to cough or external manoeuvres (back blows and chest thrusts in infants and abdominal thrusts in adults and older children) are performed to expel the foreign body.

If the patient is deteriorating, then every attempt should be taken to secure the airway. Immediate endotracheal intubation should be performed, and if the foreign body is seen in the upper airway and can be removed, avoid blind finger sweeps at all times. If intubation fails due to upper airway obstruction from foreign object or airway oedema, difficult airway society (DAS) guidelines should be followed and cricothyroidotomy should be performed.

List the indications for tracheostomy.

- Prolonged ventilation/weaning
- Failed intubation/extubation
- Bronchial toilet/reduce retention of secretions
- Airway protection in neurological dysfunction, e.g. bulbar palsy
- Domiciliary ventilation in patients with chronic conditions
- Reduction of airway complications of long-term intubation

What are the contraindications to bedside tracheostomy?

- Absolute – patient refusal, local sepsis, tumour, midline neck swelling or mass
- Relative – severe coagulopathy, thrombocytopenia or platelet dysfunction, aberrant vessels in the surgical field, difficult anatomy – short fat or immobile neck or unstable C-spine injury, tracheomalacia

When do you decide about tracheostomy for weaning in ICU?

The timing of tracheostomy in cases of predicted prolonged mechanical ventilation is still controversial. The TracMan (2014) study demonstrated a reduction in days of sedation but this was not translated into a reduction in mortality, hospital stay or ICU stay. In summary, there is no demonstrated advantage to early tracheostomy in those patients that will predictably need prolonged ventilation, therefore each case is dealt with individually.

How will you perform a percutaneous tracheostomy?

- Consent
- Assessment of neck (ultrasound may be useful)
- Monitoring including capnography; trained assistant; equipment
- 100% oxygen
- Patient positioning – reverse Trendelenburg, neck extension
- Sedation and paralysis
- Bronchoscopy to visualise larynx above level of carina
- Palpation and local anaesthetic infiltration below second or third tracheal rings
- Seldinger technique to insert percutaneous tracheostomy (Note: there are multiple techniques, see below. Choose one that you are familiar with.)
- Secure airway device
- X-ray to rule out complications and confirm positioning

What are the potential complications of tracheostomy?

- Immediate – cuff herniation, vascular damage resulting in bleeding, tracheal trauma, loss of airway, other neck trauma (thyroid), surgical emphysema and pneumomediastinum
- Early – haematoma formation, pneumothorax, haemothorax, infection, false passage formation, tracheostomy displacement, blockage and tracheo-oesophageal fistula
- Late – recurrent laryngeal nerve damage, tracheal stenosis, tracheal granulomata, swallowing difficulties and tracheomalacia

What techniques are available for insertion of a percutaneous tracheostomy?

- Percutaneous dilatational method with multiple dilators for graduated dilatation (Ciaglia)
- Percutaneous dilatational technique with single dilator (Rhino)
- Guidewire and dilating forceps (Grigg's forceps)
- Other (Portex ULTRAperc, etc.)

What are the anaesthetic considerations for a patient with long-term tracheostomy?

This can be discussed under the following headings.

- Reason for tracheostomy – difficult airway, pulmonary toilet, prolonged ICU stay and neurological dysfunction
- Presence of co-morbid diseases – ICU patient with multi-organ failure, sepsis, lung injury, neuromuscular disorders and chronic high spinal cord injury
- Dealing with the potential complications of long-term tracheostomy (as discussed earlier)

- Risk of loss of airway – various sizes of cuffed/uncuffed tracheostomy tubes, suction catheters, graspers, ambu bag and ties should be available in case of loss of airway. Additionally, a difficult airway trolley should be available for rescue.
- Practical tracheostomy management – suction prior to induction, removal of inner tube, connection to breathing circuit for preoxygenation +/– gas induction, inspection of $EtCO_2$ and spirometry loops

Bronchial Tree

The right and left main bronchi originate at the carina. The right main bronchus is shorter (2.5 cm vs 5 cm), wider and more vertical to the midline (25° vs 45°). This structure has a couple of clinical implications in anaesthesia (Figure 2.4).

- Endobronchial intubations are, more often than not, on the right side.
- Foreign bodies traversing the trachea are more likely to enter the right side.
- During use of a right-sided double lumen tube, careful positioning and confirmation with a fibreoptic scope is necessary to prevent occlusion of the right upper lobe bronchus arising at 2.5 cm.

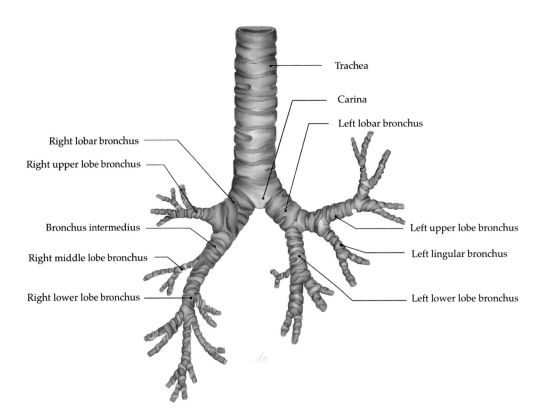

Figure 2.4   Tracheobronchial tree.

The bronchi undergo 23 divisions (16 – conducting zone or a conduit where there is no gas exchange; 7 – respiratory zone) and it is listed in Table 2.2.

Table 2.2   Generations of the Tracheobronchial Tree

Function	Structures	Generation
Conducting zone	Trachea	0
	Main bronchi - Right and left	1
	Lobar bronchi Right – upper, middle and lower Left – upper and lower	2
	Segmental bronchi (ten each side)	3
	Bronchioles to terminal bronchioles	4–16
Respiratory zone	Respiratory bronchioles	17–19
	Alveolar ducts	20–22
	Alveolar sacs	23

Lung

Lungs are conical structures, where the right is heavier and larger but shorter than the left. The apex of the lung lies at the root of neck with the tip extending 4 cm above the medial one third of the clavicle making it prone to iatrogenic damage whilst performing supraclavicular brachial plexus blocks or subclavian venous cannulation. The base of the lung rests on the diaphragm and the right base is placed higher than the left by the presence of the liver.

Fissures

The right lung is divided into three lobes by the oblique and horizontal fissures whilst the left has two lobes formed by the oblique fissure.

- *Oblique fissure* – divides the lower lobe from the upper and middle lobes

  Posteriorly – starts at T5 vertebral body, then follows the direction of the fifth rib

  Anteriorly – ends at sixth costochondral junction (T5 → 5th rib → 6th CC junction)
- *Horizontal fissure* – delineates the upper and middle lobe

  Anteriorly – starts at right fourth costochondral junction and runs transversely backwards and meets the oblique fissure in the midaxillary line at the level of the fifth rib (4th CC junction → 5th rib)

Broncho pulmonary segments

The bronchopulmonary segments (ten segments on each side) are well defined functional areas of lung supplied by a segmental or tertiary bronchus. Each segment is pyramidal in shape serving as an individual respiratory unit with its own pulmonary arterial supply; the pulmonary venous circulation running in the intersegmental plane (Figure 2.5).

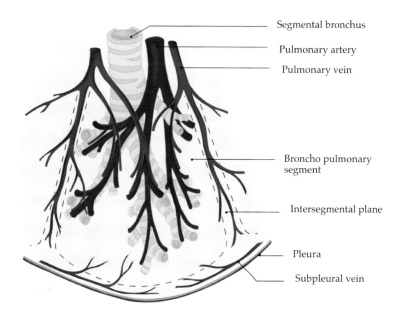

Figure 2.5   Bronchopulmonary segment.

The clinical importance of these segments are listed below.

- Segmental resection can be carried out with minimal disruption to the surrounding lung tissue.
- Visualisation with bronchoscopes can delineate the affected lung when the disease process is limited to particular segments.

Root of lung

The root or stalk connects the lung to the heart and trachea and hilum is the opening in the pleural sheath that transmits the structures constituting the root (pulmonary artery, pulmonary veins, the bronchi, bronchial vessels, lymph nodes and autonomic nerves).

Relations at the lung hilum

- Anterior – phrenic nerve, superior vena cava, anterior pulmonary plexus and part of right atrium (right lung)
- Posterior – vagus nerve and posterior pulmonary plexus
- Superior – aortic arch and azygos vein
- Inferior – pulmonary ligament

How is the right hilum different from the left?

The relationships of the roots of the right and left lung are different because of the structures that make them and their position at the hila (Figures 2.6, 2.7 and Table 2.3).

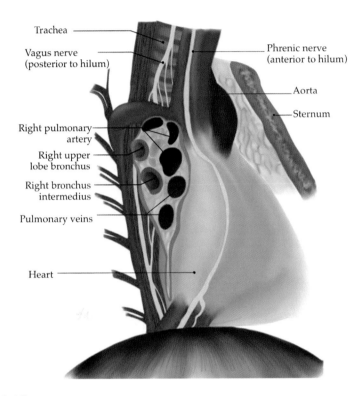

Figure 2.6 Right hilum.

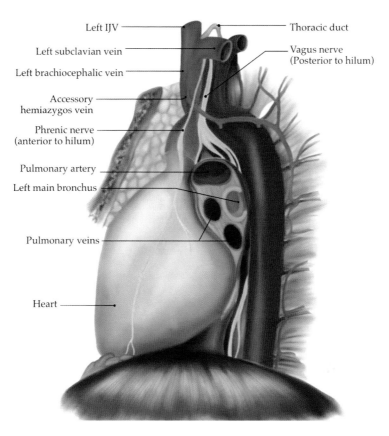

Left IJV

Left subclavian vein

Left brachiocephalic vein

Accessory
hemiazygos vein

Phrenic nerve
(anterior to hilum)

Pulmonary artery

Left main bronchus

Pulmonary veins

Heart

Thoracic duct

Vagus nerve
(Posterior to hilum)

Figure 2.7   Left hilum.

Table 2.3   Comparison of the Right and Left Lung Hilum

Right hilum	Left hilum
One pulmonary artery (anterior and above)	One pulmonary artery (anterior and above)
Two pulmonary veins (below the artery)	Two pulmonary veins (below the artery)
One upper lobar bronchus (ep-arterial or above pulmonary artery) One bronchus intermedius (hyp-arterial or below pulmonary artery)	One main bronchus (hyp-arterial or below pulmonary artery)
One bronchial artery (posterior to bronchi)	Two bronchial arteries (posterior to bronchus)
Other structures Bronchial veins, anterior and posterior pulmonary nerve plexus, areolar tissue and bronchopulmonary lymph nodes	Other structures Bronchial veins, anterior and posterior pulmonary nerve plexus, areolar tissue and bronchopulmonary lymph nodes

What type of nerves supply the lung tissue?

Sensory

- Fibres sensitive to stretch of lung (vagus nerve)
- Pain fibres from parietal pleura (phrenic and intercostal nerves)

Sympathetic

- Bronchodilatory fibres (T2–T4)

Parasympathetic

- Bronchoconstrictor fibres (Vagus)
- Secretomotor fibres to the mucous glands

Discuss the blood supply to the lung and adjoining connective tissue.

The blood supply to the lung is via the bronchial circulation which, as previously discussed, forms part of the systemic circulation. It comprises 1–2% of the total cardiac output.

- **Bronchial arteries**

  Left bronchial arteries – there are two left-sided bronchial arteries (superior and inferior) which arise from the thoracic aorta at the level of the T5 and T6 vertebrae.

  Right bronchial artery – the origin of the single right bronchial artery may vary. It may arise directly from the thoracic aorta, from a common trunk shared with the left bronchial artery, or from a right-sided posterior intercostal artery.

  The bronchial arteries supply blood to the bronchi and connective tissue of the lungs. They terminate at the level of the respiratory bronchioles by way of an anastomosis with the pulmonary arteries and together, they supply the visceral pleura.

- **Bronchial veins**

  The bronchial veins run alongside the bronchial arteries, but they only carry ~13% of the bronchial venous blood to the systemic venous circuit.

  Two types of bronchial veins that exist are the deep and the superficial veins and both communicate freely with the pulmonary veins. The superficial bronchial veins from the larger airways and hilum drain into the systemic veins (azygos vein, left superior intercostal vein and the accessory hemiazygos vein) and then into the right atrium. The deep veins originate from the terminal bronchioles and drain into the left atrium directly or via the pulmonary veins constituting the 'anatomical shunt' (1–2% of cardiac output) desaturating the left atrial blood to 99%.

- **Pulmonary circulation**

  There are two pulmonary arteries (left and right) that carry deoxygenated blood from the right ventricle to the lung and four pulmonary veins that carry oxygenated blood to the left atrium.

Two main pulmonary veins emerge from each lung hilum, receiving blood from bronchial veins and draining into the left atrium. An inferior and superior pulmonary vein drains each lung, giving four main pulmonary veins in total.

At the root of the lung, the right superior pulmonary vein lies anterior to the pulmonary artery; the inferior is situated at the lower most part of the lung hilum. The right main pulmonary veins pass posterior to the right atrium and superior vena cava; the left anterior to the descending thoracic aorta.

Please see the section on Pulmonary Circulation for further reading.

What is suprapleural membrane (Sibson's fascia) and what is its importance?

The suprapleural membrane is the dense fascial structure that is said to be flattened tendon of the scalenus minimus muscle. Its function is to provide rigidity to the thoracic inlet and prevent the changes in intrathoracic pressure during respiration causing distortion of neck structures. Also, it protects the underlying cervical pleura, and the apex of the lung beneath it. The subclavian vessels lie above the fascia.

Attachments

- Anterior – inner border of the first rib and costal cartilage
- Posterior – C7 transverse process
- Medial – mediastinal pleura
- Lateral – medial margin of the first rib
- Inferior – blends with the dome of cervical pleura

Pleura

Pleurae refer to the serous membranes covering the lung, mediastinum, diaphragm and the inside of the chest wall.

Two layers, visceral and parietal membranes, meet at the lung hilum.

- Visceral: attached closely and adheres to the whole surface of the lung, enveloping the interlobar fissures
- Parietal: the outer layer, which is attached to the chest wall and the diaphragm and named as mediastinal, diaphragmatic, costal and cervical pleura, as per the association with the adjacent structures

The potential space between the two layers is called pleural space and is filled with a small amount of fluid amounting to around 0.2 ml/kg (5–10 ml). This is determined by the net result of opposing Starling's hydrostatic and oncotic forces and lymphatic drainage. Pleural fluid as little as 1 ml serves as a lubricant and decreases friction between the pleurae during respiration.

What are the constituents of pleural fluid?

Pleural fluid is a clear ultrafiltrate of plasma.

- Quantity: 0.2 ml/kg (8.4 +/– 4.3 ml)
- Cellular contents: 75% macrophages and 25% lymphocytes
- Biochemistry: compared to plasma, the pleural fluid is alkaline (pH @ 7.6) with higher albumin content but lower sodium, chloride and LDH.

What is the blood supply of pleura?

Visceral pleura is supplied by the bronchial arteries and drains into the pulmonary veins. Parietal pleura gets its supply from systemic capillaries including intercostal, pericardiophrenic, musculophrenic and internal mammary vessels. Venous drainage is via the intercostal veins and azygos veins, finally draining into the SVC and IVC.

How is pleura innervated?

The visceral pleura does not have pain fibres but responds to stretch and is supplied by the pulmonary branch of vagus nerve and the sympathetic trunk.

The parietal pleura receives an extensive innervation from the somatic intercostal and phrenic nerves.

Explain Starling's forces and describe the pathogenesis of pleural effusion.

The movement of pleural fluid between the pleural capillaries and the pleural space is governed by Starling's law of transcapillary exchange.

$$\text{Net filtration } = \text{ Kf } \left[(\text{Pc } - \text{ Pi}) - \sigma(\pi c - \pi i) \right]$$

Kf: filtration coefficient dependent on area of capillaries and permeability to water.

Pc and Pi: hydrostatic pressure in capillary and interstitium, respectively.

σ: reflection coefficient depicting the ability of the membrane to restrict passage of proteins.

πc and πi: osmotic pressure in capillary and interstitium, respectively.

Pathogenesis of pleural effusion
Increased formation

- Increased interstitial fluid in the lung – LVF, PE and ARDS
- Increased pressure in capillaries – LVF/RVF and pericardial effusion
- Increased interstitial pressure – para pneumonic effusion
- Decreased pleural pressure – lung atelectasis
- Increased fluid in peritoneal cavity – ascites and peritoneal dialysis

Decreased reabsorption

- Obstruction of lymphatics – pleural malignancy
- Increased systemic vascular pressures – RVF

Light's criteria differentiate an exudate from transudate.

The pleural fluid is an exudate if one or more of the following criteria are met

- Pleural fluid: serum protein ratio >0.5
- Pleural fluid: serum LDH ratio >0.6
- Pleural fluid LDH is more than two-thirds the upper limits of normal serum LDH (Table 2.4).

Table 2.4   Causes of Exudative and Transudative Pleural Effusion

Exudates	Transudates
Due to local pleural and pulmonary disease	Due to factors that influence formation and reabsorption of pleural fluid
Causes	Causes
Malignancy	Left ventricular failure
Parapneumonic effusions	Liver cirrhosis
Pulmonary infarction	Hypoalbuminaemia
Rheumatoid arthritis	Peritoneal dialysis
Autoimmune diseases	Nephrotic syndrome
Pancreatitis	Mitral stenosis
Post myocardial infarction syndrome	Pulmonary embolism

What drugs are known to cause pleural effusion?

Amiodarone, phenytoin, methotrexate, carbamazepine, propylthiouracil, penicillamine, cyclophosphamide, bromocriptine

What are the effects of pneumothorax on pleural pressure?

Basic concepts

1. At FRC, due to the tendency of the lung to collapse and the chest wall to expand, the pleural pressure remains negative thus holding the alveoli open.
2. Also due to gravity, the pleural pressure at the base of the lung is less negative than that at the apex.

If the chest wall is pierced (open pneumothorax) or the visceral pleura is breached (closed pneumothorax), air leaks into the pleural cavity causing a pneumothorax until the pressure gradient no longer exists. Because the thoracic cavity is below its resting volume and lung above its resting volume, with a pneumothorax, the thoracic cavity enlarges and the lung becomes smaller and hence collapses.

The pleural pressure is the same throughout the entire pleural space, as per point (2), with the upper lobe being more affected than the lower lobe.

In tension pneumothorax, air enters into the pleural cavity with inspiration but cannot leave due to a flap of tissue acting as a one-way valve. The developed pressure collapses the affected lung and if high enough can cause a mediastinal shift.

What are the indications of intercostal drain in pneumothoraces and pleural effusions?

Pneumothorax

- In any ventilated patient
- Tension pneumothorax after initial decompression
- Persistent or recurrent pneumothorax

Pleural effusion

- Large and symptomatic effusion
- Malignant pleural effusion, chylothorax, empyema
- Traumatic haemopneumothorax
- Postoperative, for example, thoracotomy, oesophagectomy, cardiac surgery

What is the role of ultrasound in chest drain insertion?

Pleural procedures and thoracic ultrasound: British Thoracic Society Pleural disease guideline 2010.

Ultrasound guided pleural aspiration is strongly recommended to increase success rates and reduce the risk of complications, particularly pneumothoraces and inadvertent organ puncture, but may not decrease the incidence of laceration of the intercostal vessels.

The evidence concludes that site selection for all pleural aspiration should be ultrasound guided, with more emphasis when aspirating small or loculated pleural effusions or when a clinically guided attempt has been unsuccessful.

Describe the anatomy relevant to the insertion of chest drain.

- Site

  '*Safe triangle*' is bounded by the pectoralis major anteriorly, latissimus dorsi laterally, and fifth intercostal space inferiorly. The base of the axilla forms the apex of the triangle. This area is considered safe as it minimises the risk to the underlying viscera, muscles and internal mammary artery. Also, the diaphragm rises to the fifth rib on expiration, and thus chest drains should be placed above this level. Occasionally the second intercostal space in the mid clavicular line is chosen especially in apical pneumothoraces but routine use is precluded due to disruption to the internal mammary vessels. US imaging can guide in loculated effusions.

- Intercostal space

  Choose the upper surface of the rib to avoid the intercostal neurovascular bundle.

- Direction of drain

  Tip of the drain is directed apically to drain air and basally for fluid.

- Chest drain system

  The chest drain is connected to a series of bottles containing a valve mechanism (Heimlich or underwater seal) to prevent fluid or air from entering the pleural cavity. If the patient breathes spontaneously, the air/fluid is expelled during expiration and in mechanical ventilated patients it exits during inspiration.

One-bottle system

Used in simple pneumothoraces.

During inspiration the water in the bottle is sucked back up the tube to a height equal to the negative intrathoracic pressure generated. So a bottle is placed 100 cm below the patient's chest and the length of the tube under water should be limited to 2–3 cm to reduce resistance to drainage.

Two-bottle system

In pleural effusion, drainage of fluid increases the depth of fluid in the bottle and increases resistance to air flow. Hence a two-bottle system is used, where the first bottle serves simple drainage and the second stage functions as an underwater seal that is not affected by the amount of fluid collected in the first chamber.

Three-bottle system

In persistent pneumothoraces, if suction is required it is provided by use of an underwater seal at the level of 10–20 cm H_2O or a low-pressure suction. The depth of the fluid in the third bottle determines the amount of negative pressure that can be transmitted to the chest. For example, to obtain a suction of 20 cm H_2O the tube should be 20 cm below the fluid surface.

What do you know about interpleural block?

Interpleural (or intrapleural block) is the administration of local anaesthetic solution between the two layers of pleura.

Indications of interpleural block

- Acute pain
  - Non-surgical pain – rib fractures, pancreatitis
  - Postoperative analgesia – mastectomy, cholecystectomy, chest and abdominal operations
- Chronic pain
  - Chronic pancreatitis
  - Cancer pain
  - CRPS of upper limb

Mechanism of action

- The local anaesthetic injected in the interpleural space reaches the intercostal nerves, brachial plexus and cervical sympathetic chain through diffusion through the parietal pleura
- Direct action of nerve endings in pleura
- Deposition of local anaesthetic in the paravertebral space aided by gravity

Technique

- Position – supine or lateral (operated site uppermost)
- Site – 10 cm from the posterior midline at the level of T6 and T8
- Needle – 16G Tuohy needle
- Procedure – following skin puncture, using a loss of resistance technique, the needle and syringe are advanced through the intercostal space and then through the parietal pleura, often signified by a 'click'. The syringe is removed and a 5–6 cm length of an epidural-type catheter is inserted through the needle into the pleural space.
- Drug – 10–20 ml of 0.25% bupivacaine as single injection or an infusion of 0.125% at 10 ml/hr

Complications

- Pneumothorax
- Local anaesthetic toxicity
- Horner's syndrome
- Phrenic nerve palsy
- Intrabronchial injection
- Bronchopleural fistula

Bibliography

Altinok, T., & Can, A. (2014). Management of tracheobronchial injuries. *The Eurasian Journal of Medicine*, *46*(3), 209.

Des Jardins, T. (2012). *Cardiopulmonary Anatomy & Physiology: Essentials of Respiratory Care.* Nelson Education.

Grewal, H. S., Dangayach, N. S., Ahmad, U., Ghosh, S., Gildea, T., et al. (2019). Treatment of tracheobronchial injuries: A contemporary review. *Chest*, *155*(3), 595–604.

Hunt, K., & McGowan, S. (2014). Tracheostomy management. *BJA Education*, *15*(3), 149–153.

Wang, K., Harnden, A., & Thomson, A. (2010). Foreign body inhalation in children. *BMJ*, *341*, c3924.

Mediastinum

The mediastinum lies between the right and left pleura. It extends from the sternum in front to the vertebral column and contains all the thoracic viscera except the lungs (Figure 2.8).

Superior mediastinum **is located above the manubriosternal angle**

- Boundaries – posteriorly by T1–T4; above it is continuous with the neck; below it is continuous with both anterior and posterior mediastina
- Contents
  - Structures – thymus, oesophagus, thoracic duct, trachea and bronchi
  - Vessels – aortic arch and brachiocephalic trunk, SVC and both brachiocephalic veins, left common carotid artery and left subclavian artery
  - Nerves – phrenic nerves and vagi, left recurrent laryngeal nerve

Anterior mediastinum **– located between the sternum and the pericardial sac**

- Boundaries – T4 superiorly to T9 inferiorly; sternum anteriorly to pericardium posteriorly
- Contents – sternopericardial ligament, remnants of the thymus and lymph nodes

Middle mediastinum **is located between anterior and posterior mediastinum**

- Boundaries – T4 superiorly to T9 inferiorly; between anterior and posterior layers of the pericardium
- Contents
  - Structures – heart and pericardium
  - Vessels – pericardiaco-phrenic vessels, superior vena cava, origin of aorta and pulmonary trunk
  - Nerves – phrenic nerves

Posterior mediastinum **is located between the pericardial sac and vertebral bodies**

- Boundaries – T4 (superior) to T12 (inferior); posterior aspect of pericardium (anterior) to spine (posterior)
- Contents
  - Structures – oesophagus, thoracic duct and lymph nodes
  - Vessels – descending aorta and azygos system of veins
  - Nerves – vagus nerve, greater, lesser and least splanchnic nerves

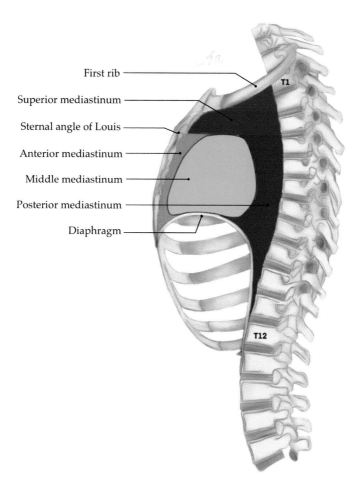

First rib — T1

Superior mediastinum —

Sternal angle of Louis —

Anterior mediastinum —

Middle mediastinum —

Posterior mediastinum —

Diaphragm —

T12

Figure 2.8   Mediastinum.

Which cranial nerve traverses through the neck, chest and abdomen?

Cranial nerve X – the vagus nerve

Where does it lie in the neck, chest and abdomen?

- Neck – within carotid sheath along the tracheo oesophageal groove
- Chest
  - Right – passes behind the right brachiocephalic vein, crosses right subclavian artery, is crossed by azygos vein and travels posterior to the hilum of the right lung
  - Left – behind left brachiocephalic vein, crosses aortic arch and travels posterior to the hilum of the left lung
- Abdomen
  - Right – enters abdomen via the oesophageal hiatus of the diaphragm, right and posterior to the oesophagus, runs along left gastric artery to the coeliac plexus
  - Left – lies left and anterior to the oesophagus in the hiatus, runs along the lesser curvature of the stomach and pylorus

Tell me about the oesophagus.

The oesophagus is a muscular tube which conveys substances from the pharynx to the stomach. It is 25 cm long and starts at C6 and ends at T11/T12.

It descends through the neck, superior and posterior mediastinum following the curvature of vertebral column. It then pierces diaphragm at the level of T10 just to the left of the median plane.

Relations

Anterior – trachea, heart, great vessels and oesophageal plexus

Posterior – vertebrae and aorta

Lateral – pleural sacs, arch of aorta, phrenic nerve and vagus nerve (including recurrent laryngeal)

- Arterial supply

  Inferior thyroid artery, bronchial arteries, branches of the aorta and phrenic arteries and the left gastric artery
- Venous supply

  Proximal and distal oesophagus drains into the azygous vein whilst the middle oesophagus drains into the left gastric vein, a branch of the portal vein
- Lymphatic drainage

  The lymphatic drainage is again segmental, and is drained by the cervical, coeliac, mediastinal and gastric lymph nodes
- Nerve supply

  Sympathetic supply – inferior cervical and thoracic ganglia provide sympathetic innervation to oesophageal sphincters

  Parasympathetic supply – peristatic movements are controlled by the vagus nerve

Why is the oesophagus important to anaesthetists?
- Mode of feeding – placement of NG tube
- Mode of monitoring – doppler/TOE/temperature probe
- Inadvertent injury – during insertion of bougie, tracheostomy
- Insufflation of air into stomach during bag-mask ventilation especially in children – increases regurgitation risk
- Inadvertent oesophageal intubation

What are the specific areas in the oesophagus where food bolus can get stuck?

Physiological narrowing

1. Upper oesophageal sphincter that includes the cricopharyngeus muscle – common in children
2. Middle oesophagus where it crosses over the aortic arch (aorto-bronchial constriction)
3. Lower oesophageal sphincter – common in adults

Pathological narrowing

Stenosis due to benign oesophageal Schatzki rings, peptic strictures, webs, extrinsic compression, esophagitis and motor disorders such as achalasia.

Possible clinical application questions...

1. How would you anaesthetise for food bolus removal or ingested foreign body?
2. What are the anatomical abnormalities of the oesophagus that increase the risk of aspiration?

Heart

'Heart' is dealt with in few different ways in Final and Primary FRCA OSCE.

Final FRCA

- All about coronary circulation and the chronological changes in the ECG with ischaemia and more physiology about supply and demand
- Autonomic nerve supply of the heart and further questions about anaesthesia in a patient with a transplanted heart

Primary OSCE

- Structure of the heart with special mention to the sinuses of Valsalva, papillary muscle, etc.
- Coronary circulation – arterial and venous! This can be in the form of a diagram with coronary vasculature or a coronary angiogram

The heart is a cone-shaped muscular organ weighing around 250 g situated in the middle mediastinum. It consists of four chambers, the right and the left atria separated by a thin interatrial septum and the right and left ventricles separated by a thick interventricular septum (Figure 2.9).

Borders and surfaces of the heart

Table 2.5   Borders and Surfaces of the Heart

Right border
Entirely by the right atrium
Left border
Predominantly by the left ventricle
Auricular appendage of the left atrium
Inferior border
Predominantly by the right ventricle
Lower part of the right atrium
Apex of the left ventricle
Anterior surface
Predominantly by the right ventricle
Posterior surface
Predominantly by the left atrium and pulmonary veins
Small area by the right atrium

Pericardium

The heart is enclosed in a double-walled sac of pericardium.

- The outer fibrous layer invests the great vessels superiorly and attaches inferiorly to the diaphragm.
- The inner serous pericardium consists of parietal and visceral layers forming the pericardial sac. The parietal layer is sensitive and is supplied by the phrenic nerve. The visceral layer of serous pericardium is continuous with the parietal layer at the root of the great vessels and is adherent to the outer surface of the heart and forms the epicardium.

Layers of the heart

Table 2.6   Layers of the Heart

Epicardium
Visceral layer of serous pericardium
Comprised of mesothelial cells, fat and connective tissues
Myocardium
Muscle layer
Contains cardiomyocytes
Endocardium
Lines inner surface of heart chambers and valves
Consists of endothelial cells and subendocardial connective tissue

Chambers of the heart

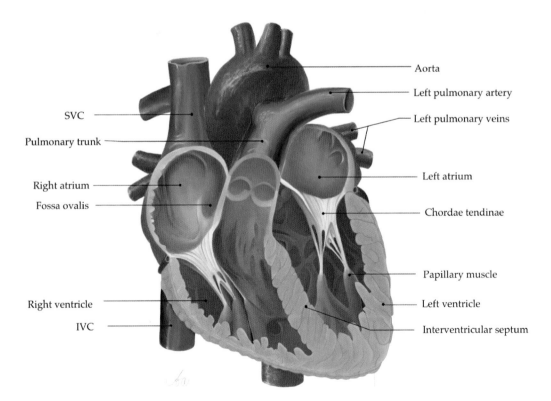

Figure 2.9   Heart – structure.

Right atrium

- The right atrium receives venous blood via the superior and inferior venae cavae, coronary sinus and the anterior cardiac vein
- The septal wall has the fossa ovalis, a shallow depression which indicates the site of the foramen ovale
- The crista terminalis is a ridge that runs vertically downwards between the venae caval openings and marks the boundary between the smooth-walled posterior part of the atrium and the trabeculated anterior portion (formed by pectinate muscles)

Right ventricle

- The right ventricle joins the right atrium through the tricuspid valve and the pulmonary artery through the pulmonary valve
- The infundibulo-ventricular crest separates the inflow and outflow tracts of the ventricle
- The inflow tract is marked by irregular muscle elevations, the trabeculae carneae, which give rise to projections called the papillary muscles. These attach to the free edges of the cusps of the tricuspid valve by means of the chordae tendinae. The importance of this *papillary muscle-chordae tendinae-valve cusp complex* is to prevent valve regurgitation during ventricular contraction when the chordae tendinae are held taut by the contracting papillary muscle
- The outflow tract of the right ventricle is smooth walled

Left atrium

- Left atrium is smaller but thick walled compared to the right atrium and the surface is ridged due to pectinate muscles
- Characterised by the opening of the four pulmonary veins at the upper part of the posterior wall and fossa ovalis on the septal wall

Left ventricle

- The left ventricle has a muscular wall and is thicker than the right ventricle correlating with the much higher pressure produced by the left ventricle
- It connects to the left atrium via the bicuspid mitral valve and to the aorta through the aortic semilunar valve
- *The papillary muscle-chordae tendinae-valve cusp complex is also functional to prevent mitral valve regurgitation*
- Immediately above the aortic valve cusps, the aorta bulges forming the dilated aortic sinuses of Valsalva marking the origin of the coronary arteries (Figure 2.10)

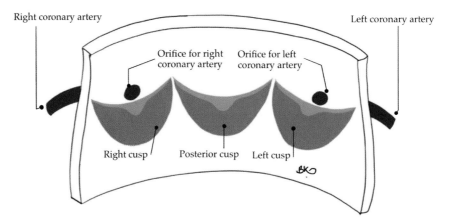

Figure 2.10   Sinuses of Valsalva.

Conducting system

The conducting system is the unique tissue specific to the heart and has specialised cardiac muscle. It generates and transmits impulses that regulate cardiac contraction.

- The *sinoatrial node* (SA node) is situated in the upper part of the crista terminalis, within the myocardium, to the right of the SVC opening. It is also called the pacemaker of the heart as it initiates and modulates the heart rate and transmits impulses to the atria and the ventricles.

- The *atrioventricular node* (AV node) is situated in the endocardium, near the atrial septum, immediately above the opening of the coronary sinus. It receives electrical impulses that originate in the SA node and transmits them to the bundle of His.

- The *atrioventricular bundle of His* transmits impulses to the walls of the ventricles. It first transits along the membranous part of the interventricular septum and then divides at the junction of the muscular and membranous parts of the interventricular septum. The subendocardial branches are the Purkinje fibres, specialised cardiac fibres, which then ascend within the muscular walls of the ventricles.

What is the normal QT and QTc interval?

The QT interval is the time from the start of the Q wave to the end of the T wave, thus representing the time taken for ventricular depolarisation and repolarisation.

- The maximum slope intercept method defines the end of the T wave as the intercept between the isoelectric line with the tangent drawn through the maximum down slope of the T wave.

- Normal value: 380–440 ms

   It is inversely proportional to heart rate, thus changing with higher and lower heart rates. Hence the corrected QT interval (QTc) is used to estimate the QT at a standard heart rate of 60/min to improve recognition of patients at increased risk of arrhythmias.

How can you calculate it?

Bazett's formula: $QTC = QT/\sqrt{RR}$

Fridericia formula: $QTC = QT/RR^{1/3}$

Framingham formula: $QTC = QT + 0.154\,(1-RR)$

Hodges formula: $QTC = QT + 1.75\,(\text{heart rate} - 60)$

$(RR\ \text{interval} = 60/\text{heart rate})$

What are the causes of a prolonged QT interval?

- Congenital long QT syndrome
- Electrolyte abnormalities – hypokalaemia, hypomagnesaemia, hypocalcaemia, hypothermia
- Cardiac ischaemia, myocarditis
- Raised intracranial pressure, subarachnoid haemorrhage
- Drugs – ondansetron, phenothiazines, atypical antipsychotics, quinolones, macrolides

Causes of short QT interval

- Hypercalcaemia
- Congenital short QT syndrome
- Digoxin

What are the possible consequences of a prolonged QT interval?

Increased risk of torsades de pointes and sudden cardiac death.

Bibliography

Burns, D. (2019). QT interval • LITFL medical blog • ECG library basics. Retrieved 24 August 2019 from https://litfl.com/qt-interval-ecg-library/.

Diaphragm

The diaphragm is a musculo-tendinous organ that separates the thoracic from the abdominal cavity. It is a muscle of respiration accounting for 70% of tidal volume in the erect position, increasing to 90% of tidal volume when supine, rendering the patients with diaphragmatic paralysis severely dyspnoeic in the supine position.

The diaphragm originates from the xiphoid process and the costal cartilages anteriorly and from the lumbar vertebral bodies and the fascia of the back muscles posteriorly (Figure 2.11).

- Sternal part – muscle fibres arise as two muscular slips from the posterior surface of the xiphoid process
- Costal part – muscle fibres arise from the lower six costal cartilages and adjoining ribs bilaterally
- Lumbar part – in the form of crura and arcuate ligaments
  - Crura – arise from the lumbar vertebral bodies (right crus – L1, L2, L3; left crus – L1, L2) and adjoining intervertebral discs. The crura are united by the median arcuate ligament. The course of these crural fibres form a muscular sphincter for the oesophagus.
  - Arcuate ligaments – the posterolateral portions of the diaphragm are reinforced by the medial and lateral arcuate ligaments which are thickenings of the fascia covering the psoas major and quadratus lumborum respectively (medial – major; lateral – lumborum).

Arterial supply

- Superior and inferior phrenic arteries
- Pericardiophrenic and musculophrenic arteries

Venous drainage

- Azygos vein (or IVC) via superior and inferior phrenic and intercostal veins

Nerve supply

- Sensory – phrenic nerve (C3, C4, C5) to the central portion of the diaphragm and lower intercostal nerves to the peripheral areas of the diaphragm
- Motor – phrenic nerve

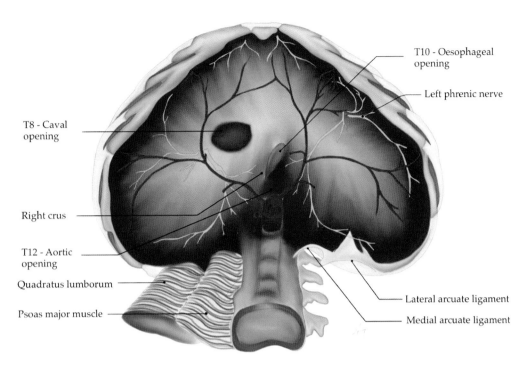

T10 - Oesophageal opening

Left phrenic nerve

T8 - Caval opening

Right crus

T12 - Aortic opening

Quadratus lumborum

Psoas major muscle

Lateral arcuate ligament

Medial arcuate ligament

Figure 2.11   Diaphragm.

At what levels are the major diaphragmatic apertures present? What structures pass through them?

All structures that pass from the thorax to the abdomen have to traverse the diaphragm.

There are three major openings and lots of small apertures. Table 2.7 shows the important structures that pass through the diaphragm.

Table 2.7   Structures Passing Through the Diaphragm at Different Levels

Level	Structures
T8 – caval hiatus	Inferior vena cava, right phrenic nerve
T10 – oesophageal hiatus (LOV)	Left gastric vessels, oesophagus and vagus nerves
T12 – aortic hiatus (ATA)	Descending aorta, thoracic duct, azygos vein
Right crus	Lesser and greater splanchnic nerves
Left crus	Hemiazygous vein, lesser and greater splanchnic nerves
Lumbocostal arch	Sympathetic trunk
Sternocostal foramen (foramen of Morgagni)	Superior epigastric branch of the internal thoracic artery, lymphatics

What are the muscles of quiet and forced respiration?

Inspiration

- Quiet – diaphragm, external intercostals
- Forced – diaphragm, external intercostal and accessory muscles (scalenes, pectoralis, sternocleidomastoid, serratus anterior and latissimus dorsi)

Expiration

- Quiet – relaxation of diaphragm and external intercostals (not an active process)
- Forced – internal and innermost intercostals and abdominal muscles

What is the cause of shoulder-tip pain post laparoscopy? What are the possible treatment options?

The incidence of shoulder-tip pain varies from 35% to 80% and can last for more than 72 hours after surgery.

The hypothesis of postoperative shoulder-tip pain is that phrenic nerve irritation is induced by carbon dioxide retention under the diaphragm which causes referred pain to C4. It is more common on the right side as there is a higher chance of carbon dioxide trapping between right diaphragm and the liver.

Management

Simple analgesics to opioids have been used to relieve the pain as sometimes this is more debilitating than the surgical pain. A recent randomised controlled trial has looked at the use of two methods that could be used to prevent or reduce shoulder-tip pain post surgery. The pulmonary recruitment manoeuvre (PRM) and intraperitoneal normal saline infusion (INSI) assist the expulsion of abdominal residual carbon dioxide by increasing the intraperitoneal pressure to facilitate the removal of residual carbon dioxide at the end of operation. INSI has an advantage as it offers a physiologic buffer system to dissolve excess carbon dioxide.

Ribs

The ribs play an important role in the protection of thoracic organs as well as in respiration via the 'bucket handle mechanism'.

Ribs 1, 2, 10, 11 and 12 are said to be atypical as they look different and have distinctive features compared to the 'typical' ones (ribs 3–9). This should not to be confused with 'true' ribs or the vertebrosternal ribs (1–7), 'false' ribs or vertebrochondral ribs (8–10) and floating ribs (11–12).

- First rib

  The first rib appears shorter, flatter, wider and more curved than the typical rib. There is no vertebral body above the first rib and hence the head has a single facet which articulates with body of T1. Scalenus anterior muscle is attached to the scalene tubercle which is located at the inner side of the rib and scalenus medius is attached to the shaft posterolaterally. The groove present on the superior surface between the attachment of the two scalene muscles houses the subclavian artery and the brachial plexus (trunks). The subclavian vein lies anterior to the scalene tubercle and serratus anterior is attached to the lateral border (Figures 2.12 and 2.13).

- Typical rib

  The ribs are flat and curved and they have two articular facets at the head (one facet articulates with the corresponding vertebrae and the other with the vertebrae above). There is a third facet for articulation of the corresponding transverse process. The groove for the neurovascular bundle is present at the inner surface of the shaft at the lower border (Figure 2.14).

You might be given the first and typical rib and asked to identify which side the rib belongs to...

- First rib: the scalene muscles and the neuro vasculature is present between the clavicle above and the superior surface of the first rib below. This gives the superior surface a rugged appearance. The broader flat end is anterior and the pointy end is posterior.
- Typical rib: the costal groove lies along the inferior border and therefore always points downwards towards the feet. Another method is to simply place the rib on the table. It is said to be in the correct vertical orientation if the head points up. Locate the head of the rib and point this posteriorly as if it was to articulate with the spinal column.

Possible clinical application questions...

1. Clinical features of tension pneumothorax and immediate management
2. Intercostal nerve block

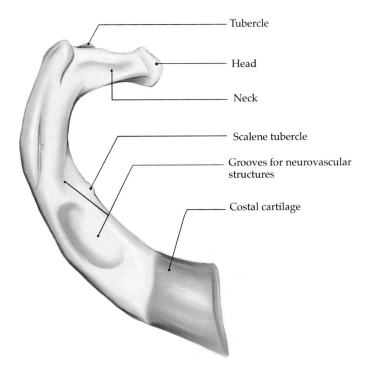

Figure 2.12   First rib.

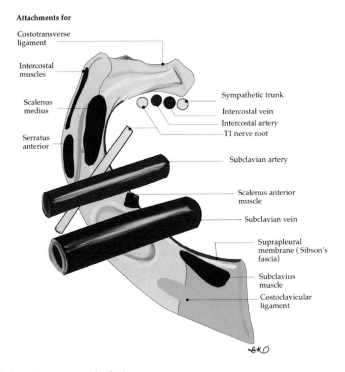

Figure 2.13   First rib – structures and relations.

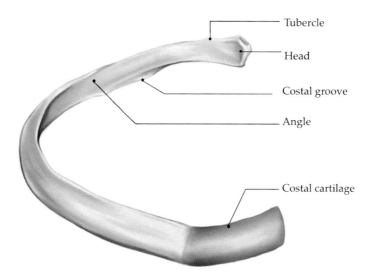

Tubercle

Head

Costal groove

Angle

Costal cartilage

Figure 2.14   Typical rib.

Circulation

- Lung
- Heart

Pulmonary Circulation

The pulmonary circulation begins when blood crosses the threshold of the pulmonary valve in the right ventricle and enters the pulmonary trunk where it divides into left and right pulmonary arteries. (A common mistake is to confuse the pulmonary arteries and veins – remember that arteries take blood <u>away</u> from the heart and veins take blood <u>towards</u> the heart. The pulmonary circulation transports deoxygenated blood from the right heart to the alveoli, where carbon dioxide is removed and oxygen is added). Pulmonary arteries transition to a rich network of pulmonary capillaries at the level of the alveolar ducts, draining into pulmonary veins, which carry oxygenated blood back to the left atrium.

Describe the anatomy of pulmonary and bronchial circulations.

The pulmonary and bronchial circulations are two distinct entities, which may be easily overlooked as both circulations involve the respiratory system (Table 2.8).

Table 2.8   Differences between Pulmonary and Bronchial Circulation

	Pulmonary circulation	Bronchial circulation
Function	Gas exchange	Nutrition and source of oxygen to lung parenchyma
Pressure and flow	*Low-pressure and high-flow system* Low-pressure: 25/8 mmHg High-flow: entire cardiac output enters the pulmonary circulation	*High-pressure and low-flow system* High-pressure: equivalent to systemic pressure Low-flow: 1% of cardiac output constitutes bronchial circulation
Origin and drainage	Arterial supply – driven by right ventricle into the pulmonary trunk Venous drainage – left atrium after passing through the lung for oxygenation	Arterial supply – thoracic aorta or intercostal arteries Venous drainage – 2/3 – into pulmonary veins constituting to physiological shunt 1/3 – into systemic circulation via azygos and hemiazygos veins

How does pulmonary circulation differ from systemic circulation?

These are parallel circuits that work in specific ways to deliver oxygenated blood most efficiently to the tissues that require it (Figure 2.15).

The pulmonary circulation operates at approximately one tenth of the systemic pressure. Pulmonary arterial pressure is 25/8 mmHg (MAP 15 mmHg) compared to 120/80 mmHg (MAP 100 mmHg) in the systemic circulation.

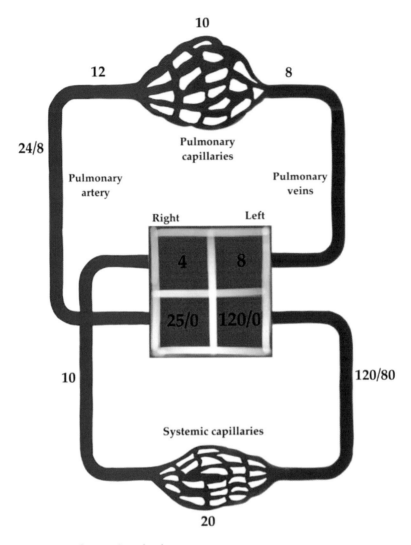

Figure 2.15 Comparison of systemic and pulmonary pressures.

The pressure is high in **systemic** circulation as it ensures

- Flow to different organs at different times with the help of resistance vessels
- Flow to organs at levels above the heart

On the contrary, the **pulmonary** circulation

- Accepts 100% of cardiac output and the thin-walled vessels make the system highly compliant

- Minimises extravasation of fluid – however, extravasation of fluid occurs when pulmonary artery pressure is even minimally increased (Table 2.9).

Table 2.9   Typical Values for Starling's Forces in Pulmonary Capillaries

Capillary hydrostatic pressure	16 mmHg (arteriolar end) 6 mmHg (venous end)
Capillary oncotic pressure	25 mmHg
Interstitial hydrostatic pressure	0 mmHg (may be slightly negative)
Interstitial oncotic pressure	17 mmHg

What is pulmonary vascular resistance and how is it maintained?

The pulmonary circuit functions on the basis of Ohm's Law

$$\text{Voltage} = \text{Current flow} \times \text{Resistance} \ (V = IR)$$

(Translated into vascular circulatory terms: Pressure = Flow × Resistance)

$$\text{Vascular Resistance} = P_{In} - P_{Out} / \text{Flow}$$

Determinants of pulmonary vascular resistance are
- **Pulmonary artery pressure (PAP)**

  Increased PAP causes a decrease in PVR as a result of

  ○ Recruitment – previously closed pulmonary capillaries are recruited when their critical opening pressure is reached, especially when MPAP is low.

  ○ Distension – vessels distend at higher pressures. This is applicable when PAP is high.

- **Lung volume**

  Lung volume has a variable effect on PVR.

  ○ At large lung volumes
    - Resistance in large extra-alveolar vessels decreases as the vessels are opened by distension of elastic tissues.
    - Resistance in small intra-alveolar vessels increases as they are compressed by the high lung volumes.

  ○ At small lung volumes, the reverse occurs.

- **Hypoxic pulmonary vasoconstriction (HPV)**

  Low P_AO_2 causes a vasoconstriction in the vessels supplying that alveolus, increasing PVR thereby diverting blood to better ventilated alveoli and improving V/Q matching.

  ○ Low alveolar PO_2 is the primary determinant and low mixed venous PO_2 also contributes.

  ○ Constriction begins when P_AO_2 falls below 100 mmHg, and becomes prominent below 70 mmHg. This is important in conditions like fetal circulation, alveolar consolidation and high altitude.

- **Response to substances**
  - Oxygen – the pulmonary circulation constricts when PaO_2 falls, whilst the systemic circulation dilates
  - Carbon dioxide – the pulmonary circulation constricts when $PaCO_2$ rises, whilst the systemic circulation dilates
- Other factors which affect PVR are

  Increase PVR
  - Hypercarbia
  - Hypothermia
  - Acidaemia
  - Pain

  Decrease PVR
  - Bronchodilators
  - Volatiles
  - Nitric oxide, prostacyclin (PGI_2)

How does perfusion of the lung differ in the upright vs the dependent lung?

The lung is subjected to the effects of gravity causing perfusion of the lung to be separated into three physiological zones called **West Zones**. The distribution of blood flow in these zones depends upon three factors: alveolar pressure (PA), pulmonary arterial pressure (Pa) and pulmonary venous pressure (Pv).

1. **Zone 1** – PA > Pa > Pv (no arterial blood flow = physiological dead space)
2. **Zone 2** – Pa > PA > Pv
3. **Zone 3** – Pa > Pv > PA

The alveolar partial pressure of oxygen and carbon dioxide are determined by the ratio of ventilation (V) to perfusion (Q). Ventilation and perfusion both increase from top to bottom in the lungs, with perfusion increasing more in comparison to ventilation.

The V/Q gradient occurs in the vertical axis of the lung fields irrespective of body positions (i.e. if patient is in upright posture, apex has more ventilation while base has more perfusion. If a patient is in the lateral position, the nondependent lung gets more ventilation while the dependent lung gets more perfusion).

Bibliography

Patwa, A., & Shah, A. (2015). Anatomy and physiology of respiratory system relevant to anaesthesia. *Indian Journal of Anaesthesia, 59*(9), 533–541. doi:10.4103/0019-5049.165849.

Terry Des Jardins. (2008). *Cardiopulmonary Anatomy & Physiology: Essentials for Respiratory Care*, 5th Edition. Clifton Park, NY: Thomson Delmar Learning.

West, J. B., & Luks, A. M. (2016). *West's Respiratory Physiology: The Essentials*, 10th Edition. Wolters Kluwer Philadelphia, PA.

www.partone.lifeinthefastlane.com/pulmonary_circulation.html.

Coronary Circulation

The total coronary blood flow is about 250 ml/min, which equates to 5% of the cardiac output. It is important to note that the blood flow increases by five times in strenuous exercise.

The heart receives its blood supply from the right and left coronary arteries (Figure 2.16).

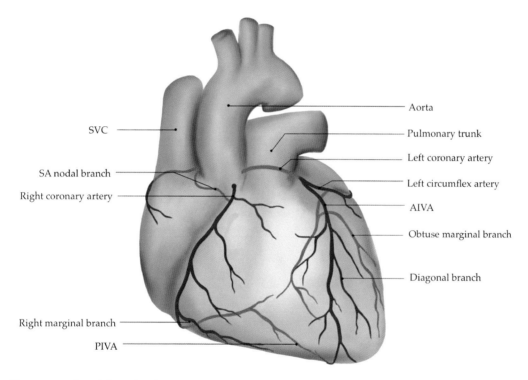

Figure 2.16   Arterial supply – heart.

Right coronary artery: arises from the right aortic sinus, runs between the right atrium and the pulmonary trunk to descend in the right atrioventricular groove. It winds around the inferior border to reach the diaphragmatic surface of the heart and runs backwards and left to reach the posterior interventricular groove. It terminates by anastomosing with branches of the left coronary artery.

- *Right marginal branch*
- *Posterior interventricular artery* (PIVA): this anastomoses with the AIVA in the posterior interventricular groove. ***It is the PIVA that determines the dominance of the arterial system.*** In this case the right coronary is dominant. If it arises from the left coronary or the left circumflex, then there is left coronary dominance.

- *Branch to the sino-atrial node*
- *Branch to the atrioventricular node*

Left coronary artery: after originating from the left aortic sinus, it passes forwards and to the left and emerges between pulmonary trunk and the left atrium and gives off two main branches.

- *Anterior interventricular artery* (AIVA), also known as the left anterior descending artery (LAD), runs downwards in the anterior interventricular groove and anastomoses with the PIVA. This is the major branch, as it supplies most of the muscle bulk. During its course, the AIVA gives off one or two large diagonal branches.
- *Circumflex branch*, which runs to the left in the left atrioventricular sulcus, winds around the left border of heart and terminates by anastomosing with right coronary artery. The left marginal artery is the large branch of the circumflex.

What are the structures supplied by the left and right coronary arteries and its branches?

Right coronary artery and branches

- Right coronary artery supplies right atrium
- Marginal branch supplies lateral walls of the right atrium and right ventricle
- PIVA supplies posterior wall of both ventricles

Left coronary artery and branches

- Circumflex artery supplies left atrium and posterior wall of left ventricle
- AIVA supplies anterior walls of both ventricles and interventricular septum

The innermost endocardium is supplied by blood within chambers. A summary of coronary blood supply can be seen in Table 2.10.

Table 2.10   Summary of Coronary Blood Supply

Right coronary artery	Left coronary artery
Right atrium, right ventricle, part of the interventricular septum	Left atrium, left and right ventricle, part of the interventricular septum
SA node in 65% of population	SA node in 35% of population
AV node in 80% of population	AV node in 20% of population
Rest of the conducting system in 80% of population	Rest of the conducting system in 20% of population

Describe the venous drainage of the heart.

Two-thirds of the venous drainage are by veins that accompany the coronary arteries and open into the coronary sinus in the right atrium. The remaining one third drains the endocardium and inner myocardium directly into the cardiac cavity (Figure 2.17).

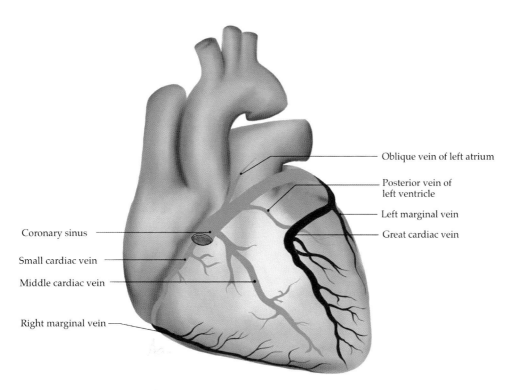

Figure 2.17   Venous drainage – heart.

- The ***coronary sinus*** lies in the right atrium between the superior and inferior vena caval openings. The main veins draining into the coronary sinus are
  - *Great cardiac vein*, which accompanies the AIVA
  - *Middle cardiac vein*, which lies in the inferior interventricular groove near the anastomosis of circumflex and right coronary arteries
  - *Small cardiac vein*, which accompanies the marginal branch of the right coronary artery
  - *Oblique vein*, which drains the posterior half of left atrium
- The ***anterior cardiac vein*** drains most of the anterior surface of the heart and opens into the right atrium directly
- The ***venae cordis minimae*** (Thebesian veins) drain the endocardium and inner myocardium directly into the cardiac cavity and is an example of physiological shunt as venous blood enters the left heart

Coronary angiogram

This is an invasive procedure performed as the gold standard to study the extent of coronary artery disease. After radial or femoral arterial access, coronary artery cannulation is performed, and a radiocontrast agent is injected with continuous fluoroscopy. The image intensifier is rotated to allow multiple views to optimally visualise the diseased vessels. The commonly used projections are

Right coronary artery

1. Right anterior oblique (RAO)
2. Left anterior oblique (LAO)

Left coronary artery

1. RAO caudal
2. LAO caudal
3. RAO cranial
4. LAO cranial
5. LAO straight

Each view is best for demonstrating a specific vessel which is beyond the scope of this book. Some examples are given below (Figures 2.18 and 2.19).

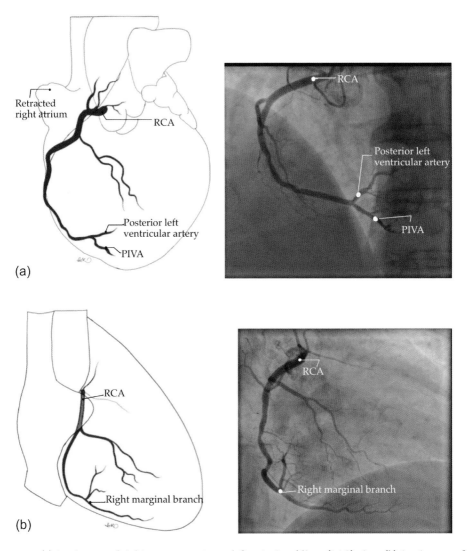

Figure 2.18   (a) Angiogram of right coronary artery – left anterior oblique (LAO) view; (b) Angiogram of right coronary artery – right anterior oblique (RAO) view.

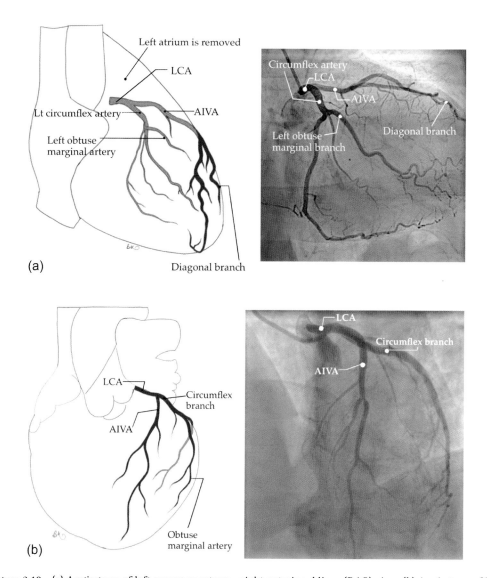

(a)

(b)

Figure 2.19 (a) Angiogram of left coronary artery – right anterior oblique (RAO) view; (b) Angiogram of left coronary artery – left anterior oblique (LAO) view.

Below is the coronary angiogram of a patient who had been admitted with a history of chest pain (Figure 2.20).

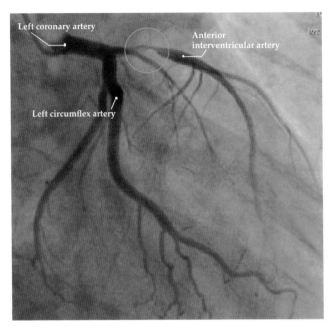

Figure 2.20   Angiogram of left coronary artery showing lesion of the proximal AIVA.

What is your diagnosis?

The coronary angiogram shows significant lesion of the proximal AIVA (LAD).

What is characteristic of chest pain in these patients? Why does coronary ischaemia cause pain?

Angina is usually described as a heavy pressure, squeezing or a burning feeling. The discomfort or pain often radiates to the left shoulder, neck or arm.

Coronary stenosis causes a mismatch in myocardial oxygen demand and supply resulting in increased levels of adenosine. This further activates afferent cardiac sympathetic neurons and gives rise to the typical visceral pain characteristic of angina.

Its poor localisation and wide variation in the type of pain can be due to the fact that the autonomic inputs converge with the common pathway ending in the sensory cortex which are used by both visceral and somatic afferents.

Discuss the management of ST elevation myocardial infarction (STEMI) in a patient.

This answer is based on 2017 ESC Guidelines for the management of acute myocardial infarction in patients presenting with ST-segment elevation.

Diagnosis

- Persisting symptoms (i.e. chest pain) consistent with myocardial ischaemia
- Persisting signs (ST elevation $\geq$ 2 mm in V2–V3 leads and/or $\geq$ 1 mm in all other leads including V3R and V4R (right ventricle MI) and/or $\geq$ 0.5 mm in V7–V9 (posterior MI) on a 12-lead ECG

General management

- Pain relief is paramount to overcome vasoconstriction and increased workload by blunting sympathetic activation. This is done with sublingual nitrate spray and/or intravenous opioids titrated to effect. Anxiolytics and reassurance are used if necessary
- Oxygen is indicated only in hypoxic patients (SaO_2 <90%)

Definitive management

- Primary PCI is the preferred reperfusion strategy in patients with STEMI within 12 h of symptom onset, provided it can be performed expeditiously (i.e. 120 min from STEMI diagnosis)
- If the reperfusion strategy is fibrinolysis, the goal is to receive the bolus of fibrinolytics within 10 min from STEMI diagnosis
- A primary PCI strategy is adopted in patients with
  - Clinical presentation compatible with acute MI and a non-interpretable ST-segment on the ECG, e.g. bundle branch block or ventricular pacing
  - Symptoms lasting >12 h in the presence of ongoing symptoms suggestive of ischaemia, haemodynamic instability or life-threatening arrhythmias

Pharmacological agents

- Platelet inhibition via dual anti platelet therapy (DAPT): DAPT is a combination of aspirin and a $P2Y_{12}$ inhibitor (prasugrel or ticagrelor) or aspirin and clopidogrel for over 12 months if not contraindicated
- Anticoagulation with unfractionated or low molecular weight heparin or bivalirudin is recommended for all patients in addition to antiplatelet therapy during primary PCI
- Beta blockers intravenously during presentation and orally thereafter is highly recommended if not contraindicated
- Statin therapy (as early as possible and continued long-term) unless contraindicated
- ACE inhibitors/ARBs are recommended unless contraindicated
- Mineralocorticoid receptor antagonist (MRAs) are indicated in patients with an LVEF $\leq$ 40% and heart failure or diabetes, who are already receiving an ACE inhibitor and a beta blocker

Miscellaneous measures

- Smoking cessation
- Cardiac rehabilitation

What are the ECG changes associated with myocardial infarction in increasing chronology?

- *Hyperacute* changes (within minutes) – tall T waves and progressive ST elevation
- *Acute* changes (minutes to hours) – ST elevation and gradual loss of R wave
- *Early* changes (hours to days)
  - ○ <24 hours: inversion of T wave and the resolution of ST elevation
  - ○ Within days: pathological Q wave begins to form
- *Indeterminate* changes (days to weeks) – Q waves and persistent T wave inversion
- *Old* changes (weeks to months) – persisting Q waves and normalised T waves

Other possible questions ...

What are the differences between systemic and coronary circulation?

What are the determinants of coronary circulation?

What are the determinants of myocardial oxygen supply and demand?

What are the anaesthetic considerations for a patient presenting for surgery with a history of heart transplant?

Bibliography

Ellis, H., Feldman, S. A., Harrop-Griffiths, W., & Feldman, S. A. (2004). *Anatomy for Anaesthetists* (pp. 105–106). Oxford: Blackwell.

Gilroy, A. M., Voll, M. M., & Wesker, K. (2017). *Anatomy: An Essential Textbook.* New York, NY: Thieme Medical Publishers, Inc.

Williams, B., Mancia, G., Spiering, W., Agabiti Rosei, E., Azizi, M., et al. (2018). 2018 ESC/ESH Guidelines for the management of arterial hypertension. *European Heart Journal, 39*(33), 3021–3104.

Nervous System

- Phrenic nerve
- Intercostal nerve block
- Thoracic wall blocks – pectoralis and serratus anterior blocks

Phrenic Nerve

Arises from the anterior primary rami of C3, C4 and C5 (principally C4) and receives contributions from accessory phrenic nerve (C5), cervical and thoracic sympathetics.

Course

In the neck
Descends between the prevertebral fascia and the anterior scalene muscle, lying posterior to the sternocleidomastoid and inferior omohyoid muscles and the carotid sheath. It is in close proximity to the brachial plexus near its origin but descends more laterally over the scalene muscle. At the root of the neck, it is between the subclavian artery and vein and enters the thorax.

In the thorax

- Right – the right phrenic nerve passes along the right side of the right brachiocephalic vein, superior vena cava and right atrium. It lies anterior to the hilum of the right lung and descends to the diaphragm along the right side of the inferior vena cava. It then passes through the caval opening and supplies the inferior surface of the diaphragm.
- Left – the left phrenic nerve has a longer intrathoracic course. It travels between the left subclavian and the left common carotid arteries and crosses the left surface of the arch of the aorta to descend anterior to the left lung hilum. It is superficial to the left atrium and ventricle and pierces the diaphragm to the left of the heart.

Function

Sensory: diaphragm, mediastinal pleura and pericardium, diaphragmatic peritoneum
Motor: diaphragm

What are the causes of phrenic nerve damage?

Iatrogenic

- Surgical – thoracic or cardiac surgery
- Anaesthetic – cervical plexus, interscalene, supraclavicular and coeliac plexus blocks, central line cannulation in neck
- Forceps delivery

Trauma

- Blunt and penetrating injury

Neurological

- Cervical spondylosis
- Multiple sclerosis
- Myopathy, e.g. muscular dystrophy

Neoplasm

- Infiltration of the nerve or destruction by tumour

Metabolic disorders

- Diabetes mellitus

Infective

- Herpes zoster
- Lyme disease

What are the clinical features of phrenic nerve damage?

In unilateral damage, patients may be asymptomatic. On CXR, damage may present as a raised hemidiaphragm, however it is important to consider other causes of a raised hemidiaphragm, such as pregnancy or intra-abdominal mass or a collapsed lung.

In severe cases or bilateral palsy, patients may complain of dyspnoea or orthopnoea, and suffer from recurrent bouts of pneumonia. On examination, there might be reduced air entry and dullness to percussion with inward movement of the epigastrium on inspiration. A restrictive picture would be seen in pulmonary function tests.

With regards to spinal cord injury, injury at C2 and C3 will result in complete loss of motor supply to the diaphragm. Damage at C4 and below results in a 75% reduction in vital capacity and damage below C6 preserves diaphragmatic function.

Intubated patients might have difficulty weaning from the ventilator, though it must be remembered that there are more common causes of difficulty weaning that should also be considered before phrenic nerve damage is diagnosed.

How can you diagnose phrenic nerve palsy?

Clinical suspicion (especially in iatrogenic causes)

Symptoms and signs

- Dyspnoea especially when supine
- Hypoventilation and lower saturations if bilateral

Investigation

- Chest radiograph – raised hemidiaphragm
- Pulmonary function test – reduction in FEV1 and FVC

- Oesophageal and gastric manometry
- Diaphragmatic electromyography
- Ultrasound of the diaphragm

What is the management?
- Treatment of underlying condition
- Symptom treatment
  - No treatment is required for asymptomatic unilateral diaphragmatic paralysis
  - In bilateral paralysis or if symptomatic, surgical options are considered such as plication and phrenic nerve stimulation (beyond the scope of this book)

Other possible questions...

How would you anesthetise a newborn for diaphragmatic hernia surgery?

How would you anaesthetise a patient with a history of hiatus hernia?

Bibliography

Dravid, R. M., & Paul, R. E. (2007a). Interpleural block–part 1. *Anaesthesia, 62*(10), 1039–1049.
Dravid, R. M., & Paul, R. E. (2007b). Interpleural block–part 2. *Anaesthesia, 62*(11), 1143–1153.

Intercostal Nerve

There are 11 paired intercostal spaces which contain intercostal muscles, membranes, nerves and vessels.

Course of intercostal nerves

The intercostal nerves pierce the posterior intercostal membrane approximately 3 cm distal to the intervertebral foramen (in adults) to enter the subcostal grove and run parallel to the rib.

- At the posterior axillary line, the intercostal nerves divide into the main branch (found near the inferior border of the upper rib) and collateral branches (follow the superior border of the lower rib).
- At the midaxillary line, the intercostal nerves give off the lateral cutaneous branches which divide into anterior and posterior cutaneous branches.

Therefore, for an effective intercostal nerve block it is important to anaesthetise the intercostal nerves at, or posterior to, the posterior axillary line. Due to overlap in innervation from adjacent nerves, blocking one or two spaces above and below the incision site is needed.

NB. Anatomical variation exists – T1 has no anterior cutaneous branch and some fibres of T2 and T3 give rise to the intercostobrachial nerve.

Lateral to the costal angle there are the external, internal and the innermost intercostal muscles which readily permit local anaesthetic diffusion. The parietal pleura is deep to the innermost intercostal muscle.

From the costal angle onwards, the main intercostal nerves and vessels are grouped as a neurovascular bundle and arranged in vein, artery and nerve (VAN) orientation from above downwards (Figure 2.21).

What are the indications for an intercostal nerve block?

- Surgical pain
  - Incisional pain from thoracic and upper abdominal surgery
  - Analgesia for thoracostomy
  - Breast surgery
  - Chronic pain post mastectomy and thoracotomy
- Trauma
  - Rib fractures
- Non-surgical pain
  - Herpes zoster or post herpetic neuralgia
  - Differentiating between visceral and somatic pain

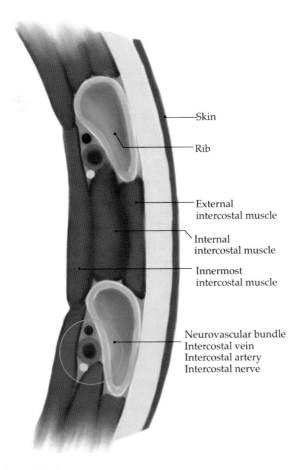

Figure 2.21   Intercostal nerve block.

What are the contraindications for intercostal nerve block?

- Patient refusal
- Disorders of coagulation
- Local infection

What are the complications of intercostal nerve block?

- General
  - Failure
- Block specific
  - Pneumothorax
  - Injury to peritoneum and viscera in lower intercostal blocks
  - Local anaesthetic toxicity because of high vascularity (arterial plasma concentration peaks in 5–10 min) and multiple level blockade

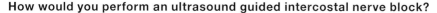

How would you perform an ultrasound guided intercostal nerve block?

With patient in the sitting position and with the hand hanging down by the side, the seventh rib is identied by scanning at the inferior angle of the scapula.

The patient is asked to reach over their contralateral shoulder to move the scapula laterally whilst scanning second to seventh intercostal space.

Transducer is then positioned oblique and lateral to the costal angle to scan the posterior intercostal space lateral to the costal angle. The intercostal nerves may not be identifiable but the vessels in the neurovascular bundle may be seen with colour flow doppler. The neurovascular bundle lies between the internal and innermost intercostal muscles. The innermost intercostal muscle is thin and may not be obvious but the parietal pleura deep to this is easily identifiable as a bright white hyperechoic line that slides with respiration.

An in-plane or out-of-plane approach may be used with the aim of 2 ml local anaesthetic deposition within the internal intercostal muscle to ensure there is no breach of the parietal pleura. Ideally, the local anaesthetic will be seen to depress the pleura.

How would you perform a landmark technique intercostal nerve block?

In the sitting position with arms forward (lateral or prone also possible), palpate and identify appropriate level of intercostal space.

The block is given lateral to the angle of the rib which is safer because of largest intercostal groove.

Identify angle of the rib (usually 7 cm from midline).

Insert a 22G, 50 mm needle at a 20-degree cephalad angle to reach the rib which is about 1 cm and then walk the needle off the rib inferiorly till a pop is felt if using a blunt needle which is usually 3 mm deep.

Inject 2–5 ml of local anaesthetic at each space making sure that maximum dosage of chosen local anaesthetic is not exceeded.

Bibliography

Felten, D. L., O'Banion, M. K., & Maida, M. E. (2015). *Netter's Atlas of Neuroscience.* Elsevier Health Sciences.

Thoracic Wall Blocks

Regional anaesthesia for breast cancer surgery offers excellent postoperative analgesia and a reduction in postoperative nausea and vomiting due to the opioid sparing.

Innervation relevant to breast surgery

- *Breast*: anterior branches of T4–T6 intercostal nerves
- *Apex of axilla*: intercostobrachial nerve (T2)
- *Pectoral muscles*: lateral pectoral nerve (C5–C7) and medial pectoral nerve (C8–T1)
- *Serratus anterior muscle*: long thoracic nerve (C5–C7)
- *Latissimus dorsi muscle*: thoracodorsal nerve (C6–C8)

Pectoralis block 1 (Pecs 1) – medial and lateral pectoral nerves

- Injection of local anaesthetic between pectoralis major and minor muscles at the level of the third rib

Advantages – unilateral breast surgery limited to pectoralis major and surgery involving anterior chest wall, i.e. pacemaker insertion and anterior thoracotomy

Disadvantages – limited axillary analgesia

Technique

Patient in supine position, a linear probe is placed inferior to the clavicle, at the level of the third rib. The pectoral muscles are identified with the axillary artery and axillary vein along with a branch of thoraco-acromial artery between the pectoral muscles. The probe is then rotated to be oblique to the spine and medial to the coracoid process and a 22G regional block needle is introduced in-plane cephalad to caudad. A minimum of 10 ml (0.2 ml/kg of 0.25% bupivacaine) of local anaesthetic is injected in the space between the pectoral muscles.

Modified Pecs 2 – medial and lateral pectoral nerve along with intercostal, intercostobrachial and the long thoracic nerves.

- Injection of local anaesthetic between pectoralis minor and serratus anterior muscles at the level of the fourth rib

Advantages – similar to Pecs 1 and also extensive procedures such as tumour resections, axillary clearances and mastectomy

Technique

After performing Pecs 1, the probe is adjusted to visualise the fourth rib and the needle is redirected to the deeper plane between the pectoralis minor and serratus anterior muscles, under the axillary suspensory ligament of Gerdy; 0.4 ml/kg of 0.25% bupivacaine or a minimum of 15 ml is suggested.

Serratus anterior plane block – lateral cutaneous branches of T2–T12 intercostal nerves

- Injection between latissimus dorsi and the deeper serratus anterior muscle

Advantages – analgesia to anterolateral chest wall, lateral rib fractures, thoracoscopy, thoracotomy, breast surgery and post-mastectomy pain syndrome

Technique

With patient supine or in the lateral decubitus position, a linear probe is placed along the midaxillary line in the transverse plane at the level of the fifth rib. After visualising the muscles, the needle is advanced in-plane at an angle of 45° towards the fifth rib. A small volume of local anaesthetic is injected to hydro-dissect the fascial layers and open the potential space between the muscle layers and then a larger volume of 30–40 ml of 0.25% bupivacaine is injected in increments. For a superficial block, the local anaesthetic is injected anterior to the serratus anterior and a deep block requires injection deeper to the serratus anterior and anterior to the rib.

Bibliography

Blanco, R. (2011). The 'pecs block': A novel technique for providing analgesia after breast surgery. *Anaesthesia*, *66*(9), 847–848.

Blanco, R., Parras, T., McDonnell, J. G., & Prats-Galino, A. (2013). Serratus plane block: A novel ultrasound-guided thoracic wall nerve block. *Anaesthesia*, *68*(11), 1107–1113.

Sherwin, A., & Buggy, D. (2018). Anaesthesia for breast surgery. *BJA Education*, *18*(11), 342–348.

ABDOMEN

3

Structures

- Spleen
- Liver

Circulation

- Mesenteric circulation

Nervous System

- Anterior abdominal wall
- Abdominal wall blocks
  - Transversus abdominis plane block
  - Rectus sheath block
  - Ilioinguinal/iliohypogastric nerve blocks
  - Quadratus lumborum block
  - Erector spinae block
  - Penile block

Structures

- Spleen
- Liver

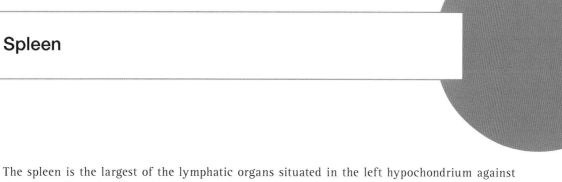

Spleen

The spleen is the largest of the lymphatic organs situated in the left hypochondrium against the 9th to the 11th ribs. In health, it weighs anywhere between 50–200 g and is non-palpable. Characteristic examination findings of a palpable spleen are the splenic notch and movement with respiration (Figure 3.1).

The spleen is related to stomach anteromedially, left kidney and splenic flexure inferiorly, pancreas medially, left ribs 9–11 posterolaterally and diaphragm superiorly and posteriorly.

Internal structure

- Fibrous capsule (outermost layer)
- Red pulp, which acts as a filter and storage for red blood cells. Blood flows through sinusoids, supported by a framework of trabeculae containing smooth muscle which helps expel blood into the circulation.
- Marginal zone, containing phagocytic macrophages
- White pulp (innermost layer), which is the immunologic layer as it is a site of antibody synthesis

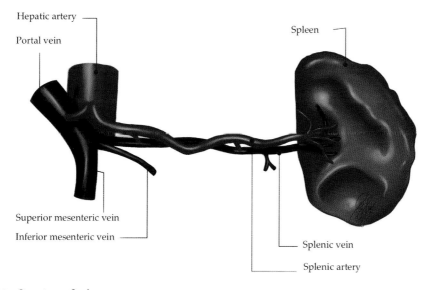

Figure 3.1   Structure of spleen.

Blood supply

- *Splenic artery* – the largest branch of the coeliac trunk
  - travels in a characteristically tortuous course along the superior border of the pancreas to reach the splenic hilum where it divides into multiple branches
  - gives off branches to the pancreas, 5–7 short gastric branches, and the left gastro-omental (gastroepiploic) artery
- *Splenic vein*
  - the splenic vein drains the spleen and meets the superior mesenteric vein behind the head of the pancreas, forming the portal vein
  - also receives the inferior mesenteric vein

Nerve supply
- Sympathetic fibres are derived from the coeliac plexus.

What are the functions of the spleen?
- *Immune* function

  The spleen is a component of the reticulo-endothelial system. It produces plasma cells and lymphocytes, therefore contributing to both humoral and cell-mediated immunity. It is also the major site of IgM production. The spleen produces opsonins, which facilitate the phagocytosis of encapsulated organisms.
- *Filtration*, storage and phagocytosis of blood cells

  The spleen receives 5% of cardiac output, stores 10% of total body red blood cells and 30% of total body platelets, along with iron storage. The spleen contains phagocytic cells which destroy aged erythrocytes and platelets.
- Extramedullary *haematopoiesis*

  In the fetus, the spleen is a site for myelopoiesis (the production of all types of blood cells). After birth, only lymphopoiesis is maintained but abnormal haematopoiesis can be reactivated in myeloproliferative disorders.

What causes splenomegaly?
- Infection – viral (e.g. infectious mononucleosis), bacterial (e.g. syphilis, infective endocarditis) or parasitic (e.g. malaria, visceral leishmaniasis)
- Malignancy – leukaemia, lymphoma, metastases
- Haematological – sickle cell disease, spherocytosis, thalassaemia, polycythaemia
- Metabolic – Gaucher disease, Niemann-Pick disease
- Other – Felty's syndrome, portal hypertension, collagen vascular diseases

What are the indications for a splenectomy?
- Trauma – commonest organ injured in blunt abdominal trauma
- Diagnostic – for histological diagnosis in idiopathic hypersplenism or splenomegaly
- Hypersplenism – hereditary spherocytosis, idiopathic thrombocytopenic purpura

- Tumour – lymphoma, leukaemia
- Surgical – en bloc with distal pancreatectomy and gastrectomy
- Others – splenic cysts, hydatid cysts, abscesses

What is overwhelming post-splenectomy infection (OPSI)?

- This is a rare, but frequently fatal, complication of infection with an encapsulated organism and occurs post splenectomy in 4% of patients without prophylaxis.
- It clinically presents as septic shock, bilateral adrenal haemorrhages and disseminated intravascular coagulopathy and is a medical emergency carrying a 50% mortality.
- It happens in the absence of splenic function and opsonisation (and therefore bacterial destruction) in a patient who is anatomically or functionally asplenic.
- The most frequent causative bacterium is Streptococcus pneumoniae. Other pathogens include Neisseria meningitidis, Haemophilus influenza type B, Listeria monocytogenes, Escherichia coli and Klebsiella sp.

What measures are undertaken to minimise the risks of infection in asplenic patients and prevent OPSI?

- Vaccination: pneumococcus, meningococcus, haemophilus type B and annual influenza vaccine. In the elective setting, these should be administered two weeks preoperatively or in the immediate postoperative period for emergency cases. These are ideally repeated every 5–10 years.
- Antibiotic prophylaxis: lifelong penicillin V or amoxicillin
- Education and awareness: patients should be educated on early signs and symptoms of infection/sepsis. They should carry an alert card and will need specialist advice on travel, especially on avoidance of malaria, animal bites and tick bites.

What is functional asplenia?

Functional asplenia occurs when splenic tissue is present but does not function properly and is characterised by the loss of phagocytosis. It occurs in autoimmune diseases, inflammatory bowel disease, sickle cell disease, beta thalassemia, chronic graft-versus-host disease and can be caused by splenic tissue infiltration by tumour cells, sickled erythrocytes, etc.

What abnormalities may be seen in the full blood count of an asplenic patient?

Blood count: poikilocytosis, siderocytosis, leucocytosis, thrombocytosis and increased NK cells

Blood smear: erythrocyte inclusions like Howell-Jolly bodies (remnants of DNA) and Heinz bodies (inclusions composed of denatured haemoglobin)

Liver

The liver is the second largest organ (second to skin) weighing around 1500 g, which accounts for 2.5% of body weight.

It contains

- Hepatocytes which are polyhedral epithelial cells arranged in sheets separated from each other by spaces filled with hepatic sinusoids
- Hepatic sinusoids which are vessels that arise at the portal triad and run between sheets of hepatocytes receiving blood from the portal triad to deliver to central vein

What is the significance of various types of divisions of the liver?

1. Surgical divisions (Corinaud's classification)
   - Total of eight segments with independent blood supply and biliary drainage, so they can be resected without damage to the adjacent segments

2. Functional classification. Liver lobule is the structural unit of liver.
   - Classic lobule
     - Based on direction of blood flow
     - Hexagonal structure with the central vein in the middle and portal triad (branches of portal vein, hepatic artery and bile duct) in the six corners. The hepatic arterial and portal venous blood flows from portal triad to the central vein.
   - Portal lobule
     - Based on direction of bile flow
     - The portal triad is in the middle and the central veins form the corners of the triangle.
   - Hepatic acinus
     - Based on changes in oxygen and nutrient content as blood flows from the portal triad to the central vein
     - It is a rhomboid tissue containing two triangles of adjacent classic lobule, with central veins at the apices.
     - Hepatocytes in the acinus are divided into three zones.
       1. Zone 1 or periportal zone, where the blood supply is the highest and is susceptible to damage by blood-borne toxins and infection
       2. Zone 2 or intermediate zone
       3. Zone 3 or centrilobular zone is closer to the central vein and is higher in CYP 450 levels but gets the least blood supply and hence is susceptible to ischaemia (Figure 3.2)

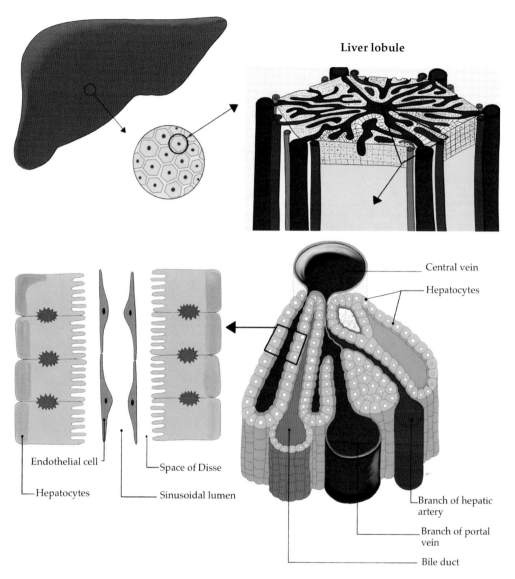

Figure 3.2   Structure of liver lobule.

What is special about the blood supply of the liver?

The liver has a *dual blood supply* and contains 10–15% of the total blood volume, and thereby acts as a powerful reservoir (Table 3.1).

Total liver blood flow = 1200 – 1400 mL/min = 25% of cardiac output

What factors determine the hepatic blood flow?

Like any other 'factors affecting blood flow' question, there is a general classification of factors. The factors listed below are in no order of importance. (It is best discussed using the Hagen-Poiseuille's equation with circulation-specific factors.)

Table 3.1   Hepatic Blood Supply

Hepatic artery	Portal vein
High-pressure/high-resistance system	Low pressure/low resistance
Branch of the coeliac trunk (branch of abdominal aorta)	Formed by the union of superior mesenteric vein and splenic vein
Carries oxygenated blood	Carries oxygen-poor but nutrient-rich blood from the abdominal viscera
20–30% of total blood supply	70–80% of total blood supply
40–50% of total oxygen supply	50–60% of total oxygen supply

- Myogenic autoregulation
  - applicable only in metabolically active liver
- Metabolic/chemical control
  - CO_2, O_2 and pH changes can alter the hepatic blood flow
  - Postprandial hyperosmolarity increases the hepatic arterial and portal venous blood flow
- Neural control
  - Autonomic nervous system via the vagus and splanchnic nerves have control of the hepatic blood flow
  - An important example is the stimulation of the sympathetic system in haemorrhage resulting in constriction of arterioles and expulsion of blood into the general circulation, thus acting as a major reservoir of blood
- Humoral control
  - Adrenaline, angiotensin II and vasopressin are the main vasoconstrictors
- Hepatic arterial buffer response (HABR)
  - Phenomenon where decrease in portal venous blood flow increases the hepatic arterial blood flow and vice versa so that a constant oxygen supply and total blood flow are maintained
  - The mechanism of HABR is unknown, but the local production of adenosine is predicted to be one of the causative factors

Other questions…

What do you understand by 'T10 level' and what structures are present at the level of T10?

Circulation

- Mesenteric circulation

Mesenteric Circulation

Blood supply to the bowel comes from three main branches of the aorta – coeliac axis, superior and inferior mesenteric arteries.

- Coeliac axis and branches – left gastric, common hepatic, splenic artery

The coeliac axis comes off at the T12 level and supplies the foregut structures such as liver, stomach, spleen, pancreas and the duodenum.

- Superior mesenteric artery (SMA) and branches – ileocolic artery, right colic artery, middle colic artery

The SMA originates at L1, and supplies the embryonic midgut structures such as the duodenum, pancreas, small bowel, caecum, ascending colon and two-thirds of the transverse colon until the splenic flexure.

- Inferior mesenteric artery (IMA) and branches – left colic artery, sigmoid artery, superior rectal artery

The IMA comes off at L3 and supplies the hindgut structures, such as the remaining one third of the transverse colon, descending colon, sigmoid and rectum (Figures 3.3 and 3.4).

What factors affect mesenteric blood flow?

The different variables that have an effect on blood flow are cardiac output, compliance of blood vessels, blood volume, blood viscosity, length and diameter of blood vessels.

This is best defined by Poiseuille's law which states that the flow of fluid is related to the viscosity of the fluid, the pressure gradient across the tubing and the length and diameter of the tubing.

What are the points of watershed blood flow?

A 'watershed' area is an area that has blood supply from the most distal branches of two large arteries. The two watershed areas in the colon are the splenic flexure and the rectosigmoid junction.

Presence of two different blood supplies is expected to maintain the blood supply to the area if there is atherosclerotic disease in one of the arteries. However, in the event of systemic hypoperfusion secondary to sepsis, heart failure, etc., these watershed areas are susceptible to ischaemia as the distal branches are least likely to receive sufficient blood.

What are the causes of mesenteric ischaemia?

Acute mesenteric ischaemia can happen because of the following reasons

- Embolus – following MI, atrial fibrillation or a mural thrombus

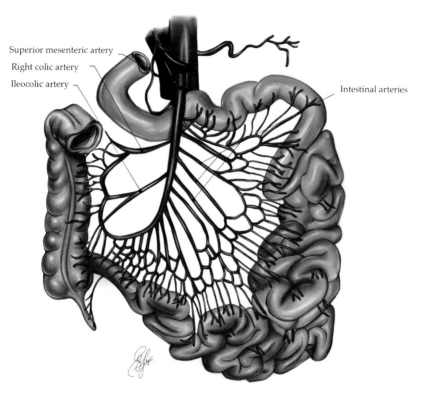

Superior mesenteric artery

Right colic artery

Ileocolic artery

Intestinal arteries

Figure 3.3   Arterial supply – small bowel.

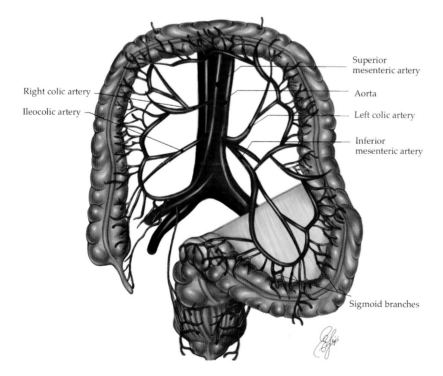

Right colic artery

Ileocolic artery

Superior mesenteric artery

Aorta

Left colic artery

Inferior mesenteric artery

Sigmoid branches

Figure 3.4   Arterial supply – large bowel.

- Thrombus – usually results from diffuse atherosclerotic disease, previous hypercoagulable states, vasculitis
- Non-occlusive thrombus – could result from hypovolaemia, spasm which result in a low flow state ultimately resulting in reduced cardiac output and decreased perfusion to the bowel

What are the symptoms and signs of ischaemic bowel?

Symptoms

- *Acute* – severe abdominal pain which is out of proportion, haematochezia, frequent and forceful bowel movement, confusion (especially in the elderly)
- *Chronic* – abdominal cramps within 30 minutes after eating, and lasting for a few hours, gradually worsening abdominal pain over weeks or months, fear of eating because of pain that follows, unintentional weight loss, diarrhoea

Signs

- Peritoneal signs – guarding, rigidity
- Circulatory signs – raised lactate, hypotension and tachycardia, new onset atrial fibrillation

How would you manage this condition?

Initial assessment

- History – be suspicious of patients with a sudden onset of severe abdominal pain
- Clinical examination – signs of peritonism and guarding are often late. The patient may have a new onset AF.

Investigations

- Blood investigations including serum lactate
- Abdominal x ray – 'gasless' abdomen (although this is no longer the investigation of choice)
- CT abdomen with IV contrast
- CT angiography/MR angiography – to look for SMA thrombus

Treatment

- ABC approach
- Volume resuscitation with vasopressors and inotropes if necessary
- Antibiotics
- Heparin, if cause of occlusion is due to a thrombus
- Urgent laparotomy and embolectomy/thrombectomy +/– resection of infarcted bowel

In patients with suspicion of acute ischaemic bowel urgent surgical intervention with early resuscitation is of paramount importance. The patient should be taken to theatre immediately for an exploratory laparotomy +/– restoration of blood flow +/– bowel resection.

Vigilance and care should be provided to prevent and treat reperfusion injury.

What is abdominal compartment syndrome?

Abdominal compartment syndrome is organ dysfunction secondary to impaired organ perfusion because of increased abdominal pressure. The normal values of intra-abdominal pressure (IAP) are 5–7 mmHg, although morbidly obese patients and pregnant women can have pressures up to 10 mmHg.

Sustained IAP of above 20 mmHg is often seen in abdominal compartment syndrome.

What are the causes of abdominal compartment syndrome?

- Primary (intra-abdominal cause) – trauma, mesenteric ischaemia, abdominal surgery and pancreatitis
- Secondary (extra-abdominal cause) – burns, sepsis

What are the risk factors for abdominal compartment syndrome?

- Diminished abdominal wall compliance
  - Abdominal surgery with tight primary closure
  - Major trauma/burns
  - Prolonged prone positioning
  - Any cause of elevated intrathoracic pressure
  - High BMI, central obesity
- Increased intraluminal contents
  - Gastroparesis and ileus
- Increased abdominal contents
  - Haemo- and pneumo-peritoneum
  - Ascites
- Capillary leak syndrome
  - Hypotension, hypothermla
  - Massive blood transfusion and fluid resuscitation
  - Coagulopathy
  - Pancreatitis

How can you measure IAP in a patient in intensive care?

Direct – by placing a sensor inside the abdomen during surgery.

Indirect – via intravesical, intragastric, intracolonic or inferior vena caval probe. The intravesical (bladder) route is the most commonly used surrogate method. IAP should be expressed in mmHg and measured at end-expiration with the subject in complete supine position after ensuring that abdominal muscle contractions are absent and with the transducer zeroed at the level of the midaxillary line.

What is intra-abdominal hypertension (IAH) and what are the grades of severity?

IAH is a sustained or repeated pathological elevation of IAP >12 mmHg.

Acute compartment syndrome is defined as a sustained IAP >20 mmHg that is associated with new organ dysfunction and failure.

According to the Burch system, IAH is graded as follows

- Grade I, IAP 12–15 mmHg
- Grade II, IAP 16–20 mmHg
- Grade III, IAP 21–25 mmHg
- Grade IV, IAP >25 mmHg

Patients with Grade III and Grade IV have a high morbidity, and decompression is essential.

What are the complications of abdominal compartment syndrome?

IAP is analogous to intracerebral pressure and an adequate abdominal perfusion pressure (APP) is necessary for normal organ function (APP is maintained above 60 mmHg).

$$APP = MAP - IAP$$

The complications could be due to direct compression or systemic effects which are outlined below.

- Cardiovascular complications
  - ↓ venous return due to compression of inferior vena cava
  - ↑ SVR and PVR
  - ↑ thrombosis due to stasis
- Abdominal complications
  - ↓ hepatic, coeliac and mesenteric blood flow leading to liver dysfunction and reduced perfusion of the bowel
  - ↓ abdominal wall blood flow causing local ischaemia and oedema
- Respiratory complications
  - ↓ pulmonary compliance, atelectasis, V/Q mismatch and respiratory failure
- Renal complications
  - ↓ blood flow to the renal vein resulting in renal derangement
  - Compression of renal vessels and bladder leading to oliguria

How is abdominal compartment syndrome managed?

The primary aim is urgent decompression which can be achieved either via a laparotomy or drainage along with supportive measures.

Bibliography

Berry, N., & Fletcher, S. (2012). Abdominal compartment syndrome. *Continuing Education in Anaesthesia, Critical Care and Pain, 12*(3), 110–117.

Cheatham, M. L. (2009). Abdominal compartment syndrome: Pathophysiology and definitions. *Scandinavian Journal of Trauma, Resuscitation and Emergency Medicine, 17*(1), 10.

Malbrain, M. L., Cheatham, M. L., Kirkpatrick, A., Sugrue, M., Parr, M., et al. (2006). Results from the international conference of experts on intra-abdominal hypertension and abdominal compartment syndrome. I. Definitions. *Intensive Care Medicine, 32*(11), 1722–1732.

World society of abdominal compartment syndrome. 2004. Retrieved 7 January 2019 from www.wsacs.org/.

Nervous System

- Anterior abdominal wall
- Abdominal wall blocks
  - Transversus abdominis plane block
  - Rectus sheath block
  - Ilioinguinal/iliohypogastric nerve block
  - Quadratus lumborum block
  - Erector spinae block
  - Penile block

Anterior Abdominal Wall

The anterior aspect of the abdominal wall is made essentially of the rectus abdominis muscle enclosed by its sheath. The anterior rectus sheath is composed of the fascial aponeuroses of external oblique muscle and the posterior sheath by the internal oblique and transversus abdominis aponeuroses. The anterior rectus sheath attaches to the muscle via transverse insertions and hence has a divided look, whereas the posterior sheath is continuous. Hence rectus sheath blocks are performed at the posterior aspect of the muscle to enhance the spread of the local anaesthetic.

The lateral side of the anterior abdominal wall has three main muscles, namely external oblique, internal oblique and transversus abdominis invested in fascial sheaths from superficial to deep. Beneath the muscles, the layers are the transversalis fascia, extraperitoneal fat and parietal peritoneum.

Innervation of the anterior abdominal wall

- Anterior rami of T7–L1
  - T7–T11 intercostal nerves
  - T12 – subcostal nerve
  - L1 – iliohypogastric nerve

The anterior divisions of T7–T11 continue from the respective intercostal grooves and enter the abdominal wall in the plane between internal oblique and transversus abdominis. The anterior ramus of T12 crosses quadratus lumborum before entering the abdominal wall and communicates with the L1, which passes behind psoas major muscle before entering the abdominal wall (Figure 3.5).

Branches of the anterior rami of the spinal nerves

- White and grey rami communicantes connecting the spinal nerves to the sympathetic ganglia
- Muscular branches to the intercostals and muscles of the abdominal wall
- Branches to periosteum of ribs, parietal pleura and the outer edge of the diaphragm
- Cutaneous branches
  - Lateral cutaneous branch at the midaxillary line which supplies the lateral abdominal wall
  - Anterior cutaneous branch near the rectus supplying the anterior abdominal wall

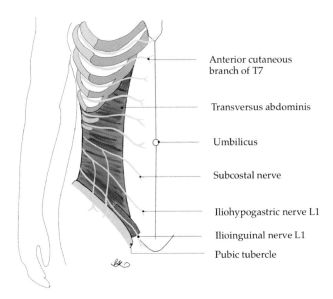

Figure 3.5   Anterior abdominal wall – nerve supply.

Blocks of the Abdominal Wall

- Transversus abdominis plane block
- Rectus sheath block
- Ilioinguinal/iliohypogastric nerve blocks
- Quadratus lumborum block
- Erector spinae block
- Penile block

Transversus Abdominis Plane Block

The nerves lie in the plane between the internal oblique and the transversus abdominis called the transversus abdominis plane (TAP).

The procedure satisfactorily blocks T7–T12, L1 to cover the somatic sensory distribution of the abdominal wall and the parietal peritoneum. It is important to note that this does not cover visceral pain and hence is an adjunct to general anaesthesia in various procedures. But it has shown to decrease opioid requirements intra- and postoperatively making it ideal for use in ambulatory surgery and all the procedures listed below (Table 3.2).

Table 3.2   Indications of TAP Block

General surgical procedures
Abdominal wall hernia, open appendicectomy
Open cholecystectomy
Colorectal procedures requiring a midline laparotomy incision
Gynaecological procedures
Hysterectomy
Caesarean section
Urological procedures
Nephrectomy
Prostatectomy
Renal transplant

Technique

Landmark method (Figure 3.6)

Landmarks: Petit's triangle bounded anteriorly by the external oblique, posteriorly by the latissimus dorsi and inferiorly by the iliac crest is the landmark for non-ultrasound guided approach. A short bevelled blunt needle is inserted perpendicular to the skin just above the iliac crest, which pierces the external oblique and internal oblique muscles and the investing fascia giving the characteristic 'two-pops' to lie in the TAP. After negative aspiration, 20 ml of the local anaesthetic is injected. The onset of analgesia is at least 45–60 minutes.

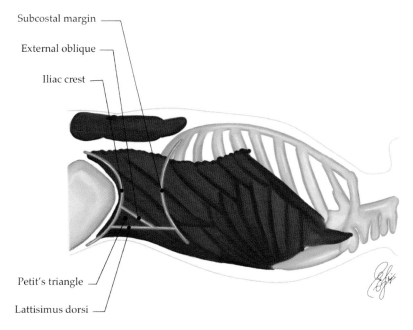

Subcostal margin

External oblique

Iliac crest

Petit's triangle

Lattisimus dorsi

Figure 3.6   TAP block – position of Petit's triangle.

Complications

Needle related – injury to the bowel and other viscera, vessels, peritoneal cavity and hepatic injury

Drug related – anaphylaxis, transient femoral nerve palsy and LA toxicity

Ultrasound guided TAP block

Although all anterior branches communicate in the TAP, each segmental nerve supplies different areas and hence there are different approaches depending on which nerves/areas need to be blocked. A linear probe is used generally but a curvilinear probe might be an option in obese patients

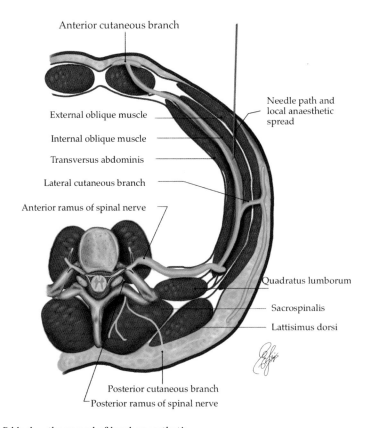

Anterior cutaneous branch

Needle path and
local anaesthetic
spread

External oblique muscle

Internal oblique muscle

Transversus abdominis

Lateral cutaneous branch

Anterior ramus of spinal nerve

Quadratus lumborum

Sacrospinalis

Lattisimus dorsi

Posterior cutaneous branch
Posterior ramus of spinal nerve

Figure 3.7   TAP block – the spread of local anaesthetic.

Table 3.3   Different Approaches to Ultrasound Guided TAP Block

Subcostal approach – anterior cutaneous branches of T6–T9 (upper TAP plexus)
Blocks upper abdominal wall just below the xiphoid and parallel to the costal margin. Probe is held parallel to the costal margin near the xiphoid process. The needle is inserted in plane. The TAP is between rectus abdominis and transversus abdominis at this location.
Lateral approach – anterior cutaneous branches of T10–T12 (lower TAP plexus)
Provides analgesia to the anterior abdominal wall at the infraumbilical area from midline to midclavicular line. Probe is placed at the midaxillary line between the costal margin and the iliac crest. The needle is inserted in plane. The LA is injected in between internal oblique and transversus abdominis.
Posterior approach – anterior and maybe lateral cutaneous branches of T9–T12
Blocks anterior abdominal wall at the infraumbilical area and possibly lateral abdominal wall between costal margin and iliac crest. The probe is held posterior to the midaxillary line between the costal margin and the iliac crest. The needle is inserted in plane. The injection site is at the TAP between internal oblique and transversus abdominis posterior to the midaxillary line.
Oblique subcostal approach – anterior cutaneous branches of T6–L1
Blocks the whole of the anterior abdominal wall. Probe in the oblique subcostal line (extending from the xiphoid toward the anterior part of the iliac crest) and needle in plane. As the oblique subcostal line is longer, a comparatively longer needle (15–20 cm) and a larger volume of LA (40–80 ml) are required.

Rectus Sheath Block

The rectus muscles originate from the pubic crest, pubic symphysis and pubic tubercle and insert onto the costal cartilages of ribs 5 to 7 and the xiphoid process. They are separated by the linea alba in the midline and the linea semilunaris along their lateral border (Figure 3.8).

The rectus muscles are enclosed in the aponeurotic rectus sheath, formed anteriorly by the external oblique aponeurosis and anterior layer of the internal oblique aponeurosis and posteriorly by the posterior layer of the internal oblique aponeurosis and the transversus abdominis aponeurosis.

The rectus sheath completely covers the upper three-quarters of the rectus muscles and the anterior portion of the lower one quarter, but the posterior one quarter is uncovered by the rectus sheath, instead being in contact with the transversalis fascia. The horizontal line that demarcates the lower limit of the posterior rectus sheath is called the arcuate line, found midway between the umbilicus and the pubic symphysis (Figure 3.9).

There are three tendinous intersections anteriorly on the rectus sheath (forming the familiar 'six pack'), but none posteriorly, allowing local anaesthetic to spread in the posterior part of the sheath.

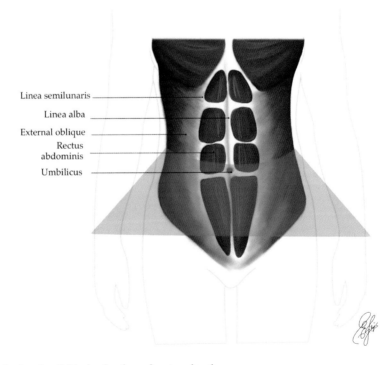

Figure 3.8   Rectus sheath block – borders of rectus sheath.

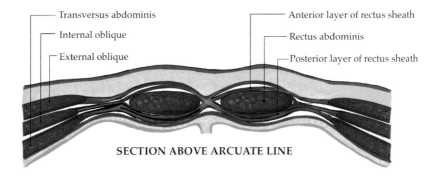

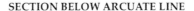

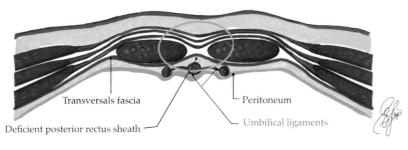

Figure 3.9   Rectus sheath block – sections above and below the arcuate line.

T7–T12 nerves continue anteriorly from the transverse plane to pierce the rectus muscle as anterior cutaneous nerves which are targeted during a rectus sheath block. Bilateral rectus sheath block has been suggested to provide analgesia in the midline from the xiphisternum to the pubic symphysis, although unreliably, and many anaesthetists feel its blockade is limited to the periumbilical area.

What are the specific indications and complications of rectus sheath block?

Specific indications

Intraoperative and postoperative analgesia for midline abdominal incision, e.g.

- Repair of umbilical, paraumbilical hernia and epigastric hernia
- Abdominoplasty
- Repair of duodenal atresia

Specific complications

- Rectus sheath haematoma from injury to superior or inferior epigastric vessels
- Perforation of peritoneum or bowel
- Major vessel puncture

How would you perform an ultrasound guided rectus sheath block?

With the patient in the supine position, a linear probe is placed just above umbilicus in the transverse plane. The linea alba is identified in the midline with the two rectus muscles either side. Scanning laterally, the semilunaris is identified on the lateral border of the rectus with the external oblique, internal oblique and transversus abdominis muscle layers seen further laterally. After identifying the rectus muscles, the anterior and posterior portions of the rectus sheath and the peritoneum (a hyperechoic line beneath the posterior rectus sheath), an in-plane approach is used.

The aim of the block is to deposit local anaesthetic between the posterior wall of the rectus sheath and the rectus abdominis muscle. Spread of local anaesthetic can be seen by turning the probe to a paramedian longitudinal plane.

Colour doppler can identify the epigastric arteries to avoid inadvertent intravascular injection or puncture.

Drug and dosage

- Adults – 10 ml on each side of 0.25% levobupivacaine (max. dose 2–3 mg/kg)
- Paediatrics – 0.1–0.8 ml/kg of 0.25% levobupivacaine
- Continuous infusion can be used at the rate of 10–15 ml/hr of 0.125–0.25% levobupivacaine

Inguinal and Iliohypogastric Nerve Blocks

These blocks provide analgesia to the abdominal wall and not abdominal viscera. They have a role in providing analgesia for incisions below the umbilicus. They can often be used when central neuraxial blockade would be contraindicated. They provide analgesia whilst maintaining haemodynamic stability.

Inguinal canal

The inguinal canal is a passageway through the inferior part of the abdominal wall, superior and medial to the inguinal canal. It begins at the deep inguinal ring and ends at the superficial inguinal ring.

Boundaries

- Floor – inguinal ligament
- Roof – transversus abdominis, internal oblique and transversalis fascia
- Posterior wall – transversalis fascia
- Anterior wall – aponeurosis of the external oblique, internal oblique laterally

Contents of the inguinal canal

- Spermatic cord in men, round ligament in women
- Ilioinguinal nerve
- Genital branch of the genitofemoral nerve

Which nerves need to be anaesthetised for an inguinal hernia repair under local anaesthesia?

- Lower intercostal/subcostal nerves
- Nerves from the lumbar plexus
  - Ilioinguinal nerve T12–L1
  - Iliohypogastric nerve T12–L1
  - Genitofemoral nerve L1–L2 (supplying inguinal cord structures)

The ilioinguinal and iliohypogastric nerves arise from the lumbar plexus, emerge at the lateral border of psoas major, pass anterior to quadratus lumborum and run in the plane between the internal oblique and transversus abdominis muscles (Figure 3.10).

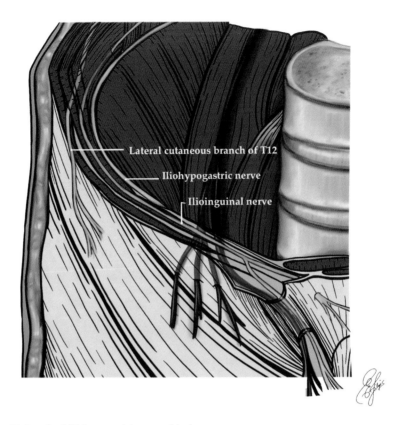

Figure 3.10 Ilioinguinal iliohypogastric nerve block.

Just lateral to the anterior superior iliac spine (ASIS), the ilioinguinal nerve pierces the internal oblique to enter the inguinal canal. It supplies the skin of the upper medial thigh, scrotum, base of penis or labia majora and mons pubis.

Just medial to the ASIS, the anterior (medial) cutaneous branch of the iliohypogastric nerve pierces the internal oblique to lie between it and external oblique. It then pierces the external oblique aponeurosis to supply the skin above the inguinal ligament and suprapubic area.

The genitofemoral nerve runs retroperitoneally on the body of psoas major dividing into its two branches. The genital branch passes through the inguinal canal, supplying the cremaster and scrotal skin or the mons pubis and labia majora. The femoral branch enters the femoral sheath, supplying the skin of the upper thigh.

What are the indications for an ilioinguinal and iliohypogastric block?

- Intraoperative and postoperative analgesia during inguinal surgery
- Inguinal hernia repair
- Orchidopexy
- Hydrocoele repair
- Varicocoele surgery

How would you perform an ilioinguinal and iliohypogastric block?

Landmark technique

- With patient in the supine position a short, blunt regional block needle is inserted 1–2 cm medial and 1–2 cm cephalad to the anterior superior iliac spine. When the needle passes through the external oblique (first pop) 5 ml local anaesthetic is inflitrated to block the iliohypogastric nerve. Through the internal oblique (second pop) infiltrate to block ilioinguinal and then fan-wise subcutaneous injection of 3–5 ml to block remaining sensory supply from the intercostal and subcostal nerves.

Ultrasound technique

- With patient supine, place a high frequency linear ultrasound probe obliquely on a line joining the anterior superior iliac spine and the umbilicus, immediately superior to the anterior superior iliac spine. Identify the peritoneum and the three muscle layers of the abdominal wall. The ilioinguinal and iliohypogastric nerves can be found between the internal oblique and transversus abdominis muscles. Using an in-plane technique, infiltrate local anaesthetic around the nerves.

What would be a suitable dose of local anaesthetic?

As these blocks are used to provide analgesia as part of a multimodal approach, often with opioid sparing benefits, a longer acting anaesthetic agent is usually chosen, e.g.

- Adults – 20 ml of 0.25–0.5% bupivacaine (total not exceeding 2 mg/kg)
- Paediatrics – 0.075 ml/kg 0.25% levobupivacaine when using an ultrasound guided technique or 0.3 ml/kg when using a landmark technique

What are the complications of an ilioinguinal and iliohypogastric block?

- Block failure
- Bowel injury – small and large bowel punctures or haematoma
- Pelvic retroperitoneal haematoma – most commonly due to inferior epigastric vessel injury
- Transient femoral nerve palsy

Bibliography

Yarwood, J., & Berill, A. (2010). Nerve blocks of the anterior abdominal wall. *Continuing Education in Anaesthesia, Critical Care and Pain, 10*(2), 182–186.

Quadratus Lumborum Block

Quadratus lumborum (QL) lies in the posterior abdominal wall posterolateral to the psoas major muscle. The ventral rami of the T7–L1 spinal nerves pass over the anterior aspect of quadratus lumborum. The thoracolumbar fascia which lines the QL is continuous with the endothoracic fascia laterally. So, it is assumed that when local anaesthetic is injected around QL, it causes blockade via thoracic paravertebral spread. Another theory is through the spread of anaesthetic drug to the coeliac ganglion.

The thoracolumbar fascia has three layers: the posterior layer surrounds the erector spinae muscle; the middle layer passes between the erector spinae muscles and quadratus lumborum; and the anterior layer lies anterior to both quadratus lumborum and psoas major muscles.

The block provides both somatic and visceral analgesia for abdominal, pelvic and retroperitoneal procedures. The list of indications is exhaustive and recent indications for hip and femur surgeries have also been published.

Technique

Patient is positioned supine, prone or lateral, and using a linear or curvilinear probe placed at the posterior axillary line below the costal margin and above the iliac crest, a short bevelled 50–100 mm block needle is inserted according to the approaches below. The block needs to be performed bilaterally and around 15–30 ml of local anaesthetic (0.2–0.4 ml/kg) is needed per side (Table 3.4).

Table 3.4   Different Approaches to the Ultrasound Guided Quadratus Lumborum Block

Lateral approach – covers T12–L1
Drug injected at the lateral margin of QL where it contacts the transversalis fascia (where transversus abdominis muscle tapers off into its aponeurosis).
Posterior approach
Local anaesthetic is injected posterior to the QL and anterior to erector spinae at the level of middle layer of thoracolumbar fascia.
Anterior or transmuscular approach
Point of injection is at anterior aspect of QL, between QL and PM. Under ultrasound guided block, this image is assumed to look like a 'shamrock' with the transverse process of L4 seen as the stem, erector spinae as posterior leaf, psoas major as anterior leaf and QL as lateral leaf.
Intramuscular approach
Injection is done in the QL muscle.

Erector Spinae Plane Block

Injection of local anaesthetic in the paraspinal fascial plane deep to erector spinae muscle at the tips of the thoracic transverse processes closer to the costotransverse foramina.

- Mechanism of blockade is secondary to diffusion of the local anaesthetic into the paravertebral space both cephalad and caudally to target the ventral and dorsal rami of spinal nerves.

It is ideal for procedures for thoracic and abdominal acute and chronic pain, i.e. breast surgery, rib fractures and shoulder surgery. It is used as an alternative to thoracic epidural and paravertebral blocks with minimal complications due to the absence of vital structures in the area. Also, the drug is injected in an avascular plane rendering little systemic absorption.

Technique

With the patient sitting, lateral or prone, a linear or curved probe is placed longitudinally to view the corresponding transverse processes (e.g. T7 for abdominal wall analgesia) and muscles (the trapezius and erector spinae). A short bevelled 80–100 mm needle is inserted at a 30–45°angle in-plane cranial to caudal aiming for the T7 transverse process. Hydro-dissection with normal saline is performed to identify the plane before injection of 20–30 ml local anaesthetic underneath the erector spinae muscle.

Bibliography

Akerman, M., Pejčić, N., & Veličković, I. (2018). A review of the quadratus lumborum block and ERAS. *Frontiers in Medicine, 5*, 44.

Mukhtar, K. 2009. Transversus abdominis plane (TAP) block. *Journal of the New York School of Regional Anesthesia, 12*, 28–33.

Onwochei, D. N., Børglum, J., & Pawa, A. (2018). Abdominal wall blocks for intra-abdominal surgery. *BJA Education, 18*(10), 317–322.

Tsai, H. C., Yoshida, T., Chuang, T. Y., Yang, S. F., Chang, C. C., et al. (2017). Transversus abdominis plane block: An updated review of anatomy and techniques. *BioMed Research International, 2017*.

Penile Block

Penile block is performed as a sole anaesthetic technique or as a postoperative analgesic option in isolated surgery of penis – circumcision, dorsal slit procedure, repair of paraphimosis and penile lacerations.

Innervation of penis

Pudendal nerve (S2 – S4) through its terminal branches – the dorsal penile and perineal nerves. The dorsal penile nerve descends below the inferior pubic ramus and continues directly within Buck's fascia next to the dorsal vessels (Figure 3.11).

Technique: effective anaesthesia is typically achieved through either a dorsal penile nerve block at the level of the pubic symphysis or a ring block at the base of the penis or a combination.

Position: supine

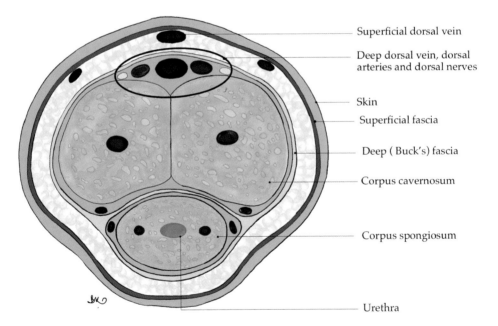

Figure 3.11   Cross section of penis – innervation.

Dorsal penile block

A 21G or 23G needle is inserted perpendicular to the dorsum of the base of the penis, slightly lateral to the midline (to avoid the dorsal vessels) until it encounters the symphysis. The needle is then withdrawn and redirected caudally and laterally to pass below the pubic symphysis, approximately 3 to 5 mm deeper. After haem-free aspiration, 5–10 ml of local anaesthetic solution without adrenaline is injected. The procedure is repeated on the contralateral side.

The block is reinforced with local anaesthetic injection at the base of the ventral penis to cover the perineal nerve.

Ring block

Local anaesthetic is injected by circumscribing the entire penis in a superficial plane.

Complications

- Pain and discomfort, if awake
- Failure due to incomplete block
- Bleeding and haematoma
- Local anaesthetic with adrenaline should never be used as penis is an end-organ with no collaterals

Bibliography

McPhee, A. S., & McKay, A. C. (2018). Dorsal penile nerve block. In: *StatPearls* [Internet]. StatPearls Publishing.

SPINE

4

Structures

- Vertebral column
- Meninges
- Spinal cord

Circulation

- Spinal cord blood supply

Nervous System

- Blocks
  - Epidural
  - Spinal
  - Caudal
  - Paravertebral block

Structures

- Vertebral column
- Meninges
- Spinal cord

Vertebral Column

The vertebral column is made up of seven cervical, 12 thoracic, five lumbar, five fused sacral and four fused coccygeal vertebrae (33 in total) separated by intervertebral discs. The primary and secondary curvatures give the classical sinusoidal pattern with cervical and lumbar lordosis, thoracic and pelvic kyphosis.

A typical vertebra has a vertebral body situated anteriorly and the vertebral arch posterolaterally thereby enclosing the vertebral canal containing the spinal cord.

- Vertebral body – anterior and weight bearing
- Vertebral arch made of
  - Two transverse processes – posterolateral projections
  - Two pedicles connecting the body to the transverse process
  - Single spinous process posteriorly
  - Two laminae – between transverse process and spinous process
- The intervertebral foramina are present between the successive pedicles and transmit the spinal nerve and radicular vessels
- Superior and inferior articular processes with their articular facets connect adjacent vertebral arches

The array of ligaments present posteriorly adjoining the vertebral arch, which are pierced by the needle during spinal anaesthetic, as shown in Figure 4.1, include

- Supraspinous ligament – connects the tips of spinous processes
- Interspinous ligament – connects the facing borders of the adjacent spinous processes
- Ligamentum flavum – connects the facing borders of adjacent laminae

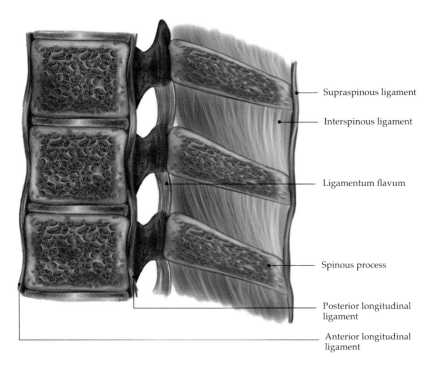

Figure 4.1   Posterior spinal ligaments.

Vertebra

There are 33 vertebrae in the human body – seven cervical, 12 thoracic, five lumbar, five sacral and four coccygeal. They are distinct in sizes and shapes, and the anatomy of a typical cervical, thoracic and lumbar vertebrae is summarised below. (See also Figure 4.2).

Comparison of cervical, thoracic and lumbar vertebrae

	Cervical	Thoracic	Lumbar
Body	Small and oval	Medium and 'heart shaped' Has facets for ribs	Large and oval
Foramen	Large	Medium	Small
Spinous process	Points inferiorly Bifid	Points inferiorly Not split	Points horizontal Not split
Transverse process	Transverse foramina present	All except T11 and 12 have facets for ribs	No articular facets

Cervical vertebra

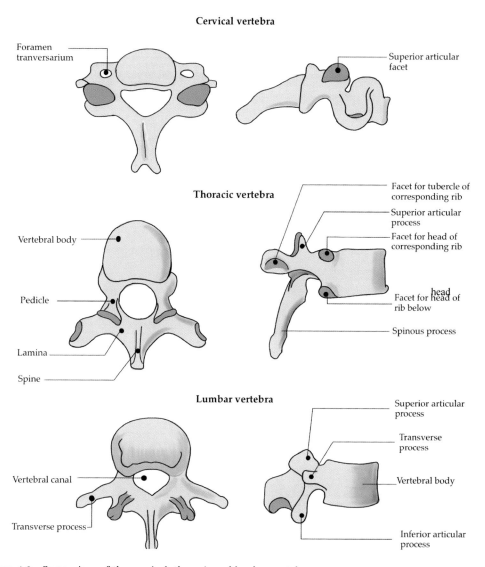

Foramen tranversarium

Superior articular facet

Thoracic vertebra

Facet for tubercle of corresponding rib

Superior articular process

Vertebral body

Facet for head of corresponding rib

Pedicle

Facet for head of rib below

Lamina

Spinous process

Spine

Lumbar vertebra

Superior articular process

Transverse process

Vertebral canal

Vertebral body

Transverse process

Inferior articular process

Figure 4.2   Comparison of the cervical, thoracic and lumbar vertebrae.

Cervical spines – C1 and C2

C1 (Atlas) has no vertebral body or spinous process. It has lateral masses bound by the posterior and anterior arch. The anterior arch contains a facet which articulates with the dens of C2 (axis) and is supported by the transverse ligament which connects the two lateral masses. The atlanto-dens interval (predendate space) is the distance between the odontoid process and the anterior arch of the atlas. A distance of >3 mm in adults (>7 mm in children) signifies atlanto-axial subluxation and hence the patient is at risk of cervical cord injury if manipulated.

Possible clinical application questions...

1. How do you clear C-spines in a multi-trauma patient?
2. What physiological changes happen with spinal cord injury?
3. How can you prevent secondary injury?

Intervertebral discs

The intervertebral discs lie between the vertebral bodies and are responsible for 25% of total height of the vertebral column. They are important in providing structural support and helping with movement.

Discs are bounded anteriorly and posteriorly by the anterior and posterior longitudinal ligaments, respectively.

The intervertebral disc comprises of

- An outer *annulus fibrosus* – made of type I and type II collagen produced by fibroblast cells, organised as lamellae
- An inner *nucleus pulposus* – formed of type II collagen and proteoglycans produced by the chondrocyte-like cells, holds water within the disc
- Two vertebral endplates – also formed by proteoglycans and type II collagen, produce a layer of the hyaline cartilage between discs and the adjacent vertebral bodies

Blood supply

- In adults, most parts of the disc are avascular. The peripheral annulus receives its nutrients from segmental arteries, which are branches of the aorta.

Nerve supply

- Recurrent sinuvertebral nerve, which arises in the dorsal root ganglion

Bibliography

Mahadevan, V. (2018). Anatomy of the vertebral column. *Surgery (Oxford), 36*(7), 327–332.

Spinal Cord and Tracts

The spinal cord is the specialised nerve tissue continuous with the medulla oblongata, enclosed circumferentially by the spinal meninges and suspended in the cerebrospinal fluid. It travels the vertebral column in the neural arch and terminates at L1/2 vertebral level in adults (L3/4 at birth) and measures about 45–50 cm in adults (Figure 4.3).

Conus medullaris: tapered end of spinal cord at its termination

Cauda equina (horse's tail): bunch of spinal nerves at the conus medullaris (contains lumbar, sacral and coccygeal spinal nerves)

Filum terminale: a thin strand of pia mater with no neural tissue that connects the conus medullaris to the coccyx.

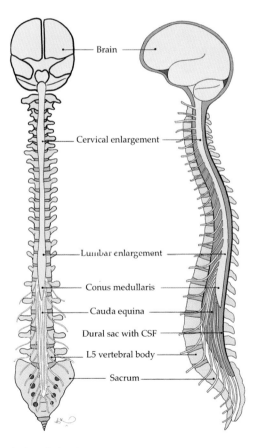

Figure 4.3a   Spinal cord – extent and structure.

Cross section of spinal cord

It is oval in shape with a deep anterior fissure and a shallow posterior septum. Anterior and posterior nerve roots arise on the lateral surface and combine to form the spinal nerves at the intervertebral foramen. They soon divide into the anterior (sensory and motor innervation to the front of the body) and posterior (sensory and motor supply to the back) primary rami. The central canal or the ependymal canal is a CSF filled space which is a continuation of the fourth ventricle and runs the entire length of the spinal cord.

The *grey matter* is H-shaped and contains cell bodies of interneurons and motor neurons, as well as neuroglial cells and unmyelinated axons. The white matter consists of bundles of myelinated axons which form the various ascending and descending tracts (Figure 4.4).

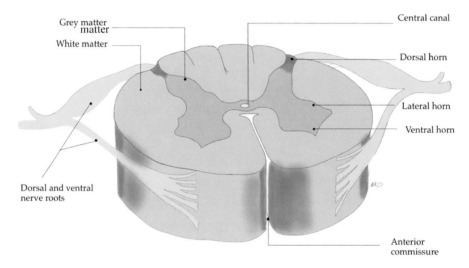

Figure 4.3b   Spinal cord – cross section.

Descending tracts (motor)

- *Lateral corticospinal tract (crossed pyramidal tract)*: fibres carry voluntary motor activity from cortex, decussate in the medulla and descend the spinal cord on the contralateral side.
- *Anterior corticospinal tract (uncrossed pyramidal tract)*: voluntary motor activity from the cortex reaches the spinal cord without decussation.
- *Tecto spinal tract*: this extrapyramidal tract causes movement of the head in response to visual and auditory stimuli from the midbrain tectum to the contralateral spinal cord.
- *Rubro spinal tract*: this extrapyramidal tract regulates voluntary movements and reflexes. Fibres originate from the red nucleus of midbrain, cross to the opposite midbrain and then descend down the spinal cord.

Ascending tracts (sensory)

- *Anterior and posterior spinocerebellar tracts*: posterior spinocerebellar tract ascends on the ipsilateral side of the spinal cord to enter the cerebellum whilst the anterior tract does a 'double cross', meaning it crosses to the contralateral side of the spinal cord initially but then crosses back to the ipsilateral cerebellum. They both carry proprioception, fine touch and vibration modality from the golgi tendon and muscle spindles.

- *Anterior and lateral spinothalamic tracts*: fibres carrying touch, pain and temperature sensation ascend for a few segments and then cross to the contralateral side of the spinal cord to reach the thalamus and cortex.

- *Posterior columns*: the medial tract of Goll (fasciculus gracilis – transmits information from the lower parts of the body – legs and trunk) and the lateral tract of Burdach (fasciculus cuneatus – transmits information from the upper parts of the body – neck, trunk and arms) carry the sensation of fine touch and position sense and reach the medulla uncrossed, but then decussate to reach the thalamus and cortex.

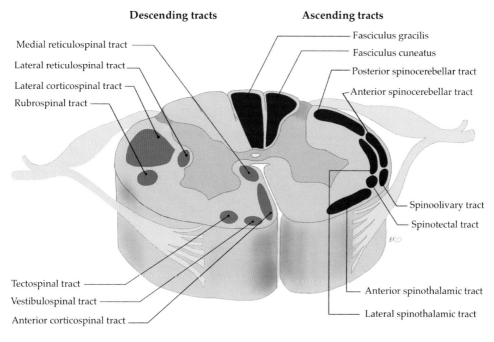

Figure 4.4   Spinal cord – ascending and descending tracts.

What are the neurological features that occur in various types of spinal cord injury?

This depends on the cause and type of injury (Table 4.1).

Table 4.1   Features in Various Types of Spinal Cord Injury

Complete transection of the spinal cord
• Loss of sensation below the transection • Flaccid paralysis below lesion initially, followed by spastic paralysis • Loss of bladder and bowel function
Hemisection of the spinal cord (Brown-Sequard syndrome)
• Loss of proprioception on the ipsilateral side • Loss of pain and temperature on the contralateral side • Paralysis on the ipsilateral side
Syringomyelia – disease of the centre of the cord
• Cystic degeneration of decussating fibres of the spinothalamic tract • Loss of pain and temperature bilaterally in the upper limbs
Tabes dorsalis – syphilitic involvement of the cord
• Loss of proprioception and ataxia due to involvement of posterior column

Bibliography

Ellis, H., & Mahadevan, V. (2018). *Clinical Anatomy: Applied Anatomy for Students and Junior Doctors.* Wiley-Blackwell.

White, J., & Seiden, D. (2017). *USMLE Step 1 Lecture Notes 2017.* New York, NY: Kaplan Medical.

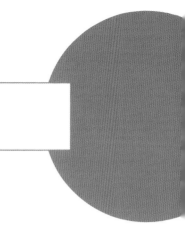

Meningeal Layers

Meninges are the connective tissue layers surrounding the spinal cord. They are

- *Duramater*: a tough, outer layer that envelops the spinal cord. Superiorly it attaches to the foramen magnum and continues as the cranial dura; inferiorly it ends at S2.
- *Arachnoid*: a delicate tissue which is avascular and terminates at S2
- *Piamater*: the innermost layer which is adherent to cord and ends with the cord at L1/2

The presence of these layers gives rise to three spaces

- *Epidural space*: situated between the vertebral canal and the dura
- *Subdural space*: potential space at the dura-arachnoid interface which is pressed against the dura due to CSF pressure
- *Subarachnoid space*: between arachnoid and pia and contains the CSF

Cerebrospinal fluid

The cerebrospinal fluid (CSF) is produced by the epithelium of the choroid plexus in the lateral, third and fourth ventricles. From the third ventricle, the CSF flows to the fourth ventricle through the aqueduct of Sylvius. It then drains into the subarachnoid space through the foramens of Magendie (medial) and Luschka (lateral) before being reabsorbed by the arachnoid villi in the dural sinuses.

The total volume is around 150 ml of which 25 ml flushes the spinal theca and the daily production is around 600 ml. The CSF pressure measures 5–10 cmH$_2$O in the lateral/supine posture which increases to 30–40 cmH$_2$O in the sitting position.

How does the composition of CSF differ from that of plasma?

Table 4.2   Differences between CSF and Plasma

	CSF		Plasma
Specific gravity	1.006		1.020
PCO_2 (kPa)	6.6	↑	4.5–5.5
pH	7.33	↓	7.4
Total protein (g/L) *	0.35	↓↓↓↓	70
Glucose (mmol/L)	3.3	↓↓	5.0
Bicarbonate (mmol/L)	24	<->	24
Sodium (mmol/L)	138	<->	140
Potassium (mmol/L)	3	↓↓	4–5
Calcium (mmol/L)	1.1	↓↓	2.2–2.6
Chloride (mmol/L)	120	↑	95–105

Because of the substantially low protein, CSF has less buffering capacity.

Bibliography

Puntis, M., Reddy, U., & Hirsch, N. (2016). Cerebrospinal fluid and its physiology. *Anaesthesia and Intensive Care Medicine, 17*(12), 611–612.

Circulation

- Spinal cord blood supply

Spinal Cord Circulation

The spinal cord derives its blood supply from a single anterior spinal artery (ASA), paired posterior spinal arteries (PSA) and by the communicating segmental arteries and the pial plexus.

ASA: single artery formed at the foramen magnum by the union of each vertebral artery. Blood flows centrifugally supplying the anterior two-thirds of the spinal cord in front of the posterior grey column.

PSA: derived from the posterior inferior cerebellar artery (PICA) or vertebral artery, with blood flowing centripetally in this arterial system. The arteries lie along the posterolateral surface of the spinal cord medial to the posterior nerve roots.

Pial arterial plexus: surface vessels branch from the ASA and PSA forming an anastomosing network that penetrates and supplies the outer portion of the spinal cord.

Segmental branches: segmental or radicular branches arise from vertebral, deep cervical, costo-cervical, aorta and the pelvic vessels. There are 20–40 pairs of radicular arteries all of which are important but the one below is the largest.

Arteria radicularis magna, or the artery of Adamkiewicz arises from the thoracolumbar part of the aorta, usually on the left, and enters the spinal cord at the level of L1 and supplies the lower thoracic and upper lumbar parts of the cord. It usually arises from a lower intercostal or a high lumbar artery but may arise as low as L4 or as high as T8. Since it makes a major contribution to the blood supply of the spinal cord, spinal injury or aortic surgery may compromise the blood supply of the lower part of the spinal cord.

Various regions of spinal cord are vascularised unevenly. The cervical and lumbosacral parts are well vascularised whereas the thoracic part of the spinal cord, especially the anterior region, derives the branches from intercostal and iliac arteries, which vary in location and numbers making it prone to ischaemic damage (Figure 4.5).

Which part of the spinal cord acts as a watershed zone?

A watershed effect occurs when two streams of blood flowing in opposite directions meet. This happens where the radicular artery unites with the ASA, where blood courses upward and downward from the entry point, thus leaving a watershed region between the adjacent radicular areas where blood flows in neither direction. The watershed effect is maximum in the mid-thoracic area due to the greater distance between the radicular arteries.

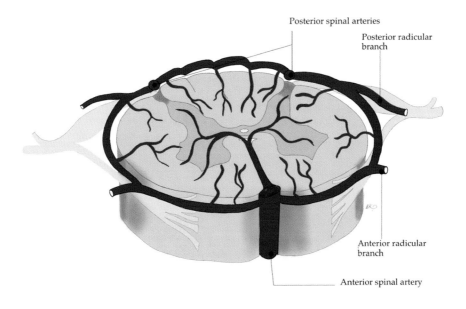

Posterior spinal arteries

Posterior radicular branch

Anterior radicular branch

Anterior spinal artery

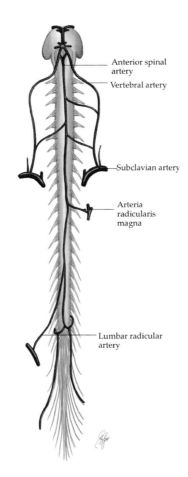

Anterior spinal artery

Vertebral artery

Subclavian artery

Arteria radicularis magna

Lumbar radicular artery

Figure 4.5   Arterial supply of spinal cord.

Describe the venous drainage. What is its importance?

Radicular and spinal veins drain into the internal vertebral venous plexus (of Batson) that later drain into the azygos system and the superior vena cava through the vertebral, intercostal and lumbar veins. The plexus communicates with the basilar sinus in the brain and with the pelvic veins and inferior vena cava. In patients with increased intra-abdominal pressure, blood is diverted from the inferior vena cava to the plexus, leading to engorgement of epidural veins. For example, in pregnant women, this increases the risk of accidental venous puncture during the conduct of epidural anaesthesia and decreases the effective epidural space volume, thereby requiring a smaller volume of local anaesthetic.

These veins can also provide a route for metastatic cancer cells to the vertebrae or the brain from an abdominal or pelvic tumour (Figure 4.6).

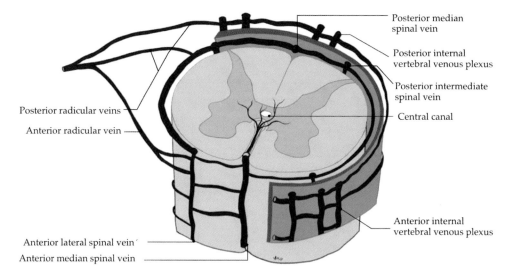

Figure 4.6   Venous drainage of spinal cord.

What are the causes of poor blood supply to the cord?

Spontaneous causes

- Aortic rupture or dissection
- Inflammation of aorta – vasculitis, collagen disorders
- Embolus from vascular atheroma or cardiac myxoma or valvular vegetation
- Degenerative spinal diseases and disc herniation
- Severe atherosclerosis and luminal narrowing
- Venous hypertension

Traumatic causes

- Any trauma jeopardising the spinal vascular supply
- Iatrogenic causes

- Vasoconstrictors or steroids in epidural space
- Surgical cross clamping of the aorta
- Coeliac plexus block
- Deliberate/accidental hypotension
- Spinal surgery resulting in microembolisation of intervertebral disc matter

What are the risk factors for spinal cord ischaemia during aortic surgery?

According to recent statistics, the incidence of spinal cord ischaemia following thoracoabdominal aortic aneurysm repair is 3–18% despite improved surgical technique, transfusion and perfusion technology. The factors that determine the neurological outcome after aortic cross clamping are

- Presence of predisposing factors, such as atherosclerosis, diabetes and renal disease
- Extent of aneurysm
- Duration of cross clamp
- Surgical difficulty
- Previous aortic surgery
- Severity of perioperative hypotension and the use of catecholamines

What are the different spinal cord protection strategies undertaken during thoracoabdominal aneurysm repair?

- Mild systemic hypothermia (32–34°C): the most reliable protective adjunct and helps by decreasing metabolic demands and attenuating inflammatory response to ischaemia
- Maintaining spinal cord perfusion pressure (SCPP) depends on the mean arterial pressure and cerebrospinal fluid pressure (CSFP). Cross clamping leads to proximal hypertension and increased cerebrospinal fluid pressure. So, controlling the arterial pressure with vasopressors or decreasing CSFP via lumbar drains plays a significant role in maintaining SCPP.

$$SCPP = MAP - CSFP$$

Cerebrospinal fluid drainage to avoid pressures above 10 mmHg for at least 48 hours postoperatively is recommended.

- Distal aortic shunting through femoro-femoral bypass and left heart bypass increases the blood flow to the distal aorta.
- Pharmacological neuroprotection: agents such as free radical scavengers, barbiturates, steroids, opiate antagonists, etc., have been evaluated in decreasing the risk of ischaemic damage of the cord.
- Monitoring spinal cord function with motor evoked potentials and somatosensory evoked potentials intraoperatively has proven effective in preventing damage by identifying a need to reimplant important radicular arteries. Postoperatively, clinical monitoring of motor and sensory function of the limbs may indicate a need to optimise the SCPP by altering MAP or CSFP.

What is anterior spinal artery (ASA) syndrome? What are the findings?

ASA syndrome: a condition characterised by critical ischaemia of the anterior part of the spinal cord due to occlusion of the anterior spinal artery.

The characteristic findings are

- Motor

Loss of motor function bilaterally below the level of lesion due to the involvement of corticospinal tracts

- Sensory

Loss of spinothalamic tract function resulting in bilateral thermoanaesthesia, BUT intact light touch, vibration and proprioception due to preservation of posterior columns

- Autonomic

Sexual dysfunction, loss of bladder and bowel function due to the effect on descending autonomic tract

A male patient underwent an open thoracic aneurysm repair under general anaesthetic. His epidural analgesia is followed up by the pain team on postoperative day 1. He presents with weakness of legs.

What are the differentials?

- Related to thoracic AAA repair
  - Incidence of paraplegia or paraparesis is 3–18% due to cross clamp leading to spinal cord ischaemia
  - Hypotension due to blood loss leading to poor spinal cord perfusion
- Related to the epidural if inserted for pain relief
  - High concentration epidural top up
  - Epidural abscess
  - Epidural haematoma
  - Migration of the catheter into the subdural/subarachnoid space
  - Direct nerve trauma
- Unrelated to both
  - Disc herniation
  - Tumours
  - Transverse myelitis
  - Vascular and neurological disease
  - Meningitis

What is the incidence of epidural haematoma? What are the risk factors for developing one?

NAP 3 (2009): the incidence of epidural haematoma in this audit was 0.85 per 100,000.

An epidural haematoma should be suspected if the effects of epidural anaesthesia persist for >8 h after the last dose of local anaesthetic and if there is backache and local tenderness. The presence of a bilateral distribution of motor and sensory abnormalities and/or disturbance of bowel or bladder function should arouse suspicion. Urgent imaging is required and, if a haematoma is present, emergency decompression is indicated as soon as possible.

Risk factors

- Bleeding tendency
- Thrombocytopaenia
- Drugs used for thromboprophylaxis
- Difficult neuraxial blocks

Bibliography

Dommisse, G. F. (1974). The blood supply of the spinal cord: A critical vascular zone in spinal surgery. *The Journal of Bone and Joint Surgery. British Volume, 56*(2), 225–235.

Willey, J. Z., Barnett, H. J., & Mohr, J. P. (2011). Spinal cord ischemia. In: *Stroke* (pp. 643–657). WB Saunders: Philadelphia, PA.

Nervous System

- Blocks
  - Epidural
  - Spinal
  - Caudal
  - Paravertebral block

Spinal and Epidural Blocks

Epidural space

The epidural space surrounds the dura from the foramen magnum to S2/S3 where the dural sac ends.

Boundaries

- Superior: foramen magnum
- Inferior: sacral hiatus and sacrococcygeal membrane
- Anterior: posterior longitudinal ligament, vertebral bodies and intervertebral discs
- Posterior: vertebral spines, interlaminar spaces filled with ligamentum flavum
- Lateral: pedicles, intervertebral foramina

Contents

Dura, spinal nerve roots, vessels, venous plexus of Batson, connective tissue, lymphatics and fat (Figure 4.7).

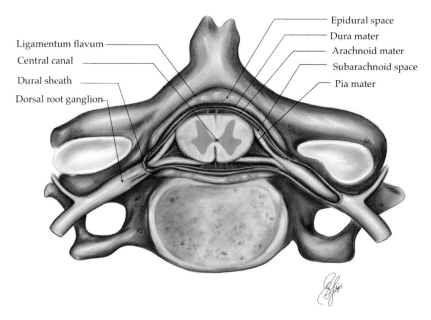

Figure 4.7   Epidural space – boundaries.

What is the depth of the epidural space in different vertebral levels?

- Lower cervical: 1–2 mm
- Upper thoracic: 3–4 mm
- Mid lumbar: 5–6 mm

What volume of local anaesthetic is required per dermatomal level?

As a rule of thumb, around 1–2 ml of local anaesthetic covers one dermatome. Epidural produces a segmental block and hence it should be sited close to the spinal level associated with the dermatomes. In a patient needing a sensory block between T6 and L1 (seven dermatomes) the epidural should be sited at least roughly in the middle (around T9–T10) and a volume of 7–14 ml would be the volume needed for successful block.

Like the volume governing the block height, the density or grade of motor block is governed by the concentration of the local anaesthetic. Adrenaline 100 mcg for an epidural top up with 20 ml of local anaesthetic (1/200,000), increases the duration of the block by decreasing systemic uptake due to local vasoconstriction.

How does spinally injected drug spread to give the desired block height?

- By displacement of CSF
- Interplay with the LA-CSF density and gravity

What factors determine the block height in spinal anaesthesia?

Table 4.3   Factors Determining the Block Height in Spinal Anaesthesia

Patient factors	• Age • CSF volume • Pregnancy • Height
Drug factors	• Baricity • Dose (volume × concentration) • Temperature
Procedure factors	• Patient position • Type of needle • Vertebral level of injection • Epidural after spinal

Patient factors

Age: older patients tend to have a higher block. This could be because of decrease in CSF volume, increase in specific gravity and increased sensitivity to local anaesthetic.

CSF volume: affects duration to peak block height and regression of sensory and motor block

Pregnancy: increased intraabdominal pressure leading to engorged epidural veins along with increased epidural fat may decrease the CSF volume and therefore increase the spread of local anaesthetic and block height.

Drug factors

Baricity: is one of the main determinants. Administration of hyperbaric local anaesthetic to patients in the lateral decubitus position will result in a preferential anaesthetic effect on the dependent side, with hyperbaric solutions 'sinking' and hypobaric solutions 'floating'. Hyperbaric solutions also produce a more reliable block with a more predictable maximal block height than isobaric solutions. It is also assumed that isobaric solutions give a prolonged sacral sensory and motor block.

Dose: most studies show that it is the *dose* rather than the *volume* of local anaesthetic injected into the subarachnoid space that determines block spread.

Temperature: increased temperature of the drug decreases its density rendering it more hypobaric.

Procedural factors

Patient position: as discussed above in relation to the relative baricity of the CSF and the drug solution used, hyperbaric solutions will 'sink' to the lowest portion, e.g. caudal in the sitting position or to the dependent side in the lateral position. It should not truly affect the spread of isobaric drug.

Needle type and position: cephalad alignment of the orifice of Whitacre needles have shown to produce greater spread in hypobaric but not hyperbaric solution.

Vertebral level of injection: a higher vertebral level of injection causes a higher spread of block using hypobaric solutions, but this is less consistent with hyperbaric solutions.

Epidural after spinal: epidural volume expansion (EVE) with saline or local anaesthetic can increase the spread.

(Injection rate and barbotage have not consistently been shown to affect block height.)

How does local anaesthetic injected into the epidural space exert an anaesthetic effect? What factors determine the block height in epidural anaesthesia?

Local anaesthetic injected into the epidural space spreads to intervertebral foramina to the dural cuff, and via the arachnoid villi into the CSF. The drug then blocks the mixed spinal nerves and the dorsal root ganglia. In theory, with an adequate volume the drug can spread to the foramen magnum and sacral foramina. It is important to note that the epidural veins absorb a significant amount of local anaesthetic with blood concentrations reaching a peak in 10–30 minutes (Table 4.4).

Table 4.4   Factors Determining the Block Height in Epidural Anaesthesia

• Volume of local anaesthetic
• Height of the patient
• Age
• Gravity

Volume: as discussed earlier. General rule is 1–2 ml per dermatome

Height: shorter patients need smaller volume

Age: smaller volume is required in increasing age to attain the same height of block. This could be attributed to the changing compliance and volume of the epidural space

Gravity: position of patient does affect spread and height of local anaesthetic although not to the extent of spinal anaesthesia

Bibliography

Ellis, H., & Mahadevan, V. (2018). *Clinical Anatomy: Applied Anatomy for Students and Junior Doctors*. Wiley-Blackwell.

White, J., & Seiden, D. (2017). *USMLE Step 1 Lecture Notes 2017*. New York, NY: Kaplan Medical.

Sacrum and Caudal Block

Sacrum (Latin for 'sacred') is believed to have played a key part in ancient pagan sacrificial rites and it was also thought to be the last bone of the body to decay and that the body will resurrect around it.

It is a triangular bone formed by the fusion of the five sacral vertebrae which is present at the lower end of the vertebral column connecting the lumbar and the coccygeal vertebrae.

On the posterior surface, the first three spinous processes fuse to form the median crest. The lamina of S4 and S5 fail to fuse giving rise the exposed dorsal surface called the sacral hiatus (Figure 4.8).

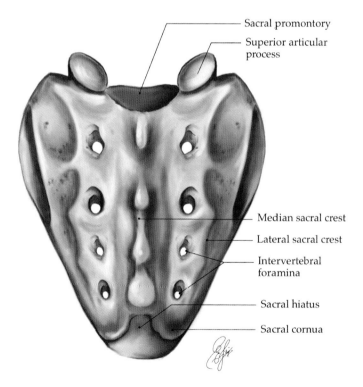

Figure 4.8   Sacrum – structure.

The *sacral canal* is a prismatic cavity which is the continuation of the lumbar spinal canal and terminates at the sacral hiatus (Figures 4.9 and 4.10).

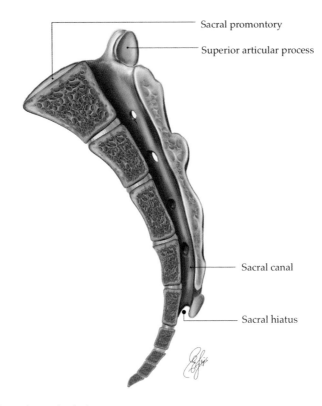

Figure 4.9   Sacral canal – sagittal view.

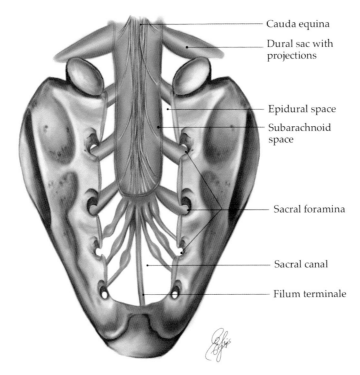

Figure 4.10   Sacral canal – boundaries.

Contents of the sacral canal

- The terminal part of the dural sac, ending between S1 and S3
- The five sacral nerves and coccygeal nerves making up the cauda equina
- Sacral epidural vessels
- Filum terminale – the final part of the spinal cord, which does not contain nerves
- Epidural fat – loose in children and fibrosed close-meshed texture in adults
- Lymphatics

The *sacral hiatus* or *caudal space* is part of sacral canal, below the attachment of dural sheath at S2 and is covered by the sacrococcygeal membrane. It is bounded above by the fused laminae of S4, laterally by the margins of the deficient laminae of S5, anteriorly by the posterior surface of the body of S5, and covered posteriorly by the dense sacrococcygeal ligament (formed from supraspinous ligament, interspinous ligament and ligamentum flavum). It is about 5 cm above the tip of the coccyx.

Four pairs of anterior and posterior sacral foramina are present lateral to the median crest and the sacral hiatus. The anterior sacral foramina transmit anterior primary rami of the sacral nerves and the posterior sacral foramina give passage to posterior primary rami.

Contents of caudal space

Fat, venous plexus, filum terminale and coccygeal nerves

What is the volume of sacral canal and caudal space in adults?

According to the morphometric and MRI studies in adults, the volume of

- Sacral canal ~35 ml
- Caudal space ~14.4 ml

How would you perform a caudal block?

Preparation: informed consent, intravenous access, monitoring, resuscitation equipment and equipment needed for the block

Full asepsis: similar to any central neuraxial block

Personnel: trained anaesthetist and skilled assistant

Calculation: calculate the local anaesthetic dose using the Armitage regimen

Drug: 0.25% L-bupivacaine

Dose:
- Lumbosacral block (e.g. circumcision): 0.5 ml/kg
- Thoraco-lumbar block (e.g. inguinal hernia): 1 ml/kg
- Midthoracic block : 1.25 ml/kg

Position: the lateral position is chosen in paediatric patients because it permits easy access to the airway when general anaesthesia has been administered. Prone position is preferable in adults, as the caudal space is made more prominent by internal rotation of the ankles.

Landmarks: locate the sacral hiatus.

The sacral hiatus forms the apex of an equilateral triangle drawn joining posterior superior iliac spines. When the curve of the sacrum is followed in the midline with the tip of the finger from the tip of the coccyx, the sacral hiatus is felt as a depression.

Procedure: a 22G short bevelled cannula is inserted at 45 degrees until a 'click' is felt, indicating the sacrococcygeal ligament has been pierced. Then the needle is directed cephalad at the angle approaching the long axis of sacral canal. Careful aspiration for blood or CSF should be performed before injection of local anaesthetic although negative aspiration does not always exclude intravascular or intrathecal placement. For this reason, many anaesthetists prefer to leave the cannula in place whilst the drugs are being drawn, thus giving adequate time for the passive flow of CSF/blood with any inadvertent puncture. After confirming position, drugs are injected slowly.

Test to confirm: introduction of small amounts of air would produce subcutaneous emphysema if the needle were superficial. A 'whoosh' sound is heard when a stethoscope is placed further up the lumbar spine in successful blocks.

Use of ultrasound and performing the block under x-ray guidance with radiocontrast dye are the other methods.

What are the additive drugs that can be used along with the local anaesthetics whilst performing a caudal block?

Preservative-free additives are used to prolong the duration of analgesia, improve the quality of the block and reduce the unwanted side effects.

Opioids – fentanyl, morphine and diamorphine: injection of opioids enables provision of analgesia due to a local action of the opioid at the spinal cord level rather than due to systemic absorption. It increases the duration of the block by up to 24 hours, but at the expense of nausea, pruritus, urinary retention and late respiratory depression.

The use of opioids has been replaced by clonidine and ketamine as they significantly prolong the duration of 'single-shot' caudal injections with minimal risk of side effects. The addition of clonidine to plain bupivacaine 0.25% can extend the duration of postoperative analgesia by 4 h, whereas ketamine and bupivacaine can provide analgesia for up to 12 h. The main side effects of epidurally administered clonidine are hypotension, bradycardia and sedation.

Clonidine (1–2 mcg/kg): α2 adrenoceptor agonist. It acts by stimulating the descending noradrenergic medullospinal pathway, thereby inhibiting the release of nociceptive neurotransmitters in the dorsal horn of spinal cord.

S(+) ketamine (0.5–1 mg/kg): NMDA receptor antagonist that binds to a subset of glutamate receptor and decreases the activity of dorsal horn neurons.

What are the complications of this block?

Serious or catastrophic complications are rare and can be related to the procedure or the drug injected.

Complications with the needle

- Subcutaneous injection
- Dural puncture – resulting in total spinal block if not recognised

- Intravenous or intraosseous injection – seizures and cardiac arrest
- Rectal perforation
- Haematoma

Complications with the drug/procedure

- Absent/patchy block
- Hypotension
- Urinary retention
- Sepsis

What are the differences in the anatomy of the caudal epidural space between adults and children?

Adults	Children
Dura ends at S2	Dura ends at S4 at birth
Presence of sacral fat pad makes it difficult to feel hiatus	No fat and thus easy anatomy
Epidural fat is dense, making it difficult to achieve a high block	Epidural fat is loose, so drug spreads well
Sympathetic blockade causes pronounced hypotension	Delay in autonomic maturation, so there is cardiovascular stability

Bibliography

Asghar, A., & Naaz, S. (2013). The volume of the caudal space and sacral canal in human sacrum. *Journal of Clinical and Diagnostic Research: JCDR, 7*(12), 2659.

Krishnachetty, B., & Sethi, D. (2016). *The Final FRCA Structured Oral Examination: a complete guide.* Boca Raton, FL: CRC Press, Taylor & Francis Group.

Neuroanatomy - TeachMeAnatomy. (2019). Retrieved 24 August 2019 from https://teachmeanatomy.info/neuroanatomy/.

Sacrum. (2019). Retrieved 24 August 2019 from www.kenhub.com/en/library/anatomy/sacrum.

Paravertebral Block

Most paravertebral blocks are performed at a thoracic level. The thoracic paravertebral space extends from T1 cranially to T12 caudally.

Boundaries of paravertebral space (Figure 4.11)

- Apex (laterally): posterior intercostal membrane and intercostal space
- Base (medially): vertebral body, intervertebral disc and the vertebral foramen with its corresponding spinal nerve
- Anterior: parietal and visceral pleura and lung parenchyma
- Posterior: transverse processes of the vertebrae, heads of ribs and costotransverse ligament

The paravertebral space communicates with epidural space through the intervertebral foramina medially and intercostal spaces laterally.

Contents

Endothoracic fascia divides the thoracic paravertebral space into an anterior subserous compartment and a posterior subendothoracic compartment.

- Neural tissue surrounded loosely by areolar and adipose tissue
- Spinal nerves: with white and grey rami communicantes
- Sympathetic chain: lies at the neck of the rib anterior to the intercostal neurovascular bundle

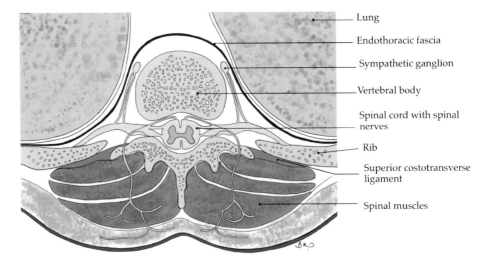

Figure 4.11 Paravertebral space – boundaries and contents.

What are the indications for a paravertebral block (PVB)?

- Acute pain
  - Surgical pain
    - Unilateral thoracic surgery – open thoracotomy, VATS, cardiac and breast surgery
    - Unilateral abdominal surgery – renal surgery and open cholecystectomy
  - Nonsurgical pain
    - Rib fracture
- Chronic pain
  - Post-herpetic neuralgia
  - Post-surgical chronic pain
  - Relief of cancer pain (e.g. mesothelioma or deposits)
- Miscellaneous
  - Control of hyperhidrosis

What are the contraindications to a PVB?

- General
  - Patient refusal
  - Local sepsis
  - Severe coagulopathy
  - Allergy to local anaesthetic drugs
- Block-specific
  - Severe respiratory disease
  - Ipsilateral diaphragmatic paresis
  - Severe spinal deformity

What are the complications of PVB?

- Adequacy of the block
  - Failure up to 5%
- Damage to surrounding structures
  - Parietal pleural puncture – intrapleural block
  - Parietal and visceral pleural puncture – pneumothorax
  - Vascular puncture – bleeding, haemothorax, local anaesthetic toxicity
  - Epidural placement
  - Dural puncture – high spinal, PDPH
- Extension of the block
  - Bilateral block – 10%
  - Stellate ganglion block (hoarseness) in high-thoracic PVB

How would you perform a paravertebral block?

Ascertain the extent of surgical procedure by discussion with the surgeon regarding the planned approach and extent of surgery to elucidate the dermatomal distribution of the incision.

As a rough guide

1. VATS procedures: T3 to T8, depending on the site of operation
2. Muscle-sparing thoracotomy: the incision is about 5–7 cm long extending vertically from T2 to T9
3. Posterolateral thoracotomy: the incision spans over at least six dermatomal levels – T3 posteriorly to T8 anteriorly, with chest drains placed at 8th/9th intercostal space
4. Total mastectomy: requires blockade extending from T1 to T6 level

Choosing the type of block – single or multiple injections.

If anaesthesia of several dermatomes is required a small volume, multiple injection technique is recommended. For example, to block T3 to T8, three injections at T3, T5 and T7 are done with 8–10 ml of local anaesthetic at each level.

Prerequisites

Consent, intravenous access, non-invasive monitoring, presence of full resuscitation facilities and trained assistant.

Procedure

The experience and local policy guide the choice of technique – landmark, nerve stimulator or ultrasound guided block.

The patient is positioned in the sitting or lateral decubitus position (with the side to be blocked uppermost) and supported by an assistant. To block T3 to T8, the skin is marked at tips of the spinous processes and at points 2.5 cm lateral to these. The parasagittal points correspond with appropriate transverse processes.

Following strict aseptic precautions, the site of injection is infiltrated with 2% lignocaine. An 18G graduated epidural needle is advanced perpendicular to the skin, until contact with the transverse process is established. A loss of resistance (LoR) syringe with saline is attached to the needle, and while continuously testing for LoR, the needle is 'walked off' the structure in a caudad and lateral direction and advanced approximately 1 cm (to a maximum of 1.5 cm).

As the costotransverse ligament is penetrated, a 'pop' is felt as the needle enters the paravertebral space. This is aptly called a 'change of resistance' rather than 'loss of resistance', as the complete LoR is experienced when the needle punctures the pleura and the saline is injected intrapleurally.

After careful aspiration to confirm that the needle tip is not intravascular or intrathecal, the predetermined dose of local anaesthetic should be administered.

What are the advantages of paravertebral block over epidural block?

PVB provides analgesia comparable to an epidural without many of the side effects. The block is equivalent to epidural in terms of success rate, postoperative pain scores and analgesic efficacy and provides better analgesia compared to intrapleural block.

- Procedure
  - Easy to teach, learn and perform
  - Can be done in anaesthetised patients
- Side effects
  - Decreased neurological complications: post-dural puncture headache, radicular pain, paraplegia and peripheral nerve lesions
  - Decreased side effects: less sedation, nausea and vomiting, as PVB is dependent on the use of local anaesthetics only
  - Decreased cardiovascular side effects: severe hypotension is rare because of the unilateral blockade
  - Decreased or no incidence of urinary retention
  - Lack of motor blockade of the lower extremities
  - Better preservation of pulmonary function
- Effects similar to epidural block
  - Inhibition of chronic pain by preventing sensitisation of the CNS by blocking the 'sensory flow'
  - Prevention of cardiopulmonary complications and decreased perioperative morbidity

Clinical questions...

1. What is a bronchopleural fistula and the anaesthetic management?
2. What are the analgesic options in corrective BPF surgery?

Bibliography

Krishnachetty, B., & Sethi, D. (2017). *The Final FRCA Structured Oral Examination: A Complete Guide.* CRC Press: Boca Raton, FL.

Tighe, S. Q. M., Greene, M. D., & Rajadurai, N. (2010). Paravertebral block. *Continuing Education in Anaesthesia Criticale Care and Pain, 10*(5), 133–137.

UPPER LIMB

5

Structures

- Antecubital fossa

Circulation

- Arterial supply
- Venous drainage

Nervous System

- Dermatomes and peripheral nerves
- Brachial plexus
- Blocks
  - Interscalene block
  - Supra and infraclavicular block
  - Axillary block
  - Median, radial and ulnar nerve blocks

Structures

- Antecubital fossa

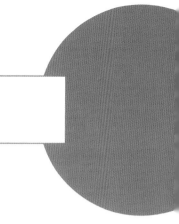

Antecubital Fossa

The cubital (antecubital) fossa is a triangular depression anterior to the elbow joint.

Boundaries

- Lateral – medial border of brachioradialis muscle
- Medial – lateral border of pronator teres muscle
- Base – imaginary horizontal line between the medial and lateral epicondyles of the humerus
- Apex – meeting point of the medial and lateral borders (brachioradialis overlaps with pronator teres)
- Floor – brachialis in the upper part and supinator in the lower part of the fossa
- Roof – superficial to deep – skin, superficial fascia and deep fascia which is reinforced by the bicipital aponeurosis

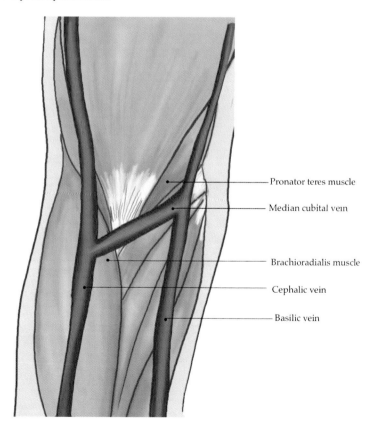

Figure 5.1   Anterior cubital fossa – superficial structures.

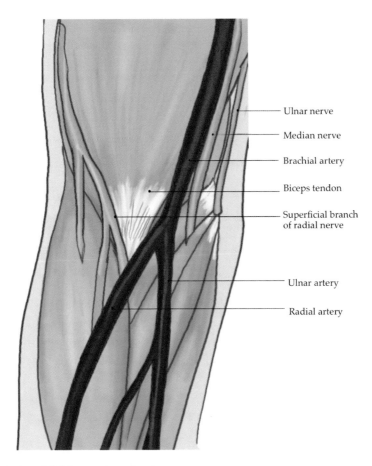

Figure 5.2   Anterior cubital fossa – deep structures.

Contents

- Biceps tendon
- Brachial artery
- Median and radial nerves
- Median cubital, cephalic and basilic veins (considered to be superficial to the fossa)

The contents of cubital fossa from the **medial to lateral** side are easily recalled by the mnemonic MBBS (Figures 5.1 and 5.2).

(M = Median nerve, B = Brachial artery, B = Biceps tendon, S = Superficial radial nerve)

Describe the course of brachial artery in the antecubital fossa.

The brachial artery normally bifurcates into radial and ulnar arteries in the apex of the fossa, although this bifurcation may occur much higher in the arm due to anatomical variation.

Which vein would you choose for the insertion of a long line at the antecubital fossa? Where might the line 'stick' and how would you negotiate it?

When placing a long line, the two main veins available in the antecubital fossa are the basilic and cephalic veins. The more medial basilic vein has a smoother and direct route to the subclavian vein. The lateral cephalic vein turns more sharply and passes through the clavipectoral fascia with valves present at its termination. These factors increase the risk of the long line not advancing into the subclavian vein when using the cephalic vein. If problems occur with advancing the line, abducting the arm to help straighten out its path might be useful. Flushing the line with saline can also help to advance a line through a valve that may be obstructing its passage.

Bibliography

Sinnatamby, C. S. (2011). *Last's Anatomy, International Edition: Regional and Applied.* Elsevier Health Sciences.

Circulation

- Arterial supply
- Venous drainage

Arterial Supply of Upper Limb

Can you describe the arterial supply to the upper limb, starting at the aorta?

The subclavian artery originates from the aorta on the left and the brachiocephalic artery on the right. The subclavian artery becomes the axillary artery which then continues as the brachial artery. The brachial artery divides into the radial and ulnar artery at the antecubital fossa between the two heads of the biceps (Figure 5.3 and Table 5.1).

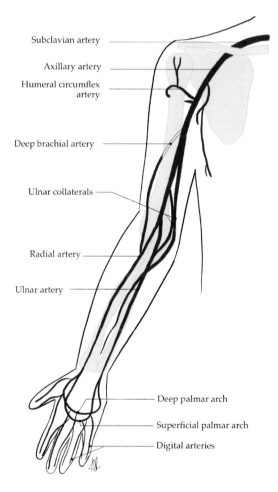

Figure 5.3   Arterial supply – upper limb.

Table 5.1   Arterial Supply of Upper Limb

Axillary artery
Course: formed at the lateral border of the first rib as a continuation of subclavian artery. It is deep to the pectoralis minor and has the cords of brachial plexus around it. It continues as the brachial artery at the lower border of the teres major muscle.
Supply: shoulder, scapula, axilla, lateral thoracic wall and associated muscles
Brachial artery
Course: begins at the lateral border of axilla and runs medial to the biceps muscle towards the antecubital fossa where it bifurcates into the terminal branches – radial and ulnar arteries
Supply: humerus, elbow and muscles of the arm
Radial artery
Course: descends from the antecubital fossa to the wrist along the lateral side of the forearm between the flexor carpi radialis and the brachialis. It crosses the anatomical snuff box on the dorsal aspect and enters the palm of the hand terminating as the deep palmar arch.
Supply: elbow, muscles of the forearm and hand
Ulnar artery
Course: the ulnar artery descends along the medial side of the forearm alongside the ulnar nerve which lies lateral to it. It travels above the flexor retinaculum at the wrist and sends a branch to the deep palmar arch and terminates as the superficial palmar arch.
Supply: elbow, muscles of the forearm and hand

What are the indications for an arterial cannula?

Blood pressure monitoring

- Patients with haemodynamic instability (critically ill or undergoing major surgery)
- Patients requiring vasoactive drugs
- Patients with burns, arrhythmia and obesity causing inaccurate non-invasive blood pressure monitoring

Blood sampling

- Frequent blood gas measurements in intensive care patients
- Regular electrolyte monitoring and in patients with difficult venous access

Interventional procedure

- Endovascular procedures, coronary angiography, intra-aortic balloon insertion
- Arterial embolisation

Continuous cardiac output monitoring

- In critically ill patients
- In major surgery, to optimise fluid therapy

What might the contraindications be?

Absolute contraindications

- Absence of collateral circulation (e.g. abnormal modified Allen's test)
- Vasculitis – Raynaud's disease, Buerger's disease
- Local vessel pathology – distorted anatomy, aneurysm, stent or vascular graft, arteriovenous malformation or fistula

Relative contraindications

- Severe peripheral vascular disease
- Recent use of thrombolytic agents
- Severe coagulopathy

Which sites in the upper limb do you use for arterial cannulation? What are the site-specific disadvantages?

The *radial artery* is commonly used as it has a fairly reliable anatomy, is easily palpated and visible with ultrasound guidance. However, it is more prone to occlusion and haematoma formation.

The *brachial* or *axillary artery* is often used in paediatric/neonatal ICU but there is significant risk of distal ischaemia and compartment syndrome if there is an arterial occlusion due to the absence of collateral circulation.

The *ulnar artery* is not routinely used in anaesthetics and there is a risk of ulnar nerve injury due to its close proximity.

How would you site a radial arterial cannula?

- Preprocedure ultrasound is useful to identify the course, presence of tortuosity and atheroma.
- Aseptic precautions
- Cannulation can be done using either 'over the needle' or 'over the wire' technique using modified Seldinger technique
- Ensuring connecting line is flushed to prevent accidental air embolus
- Securing and labelling the line once inserted to prevent accidental use of the line to administer drugs

What are the possible complications?

- Pain and swelling
- Accidental dislodgement
- Thrombotic complications with cerebral embolisation
- Nerve damage

- Limb ischemia
- Haematoma, haemorrhage
- Infection
- Formation of pseudoaneurysm and AV fistula

What is Allen's test? How is it performed?

Allen's test is a non-invasive evaluation of the arterial patency of the hand which assesses the collateral arterial blood flow. It is done prior to any radial arterial intervention (radial artery harvesting for coronary artery bypass grafting or for forearm flap elevation) or diagnostic work up for thoracic outlet syndrome.

The aim is to check the adequacy of blood flow from the ulnar artery in the event of radial artery occlusion following the procedure.

The original Allen's test tests both hands at the same time. A modified Allen's test is currently used which tests one hand at a time.

1. Elevate the hand and make a tight fist for 30 seconds
2. Occlude the ulnar and radial arteries
3. Unclench the fist which should appear pale
4. Release the ulnar pressure while maintaining radial pressure
5. Note the time to reperfusion

In a negative (normal) Allen's test, the hand will flush in 5–15 seconds indicating that the ulnar artery has a good flow.

In a positive (abnormal, *positive = persistent pallor*) Allen's test, the time to reperfusion is >15 seconds suggesting that the ulnar circulation is inadequate, in which case, the radial artery should not be cannulated.

What is Volkmann's ischaemic contracture?

The permanent contraction of the flexor compartment at the level of the wrist due to obstruction of the brachial artery is called Volkmann's ischaemic contracture. The claw-like deformity occurs due to ischaemia and necrosis of the flexor digitorum profundus and the flexor pollicis longus.

Causes include supracondylar fractures, prolonged upper arm tourniquet time, compression from a plaster cast, compartment syndrome and accidental intra-arterial injection of drugs.

What is the management of inadvertent intra-arterial injection?

Intra-arterial injection of drugs may cause acute, severe extremity ischaemia and gangrene and the main priority is to maintain distal perfusion.

The drugs which cause the most severe ischaemia and tissue death are barbiturates, ketamine and phenytoin, whilst propofol, atracurium, rocuronium and amiodarone can also cause ischaemia.

The steps in the pathophysiology are arterial spasm, direct tissue destruction by the drug and subsequent chemical arteritis leading to endothelial destruction. With certain drugs such as thiopentone, precipitation and crystal formation within the distal microcirculation lead to ischaemia and thrombosis.

Management

General measures

- Assessment of extent of the injury and early plastic surgery advice
- Elevation of affected limb to improve venous and lymphatic drainage
- Good analgesia
- Anticoagulation with heparin to limit the extent of the ischaemia as thrombosis is ultimately the cause of the tissue injury

Specific measures

- Local anaesthetic injection

  Intra-arterial injection of lignocaine through the implicated cannula may be useful in preventing reflex vasospasm. But this can cause further damage and compromise the perfusion to the affected limb.
- Sympatholysis

  Stellate ganglion blocks and lower-extremity sympathetic blocks can produce arterial and venous vasodilatation which can also be a good mode of analgesia but should be done after risk-benefit analysis.
- Other drugs

  Calcium channel blockers, thromboxane inhibitors (aspirin and methylprednisolone), prostacyclin analogues, intra-arterial papaverine have been used for their vasodilatory and platelet-inhibiting properties to varying success.

Venous Drainage of Upper Limb

The venous drainage of the upper limb can be divided into the superficial and the deep system. The superficial venous system lies in the subcutaneous tissue and drains into the deep venous system via perforating veins.

Superficial venous system

- The dorsum of the hand displays the dorsal venous network which drain into the cephalic and basilic veins on the lateral and medial side, respectively.
- The cephalic vein ascends on the lateral side of the forearm and arm and it passes through the deltopectoral groove in the shoulder before emptying into the axillary vein.
- The basilic vein runs posteromedially to pass anterior to the medial epicondyle of the humerus. In the arm, it pierces the brachial fascia and joins the paired deep brachial veins to form the axillary vein.
- The median cubital vein connects the cephalic and basilic veins anterior to the cubital fossa.

Deep venous system

- The deep veins of the upper limb lie underneath the deep fascia. Distally, paired veins lie on either side of the artery but as they continue proximally, the paired vessels merge to form a single vein.
- The axillary vein drains the shoulder, arm, forearm, hand and lateral chest wall.
- The subclavian vein, the continuation of the axillary vein, also receives the venous drainage from the scapular region and joins the internal jugular vein to ultimately form the brachiocephalic vein (Figure 5.4).

When attempting venepuncture at the antecubital fossa, which structure in particular provides a degree of protection to the brachial artery?

The bicipital aponeurosis separates the brachial artery (which lies beneath the aponeurosis) from median cubital vein thereby preventing inadvertent arterial puncture during median cubital vein cannulation.

Which superficial nerves are at risk during attempted venous cannulation at the elbow?

Medial, lateral and posterior cutaneous nerves of the forearm.

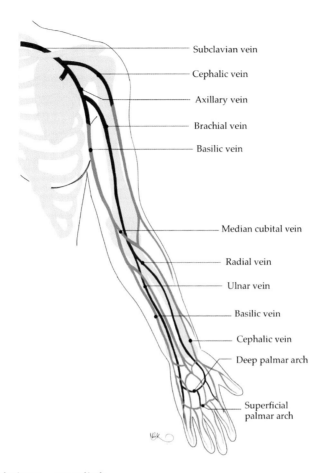

Figure 5.4   Venous drainage – upper limb.

How can the veins of the upper limb be used to provide central venous access?

Peripherally inserted central catheters (PICC) can be inserted into the upper limb using the Seldinger technique via a needle. The catheter passes through the skin and into the superior vena cava. It can be placed under ultrasound guidance or with a contrast venogram. It is an excellent method of providing medium-term venous access (e.g. feeding lines in paediatrics, long-term intravenous antibiotics).

Bibliography

Gilroy, A. M., Voll, M. M., & Wesker, K. (2017). *Anatomy: An Essential Textbook.* New York, NY: Thieme Medical Publishers, Inc.

Irwin, R. S., & Rippe, J. M. (2011). *Irwin and Rippes Intensive Care Medicine.* Philadelphia, PA: Wolters Kluwer/Lippincott Williams & Wilkins Health.

Lake, C., & Beecroft, C. L. (2010). Extravasation injuries and accidental intra-arterial injection. *Continuing Education in Anaesthesia, Critical Care & Pain, 10*(4), 109–113.

Nervous System

- Dermatomes and nerve distribution
- Brachial plexus
- Blocks
  - Interscalene block
  - Supra and infraclavicular block
  - Axillary block
  - Median, radial and ulnar nerve blocks

The upper limb is divided into the shoulder, arm (between shoulder and elbow), forearm (between elbow and wrist) and hand. The axilla, cubital fossa and carpal tunnel are important areas of transition in the upper limb.

Figures 5.5 and 5.6 show the dermatomal and peripheral nerve distribution of the anterior and posterior aspects of the upper limb.

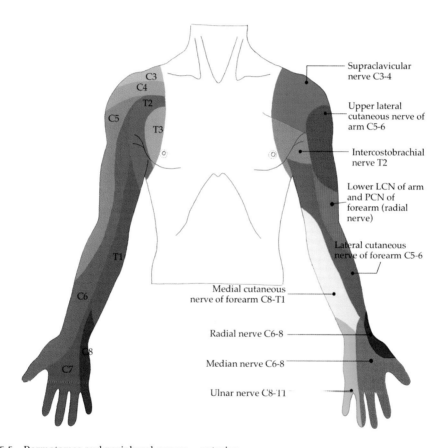

Figure 5.5   Dermatomes and peripheral nerves – anterior.

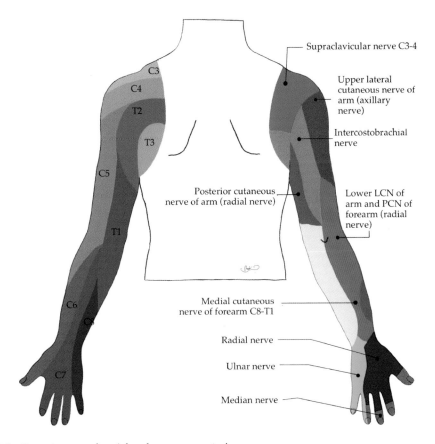

Figure 5.6   Dermatomes and peripheral nerves – posterior.

What movements are provided by the myotomes of the upper limb?

C5 – abduction of the arm at the glenohumeral joint

C6 – flexion of the forearm at the elbow joint

C7 – extension of the arm at the elbow joint

C8 – flexion of the fingers

T1 – abduction and adduction of the index, middle and ring fingers

Brachial Plexus

A complex neural network in the neck and axilla that starts from the intervertebral foramina, passes between scalenus anterior and medius, into the posterior triangle of the neck, behind the clavicle, over the first rib, posterolateral to the subclavian artery and into the axilla. The major nerves of the brachial plexus carry motor and sensory function and it is important to note that the sensory distribution from the peripheral nerves is different from the dermatomes (Table 5.2).

Table 5.2 Functional Importance of Brachial Plexus

Sensory innervation of the upper limb and most of the axilla – except for an area in the medial upper arm supplied by the intercostobrachial nerve. This is often the origin of tourniquet pain.
Motor innervation to the upper limb and shoulder girdle – except for trapezius, which is innervated by the 11th cranial nerve
Autonomic innervation to the upper limb, by communicating with the stellate ganglion at T1

Course of the brachial plexus through the neck, demonstrating its relations to the scalene muscles, subclavian artery and clavicle (Figure 5.7).

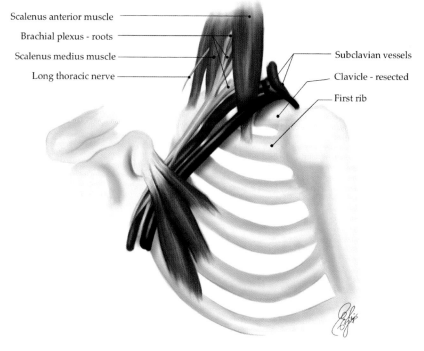

Figure 5.7 Brachial plexus – relations.

The brachial plexus is divided into Roots – Trunks – Divisions – Cords – Branches.

This can be remembered using the mnemonic Read – That – Damn – Cadaver – Book (Figure 5.8 and Table 5.3).

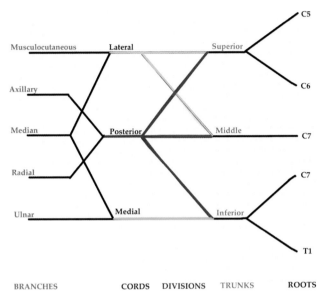

Figure 5.8   Brachial plexus – schematic diagram.

Table 5.3   Origin and Course of the Brachial Plexus

Roots
The brachial plexus is formed by the ventral rami of C5 to T1 nerve roots. The C5, C6, C7 roots lie 1–3 cm below the skin in the interscalene groove, between the scalenus anterior and scalenus medius muscles in the posterior triangle of the neck. The C7 root is deep to C6 and in close proximity to the vertebral artery, which puts the artery at risk of inadvertent puncture during an interscalene block.
Trunks
The roots combine between scalenus anterior and medius, forming three trunks which cross the base of the posterior triangle of the neck, where they can be found behind the subclavian artery. The trunks are so named according to their anatomical location. C5 and C6 combine to form the superior trunk, C7 continues to form the middle trunk and C8 and T1 combine to form the inferior trunk.
Divisions
Behind the middle third of the clavicle, each trunk divides into anterior and posterior divisions. They pass behind the clavicle and into the axilla.
Cords
The three cords are labelled lateral, posterior and medial according to their position around the axillary artery. Lateral cord – receives the anterior divisions from the superior and middle trunk Posterior cord – receives the posterior divisions from all three trunks Medial cord – receives the anterior division from the inferior trunk
Branches
The terminal branches are discussed below.

Figure 5.8 demonstrates a schematic representation of the brachial plexus that you should learn and be able to reproduce in the exam.

Viva and OSCE questions have been asked on the specifics of this without a diagram to refer to, so intimate knowledge is required. Alternatively, you may be shown a diagram of the brachial plexus and be asked to explain it. It will likely look like the one below so you should make sure you are familiar with this too (Figure 5.9).

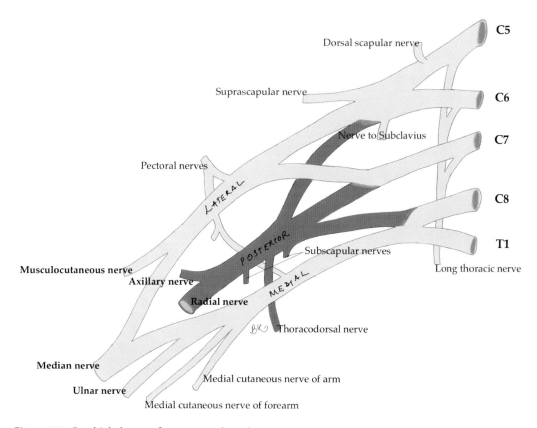

Figure 5.9   Brachial plexus – from roots to branches.

Mnemonics for the terminal branches of the cords

Medial cord – MMUMM

- ○ Median nerve
- ○ Medial pectoral nerve
- ○ Ulnar nerve
- ○ Medial cutaneous nerve of arm
- ○ Medial cutaneous nerve of forearm

Posterior cord – SSTAR

- ○ Subscapular nerve (upper)

- ○ Subscapular nerve (lower)
- ○ Thoracodorsal nerve
- ○ Axillary nerve
- ○ Radial nerve

Lateral cord – DLMM

- ○ Dorsal scapular nerve
- ○ Lateral pectoral nerve
- ○ Median nerve
- ○ Musculocutaneous nerve

What do the nerves of the brachial plexus innervate?

Table 5.4 Branches of the Brachial Plexus and Their Function

Nerve	Motor innervation	Movement	Sensory innervation
From the roots			
Long thoracic nerve	Serratus anterior	Protraction of scapula	n/a
From the lateral cord (LDMM)			
Lateral pectoral nerve	Pectoralis major	Contraction of pectoralis	n/a
Dorsal scapular nerve	Rhomboid major and minor, levator scapulae	Adduction and rotation of shoulder, elevation of scapula	n/a
Musculocutaneous nerve	Coracobrachialis, biceps brachii, brachialis	Flexion of elbow	Skin over lateral side of forearm (via lateral cutaneous nerve of the forearm)
Median nerve	All muscles in anterior compartment of the forearm **except** flexor carpi ulnaris and the medial two parts of flexor digitorum profundus, i.e. pronator teres, flexor carpi radialis, palmaris longus, flexor digitorum superficialis, the lateral two parts of flexor digitorum profundus, flexor pollicis longus and pronator quadratus. Also LOAF muscles of the hand – lateral two lumbricals, opponens pollicis, abductor pollicis brevis, flexor pollicis brevis	Flexion of first three-and-a-half fingers, opposition of thumb	Skin over radial half of palm and palmar side of radial three-and-a-half digits
From the posterior cord (SSTAR)			
Upper subscapular nerve	Subscapularis	Medial rotation of arm	n/a
Lower subscapular nerve	Subscapularis, teres major	Internal rotation, adduction of shoulder	n/a

(Continued)

Table 5.4 (Continued)   Branches of the Brachial Plexus and Their Function

Nerve	Motor innervation	Movement	Sensory innervation
Thoraco-dorsal nerve	Latissimus dorsi	Abduction of arm	n/a
Axillary nerve	Deltoid, teres minor	Arm abduction	Skin over regimental patch (via superior lateral cutaneous nerve of arm)
Radial nerve	Triceps, brachioradialis, abductor pollicis longus, extensor muscles of the wrist and fingers (extensor carpi ulnaris, extensor carpi radialis, extensor digitorum, extensor pollicis longus and brevis, extensor indicis, extensor digiti minimi)	Abduction of thumb, extension of wrist and fingers	Skin over posterior arm, forearm and hand
From the medial cord (MMUMM)			
Medial cutaneous nerve of arm	n/a	n/a	Skin over medial side of the arm
Medial cutaneous nerve of forearm	n/a	n/a	Skin over medial side of the forearm
Ulnar nerve	Arm: only two muscles in anterior compartment of the arm – flexor carpi ulnaris, medial two parts of flexor digitorum profundus. Hand: HILA muscles – Hypothenar eminence, Interossei, medial two Lumbricals, Adductor pollicis, i.e. all intrinsic muscles of the hand **except** for LOAF muscles	Flexion of the fourth and fifth fingers and thumb adduction	Skin of medial side of wrist and hand and ulnar one-and-a-half digits
Medial pectoral nerve	Pectoralis minor and major	Contraction of pectoralis	n/a
Median nerve	See above	See above	See above

Terminal Branches

Note that the terminal branches of the brachial plexus are mixed nerves. The branches that exit the brachial plexus high up are *either* sensory *or* motor nerves.

In summary,

Musculocutaneous nerve – all muscles in the anterior compartment of the arm

Median nerve – muscles in anterior compartment of the forearm, except for flexor carpi ulnaris and the medial part of flexor digitorum profundus, which are innervated by the ulnar nerve

Ulnar nerve – most intrinsic muscles of the hand, except for the thenar muscles and two lateral lumbricals, which are innervated by the median nerve

Radial nerve – all muscles in posterior compartment of the arm

What is the path of the terminal branches of the brachial plexus as they travel from the axilla?

Median nerve

In the axilla, the median nerve lies on the biceps side of the axillary artery, usually superficial to the artery. Proximally, the median nerve is lateral to the artery. As it travels down the arm, it traverses the brachial artery to lie medial to it at the antecubital fossa.

The median nerve has no major branches in the arm.

In the forearm, the median nerve lies deep to the superficial flexors, then passes through the carpal tunnel into the hand.

Ulnar nerve

In the axilla, the ulnar nerve lies on the triceps side of the axillary artery, often between the artery and axillary vein, or beneath the axillary vein. As it travels down the arm, it remains superficial, moving away from the artery, and heads to the medial epicondyle of the humerus.

The ulnar nerve has no major branches in the arm.

It passes posteriorly to the medial epicondyle, through the cubital tunnel and into the anterior compartment of the forearm between the two heads of flexor carpi ulnaris. It then runs along the ulnar side of the forearm alongside the ulnar artery to the wrist.

Radial nerve

In the axilla, the radial nerve lies deep to the axillary artery. As it travels down the arm, it dives deep towards the triceps side of the humerus with the profunda brachii artery. It travels between the two heads of the triceps, around the spiral groove of the humerus to the lateral side of the humerus.

The radial nerve has muscular (to triceps, brachioradialis, extensor carpi radialis longus) and cutaneous branches in the arm.

It divides into the superficial radial and deep interosseous nerves before passing into the forearm anterior to the lateral epicondyle of the humerus, just deep to the brachioradialis muscle.

How can you clinically examine the radial, median and ulnar nerves?

Table 5.5a   Clinical Examination of the Ulnar Nerve

Ulnar nerve	
Inspection	Claw hand
Motor	Weakness of abduction and adduction of the fingers • Test for adduction and abduction of fingers by placing a card between the patient's fingers and attempting to pull it out against resistance
Sensory	Altered sensation in the medial one-and-a-half fingers

Table 5.5b   Clinical Examination of the Radial Nerve

Radial nerve	
Inspection	Wrist drop
Motor	Weakness of wrist and finger extensors • Test by resisting wrist and finger extension
Sensory	Altered sensation on dorsum of hand including first web space and posterior aspect of the forearm

Table 5.5c   Clinical Examination of the Median Nerve

Median nerve	
Inspection	Wasting of the thenar eminence
Motor	Weakness of the LOAF muscles • Test for *thumb opposition* by asking the patient to touch thumb and little finger together while you attempt to break them apart • Test for *thumb abduction* by placing the patient's hand palm up on a surface and asking them to lift their thumb vertically against resistance
Sensory	Sensory loss over palmar aspect of the lateral three-and-a-half fingers If carpal tunnel syndrome suspected, the provocation tests may be useful: Tinel's test – tapping over the flexor retinaculum causes tingling in the median nerve distribution Phalen's test – flexion of the wrists in the reverse prayer position may produce tingling in the median nerve distribution

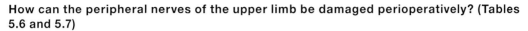

How can the peripheral nerves of the upper limb be damaged perioperatively? (Tables 5.6 and 5.7)

Mechanisms of injury include

- Compression
- Stretch ischaemia
- Direct nerve trauma
- Local anaesthetic toxicity

Table 5.6   Risk Factors for Perioperative Nerve Damage

Patient factors	Hypertension
	Diabetes
	Smoking
	Anatomical abnormalities especially in the thoracic outlet and at the elbow
Perioperative factors	Hypovolaemia
	Dehydration
	Hypotension
	Hypoxia
	Electrolyte disturbances
	Hypothermia
Surgical factors	Neurosurgery
	Cardiac surgery
	Orthopaedic surgery
	Use of tourniquets
Anaesthetic factors	General and regional anaesthesia carry higher risks as patient unable to move position
	Direct trauma in regional anaesthesia
	Poor positioning and padding

Table 5.7   Specific Factors for Upper Limb Nerve Damage

Mechanism of injury	Presentation of injury
Brachial plexus	
• Compression against the clavicle during retraction of a median sternotomy • Compression between the humeral head and the thorax in lateral position • Arm abduction, external rotation	Depending on the level of the plexus injury. • Waiter's tip position – arm adducted, medially rotated and pronated – if high roots injured • Claw hand ulnar nerve injury presentation if lower roots injured
Ulnar nerve	
• Direct pressure on the ulnar groove at the elbow • Prolonged forearm flexion	• Altered sensation in the medial one-and-a-half fingers • Weakness in adduction or abduction of the fingers • Claw hand
Radial nerve	
• Compression by blood pressure cuff or tourniquets • Compression against the arm board	• Altered sensation on dorsum of hand including first web space and posterior aspect forearm • Wrist drop
Median nerve	
• Compression around elbow or carpal tunnel	• Altered sensation on palmar aspect of lateral three-and-a-half fingers • Weakness of abduction and opposition of thumb • Weak wrist flexion

Nerve Blocks

The brachial plexus can be blocked at multiple level which are explained in separate sections.

Even if you are most familiar with using an ultrasound guided technique, exam questions have been asked on landmarks and nerve stimulator technique, so you must be able to discuss both.

Interscalene Approach

Table 5.8 Summary of Interscalene Brachial Plexus Block

Interscalene approach – block at the level of ROOTS	
Sensory block	**Specific complications**
• Shoulder, proximal humerus, lateral two-thirds of clavicle • May miss the ulnar nerve	• Phrenic nerve palsy almost universal (caution in respiratory disease) • Horner's syndrome • Subarachnoid/epidural injection • Vertebral artery injection • Recurrent laryngeal nerve block • Stellate ganglion block

Landmark and nerve stimulator technique

Winnie's approach.

Identify the clavicular head of the sternocleidomastoid muscle. By palpating behind the lateral edge of this muscle, the fingers lie on scalenus anterior.

Palpate the interscalene groove at the level of the cricoid cartilage and inject local anaesthetic between scalenus anterior and medius.

Nerve stimulation elicits motor response in the pectoralis, deltoid, triceps or biceps muscle, or twitches of the hand or forearm.

If the phrenic nerve is stimulated – needle is too anterior.

If the dorsal scapular nerve is stimulated – needle is too posterior.

• Depth 1–2 cm (very superficial)
• Needle 25–50 mm insulated
• LA 20–40 ml

Ultrasound technique

Patient supine, head turned to contralateral side.

Place transducer at level of cricoid cartilage. Identify carotid artery, internal jugular vein and sternocleidomastoid muscle. Move the transducer posteriorly to identify the nerve roots as round hypoechoic structures lying between the scalenus anterior and scalenus medius muscles.

Deposit local anaesthetic deep to the C6 root. If it spreads around C5 and C6 this will be sufficient, if not reposition the needle to achieve spread.

(Continued)

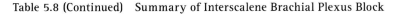

Table 5.8 (Continued)   Summary of Interscalene Brachial Plexus Block

Initially scanning the supraclavicular region to identify the 'bunch of grapes' of the plexus in the supraclavicular region and then moving the transducer up to the interscalene groove to view the 'traffic lights' appearance can be helpful.

Each nerve root is followed as it disappears into its transverse process, each of which has a particular shape to be sure which nerve root you are seeing.

Note the phrenic nerve traverses scalenus anterior and is vulnerable to being blocked by local anaesthetic. Using smaller volumes of 5–7 ml reduces this risk.

- Depth 1–4 cm
- Needle 25–50 mm
- US transverse plane
- Needle in-plane
- LA 15–20 ml

Figure 5.10a shows the probe position with marker for right interscalene brachial plexus block.

Figure 5.10b shows the ultrasound appearance of C5, C6, C7 nerve roots in the interscalene groove between scalenus medius and scalenus anterior.

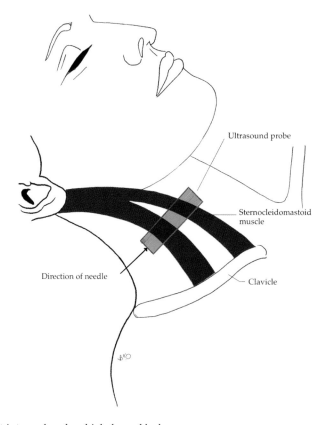

Figure 5.10a   Right interscalene brachial plexus block.

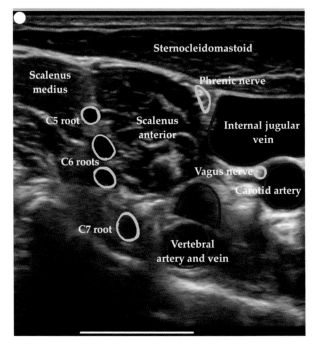

Figure 5.10b   Right interscalene brachial plexus block – ultrasound.

Supraclavicular Approach

Table 5.9 Summary of Supraclavicular Brachial Plexus Block

Supraclavicular approach – block at the level of TRUNKS and DIVISIONS	
Sensory block	**Specific complications**
• Entire arm including shoulder • May miss cutaneous innervation of shoulder	• Pneumothorax • Phrenic nerve palsy • Horner's syndrome • Vertebral artery injection • Recurrent laryngeal nerve block
Landmark and nerve stimulator technique	

Identify the point where the clavicular head of the sternocleidomastoid muscle meets the clavicle. As a safety margin, a point 2.5 cm lateral to this is marked so that the needle insertion point is not medial to it. The needle is inserted one finger's breadth superior to the safety point and directed caudally parallel with the midline.
Nerve stimulation aims to produce muscle twitch in all the fingers.
  • Depth 1–2 cm (very superficial)
  • Needle 25–50 mm insulated
  • LA 20–40 ml	

Ultrasound technique	
Patient supine, arm adducted, hand resting on abdomen, head on pillow folded under to allow enough space for dexterity. Place transducer parallel to clavicle in supraclavicular fossa. Identify the subclavian artery, the plexus posterior and superior to the artery, the first rib and pleura. Maximise the view of the first rib to minimise the chance of pleural puncture. Use colour doppler to check for the presence of blood vessels (the transverse cervical artery can often be seen amongst the plexus at this level). The plexus appears as a hypoechoic 'bunch of grapes'.	

(Continued)

Table 5.9 (Continued)   Summary of Supraclavicular Brachial Plexus Block

Some authors recommend a single injection in the 'corner pocket' between the subclavian artery and first rib – this ensures the inferior trunks and divisions are not spared. Others recommend a multiple injection technique.
- Depth 1–4 cm
- Needle 50 mm
- US coronal oblique plane
- Needle in-plane
- LA 20–40 ml

Figure 5.11a shows the probe position with marker for right supraclavicular brachial plexus block.

Figure 5.11b shows the ultrasound appearance of brachial plexus in supraclavicular fossa, resting on first rib.

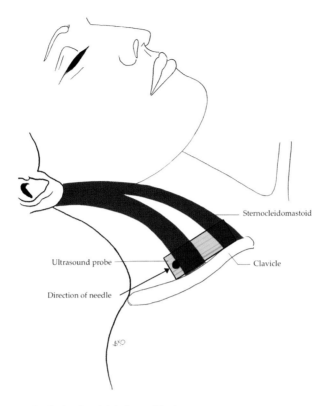

Sternocleidomastoid

Ultrasound probe

Clavicle

Direction of needle

Figure 5.11a   Right supraclavicular brachial plexus block.

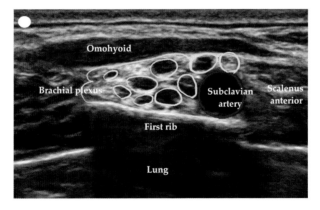

Omohyoid

Brachial plexus

Subclavian
artery

Scalenus
anterior

First rib

Lung

Figure 5.11b   Right supraclavicular brachial plexus block – ultrasound.

Infraclavicular Approach

Table 5.10   Summary of Infraclavicular Brachial Plexus Block

Infraclavicular approach – block at the level of CORDS	
Sensory block	**Specific complications**
• Forearm, wrist, hand	• Pneumothorax • Intravascular injection

Landmark and nerve stimulator technique
Vertical approach. Needle insertion is at the midpoint of a line drawn from the jugular fossa to the acromioclavicular joint, below the clavicle, at 90° to the skin. Aim to elicit muscle twitches below the elbow, ideally wrist or finger extension. If twitches are not detected, sequentially move the needle 10° caudally or cranially – never medially. • Depth 2–5 cm • Needle 50 mm insulated • LA 20–40 ml

Ultrasound technique
Patient supine, arm adducted, hand resting on abdomen. Place transducer underneath and parallel to clavicle. Identify the axillary artery, axillary vein and more deeply, the pleura, all beneath pectoralis major and minor. The cords are seen lateral to the axillary artery as multiple hypoechoic structures, often enclosed in a fascial sheath. Inject local anaesthetic to encircle the artery. Alternatively, a lateral sub-coracoid approach can be used. • Depth 4–6 cm • Needle 50 mm • US coronal oblique plane • Needle in-plane • LA 15–20 ml Figure 5.12a shows the probe position with marker for right infraclavicular brachial plexus block. Figure 5.12b shows the ultrasound appearance of brachial plexus in the infraclavicular region.

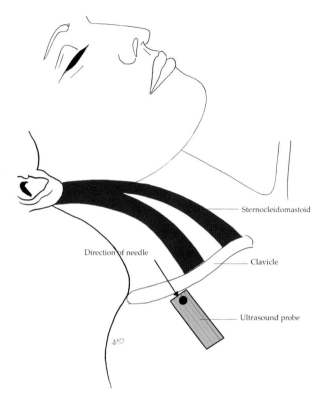

Figure 5.12a   Right infraclavicular brachial plexus block.

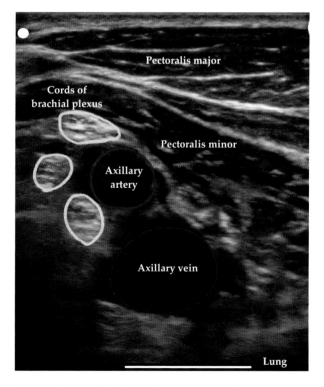

Figure 5.12b   Right infraclavicular brachial plexus block – ultrasound.

Axillary Approach

Table 5.11   Summary of Axillary Brachial Plexus Block

Axillary approach – block at the level of TERMINAL BRANCHES	
Sensory block	**Specific complications**
• Forearm, wrist, hand • May miss musculocutaneous nerve	• Haematoma • Intravascular injection • Patient may experience tourniquet pain as intercostobrachial nerve is not blocked
Landmark and nerve stimulator technique	
Transarterial technique. This technique does not use a nerve stimulator. Palpate the arterial pulse at the level of pectoralis major. Infiltrate the subcutaneous tissue with 4–5 ml of local anaesthetic to block the intercostobrachial and medial cutaneous nerves of the arm. Insert the needle through the artery and continue to insert even after aspirating blood. As the blood stops at the other side of the artery, deposit half the local anaesthetic behind the posterior wall of the artery. Withdraw the needle, again aspirating arterial blood. When the blood stops on the anterior side of the artery, deposit the other half of the local anaesthetic. Other techniques using nerve stimulation exist to avoid arterial puncture, such as the double injection technique: one injection above and one below the artery. • Depth 1–2 cm (very superficial) • Needle 25–50 mm insulated/uninsulated • LA 20–40 ml	
Ultrasound technique	
Patient supine, arm abducted and elbow flexed. Place transducer transversely across the axilla at the junction of the biceps and pectoralis muscles. Identify the axillary artery and vein. Scan proximally to identify the conjoint tendon of the latissimus dorsi and teres major muscles. Note the biceps muscle anteriorly and the wedge-shaped coracobrachialis inferior to the biceps.	

(*Continued*)

Table 5.11 (Continued)   Summary of Axillary Brachial Plexus Block

The terminal branches of the plexus surround the axillary artery and have a heterogenous honeycomb appearance.

The median nerve is superficial to the artery; the ulnar nerve is superficial and medial to the artery, usually between the artery and vein; the radial nerve is posterior to the artery; the musculocutaneous nerve lies between the biceps and coracobrachialis muscles. The nerves can be traced along their paths to confirm their identity. The location of the nerves around the artery show a large amount of patient variability.

Approach from the lateral side of the probe and infiltrate local anaesthetic around each nerve.

- Depth 1–4 cm
- Needle 50 mm
- US transverse plane
- Needle in-plane
- LA 10–25 ml

Figure 5.13a shows the probe position with marker for right axillary brachial plexus block.

Figure 5.13b shows the ultrasound appearance of the terminal nerves of the brachial plexus surrounding the axillary artery.

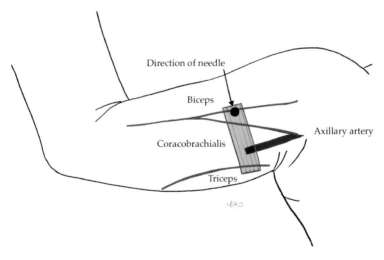

Figure 5.13a   Right axillary brachial plexus block.

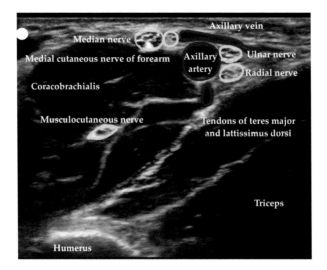

Figure 5.13b   Right axillary brachial plexus block – ultrasound.

What are the possible neurological complications of an interscalene block?

This structure could be adapted to answer a question relating to any nerve block.

General

- Compression (haematoma)
- Stretch (positioning)
- Trauma (axonal damage)
- Ischaemia
- Neuropraxia (myelin sheath damage; axon preserved)
- Local anaesthetic toxicity

Specific

- Phrenic nerve palsy
- Recurrent laryngeal nerve palsy
- Stellate ganglion block
- Subarachnoid/epidural injection
- Horner's syndrome
- Stroke from atheromatous plaque dislodgement
- Pneumothorax

Peripheral Nerve Blocks at the Level of Forearm

Table 5.12   Summary of Median Nerve Block at Forearm Level

Median nerve in the forearm
Landmark and nerve stimulator technique
Performed at the elbow crease, medial to the brachial artery. A pop is felt on piercing the bicipital aponeurosis. Aim to elicit flexion of the fingers. • Depth 1–2 cm (very superficial) • Needle 25–50 mm insulated/uninsulated • LA 5 ml
Ultrasound technique
Patient supine, arm abducted, elbow extended. Scan at the antecubital fossa and identify the nerve medial to the brachial artery. Trace the nerve distally as it departs from the artery. It can be blocked at the antecubital fossa or mid forearm where it lies between flexor digitorum superficialis and flexor digitorum profundus in the middle of the forearm. • Depth 1–2 cm • Needle 50 mm • US transverse plane • Needle in-plane or out of plane • LA 2–5 ml

Table 5.13   Summary of Ulnar Nerve Block at Forearm Level

Ulnar nerve in the forearm
Landmark and nerve stimulator technique
Performed 2 cm proximal to the ulnar sulcus at the medial epicondyle. Aim to elicit finger movement. Do not inject at the ulnar sulcus which is a tight space and can compress the ulnar nerve. • Depth 1–3 cm • Needle 25–50 mm insulated/uninsulated • LA 5 ml
Ultrasound technique
Patient supine, arm abducted, elbow extended. Scan at the ulnar side at the mid forearm. The nerve lies beneath the flexor carpi ulnaris muscle. Scanning distally, the nerve can be seen to accompany the ulnar artery. • Depth 1–2 cm • Needle 50 mm • US transverse plane • Needle in-plane or out of plane • LA 2–5 ml

Table 5.14   Summary of Radial Nerve Block at Forearm Level

Radial nerve in the forearm
Landmark and nerve stimulator technique
Performed at the antecubital fossa in the groove between the biceps tendon and brachioradialis muscle, 2 cm above the elbow crease, pointing the needle caudally and towards the lateral epicondyle. Aim to elicit extension of the thumb. • Depth 2–4 cm • Needle 50 mm insulated • LA 5 ml
Ultrasound technique
Patient supine, arm adducted and hand resting on abdomen. Scan approximately four fingers breadth above the lateral epicondyle of the humerus and trace the nerve proximally as it travels with profunda brachii artery around the spiral groove of the humerus. Surround the nerve with 2–5 ml local anaesthetic. The radial nerve can also be blocked more distally at mid forearm on the radial side of the radial artery, but it will have divided into superficial and deep radial branches and will miss the deep branch. • Depth 1–2 cm • Needle 50 mm • US transverse plane • Needle in-plane or out of plane • LA 2–5 ml

Peripheral Nerve Blocks at Level of Wrist

The nerves are small at the wrist and local anaesthetic will effectively diffuse into the nerve so circumferential spread of local anaesthetic is not essential.

Figure 5.14 illustrates the relations of the radial, median and ulnar nerves at the wrist.

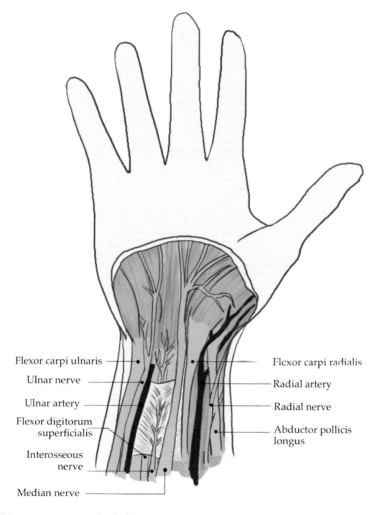

Figure 5.14   Wrist – structures and relations.

Table 5.15   Summary of Median Nerve Block at the Wrist

Median nerve at the wrist
Landmark technique
Insert the needle between the tendons of palmaris longus and flexor carpi radialis through the deep fascia. If you contact bone, draw back slightly and inject 2–3 ml local anaesthetic.
Ultrasound technique
Using a small linear or hockey stick probe, identify the tendons of palmaris longus and flexor carpi radialis (which become muscle belly when traced proximally and move when the patient moves their wrist). The median nerve lies between these tendons. The nerve can also be identified by tracing it from its proximal position. Infiltrate local anaesthetic around the nerve.

Table 5.16   Summary of Ulnar Nerve Block at the Wrist

Ulnar nerve at the wrist
Landmark technique
Inject 3–5 ml local anaesthetic under the flexor carpi ulnaris tendon above the styloid process of the ulna and inject 2–3 ml local anaesthetic subcutaneously above the tendon. Inject a 5 ml subcutaneous 'sausage' around the medial and dorsal aspect of the wrist to block the dorsal sensory branch.
Ultrasound technique
Using a small linear or hockey stick probe, identify the ulnar nerve sitting between the flexor carpi ulnaris tendon medially and the ulnar artery laterally. The tendon can be seen to move as the patient deviates their hand to the ulnar side. Infiltrate local anaesthetic around the nerve.

Table 5.17   Summary of Radial Nerve Block at the Wrist

Radial nerve at the wrist
Landmark technique
Essentially a field block as the anatomy of the radial nerve at this level is variable. Inject 5 ml local anaesthetic anterior to the radial styloid and inject 5 ml laterally. Inject 5 ml posteriorly to block the dorsal sensory branch.
Ultrasound technique
As the radial nerve has divided into its terminal branches at the wrist, identification using ultrasound is not easy. It is easier to block the radial nerve at mid forearm or elbow.

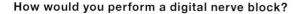

How would you perform a digital nerve block?

Used for surgery distal to the base of the proximal phalanx.

Digital nerves travel distally on either side of the phalanx and can be easily infiltrated with local anaesthetic to either side of the base of the proximal phalanx.

A 25G 25 mm (orange) needle is inserted vertically from the dorsal aspect to slide past the base of the phalanx, injecting 2–3 ml local anaesthetic on either side (i.e. two injections). Vasoconstrictors should not be used around end arteries.

Which nerves should be blocked to achieve effective local anaesthesia for shoulder surgery?

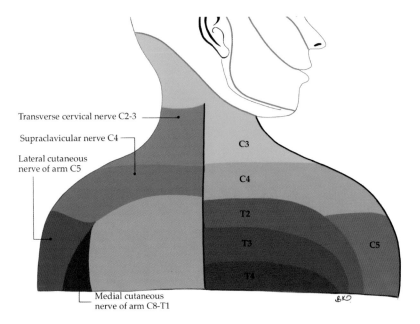

Figure 5.15   Innervation around the shoulder.

Skin around the shoulder

- From the cervical plexus
    - Transverse cervical nerve
    - Supraclavicular nerve
- From the brachial plexus
    - Axillary nerve
    - Medial cutaneous nerve of the arm
    - Intercostobrachial nerve

Shoulder joint

- From the brachial plexus
    - Suprascapular nerve – the acromioclavicular joint, capsule and glenohumeral joint

  o Axillary nerve – inferior aspect of the capsule and glenohumeral joint

  o Musculocutaneous nerve

  o Subscapular nerve

How can you block the suprascapular nerve?

With the patient sitting, choose a needle insertion point 1 cm above the midpoint of the scapular spine. If using a nerve stimulator, look for movement of the supraspinatus muscle.

Outline the measures available to reduce all types of neurological damage during shoulder surgery.

Block technique

- Asepsis – 0.5% chlorhexidine (not 2%!), air dry
- Ultrasound guidance, maintain visualisation of needle tip
- Low pressure injection
- Appropriate needle length (not too long)
- Awake block

GA

- Eye protection – taping and padding
- Avoid tying ETT, tape preferred to avoid impeding venous return

Intraoperative management

Deck chair position

- avoid excessive head extension
- avoid pressure on brachial plexus and ulnar nerve
- flex at knees, padding under knees, avoid pressure and stretch of sciatic nerve
- maintain mean arterial pressure and cerebral perfusion pressure

Postoperative management

Smooth extubation, avoid large increases in intracerebral pressure

Bibliography

Drake, R. L., Vogle, W., & Mitchell, A. W. M. (2005). *Gray's Anatomy for Students*. Canada: Elsevire Inc.

Lin, E., Gaur, A., Jones, M., & Ahmed, A. (2013). *Sonoanatomy for Anaesthetists*. Croydon: Cambridge University Press.

NYSORA (New York School of Regional Anaesthesia). (2019). *Upper Extremity Blocks*. Retrieved 12 March 2019 from www.nysora.com/techniques/upper-extremity.

Townsley, P., Bedforth, N., & Nicholls, B. (2014). *A Pocket Guide to Ultrasound-Guided Regional Anaesthesia*. London: Regional Anaesthesia – UK, Alpine Press.

LOWER LIMB

6

Structures

- Femoral triangle
- Popliteal fossa

Circulation

- Arterial supply
- Venous drainage

Nervous System

- Dermatomes and nerve distribution
- Lumbar plexus, femoral, saphenous and sciatic nerves
- Blocks
  - Lumbar plexus block
  - Femoral nerve block
  - 3-in-1 block
  - Fascia iliaca block
  - Adductor canal block
  - Sciatic nerve block
  - Popliteal nerve block
  - Ankle block

Structures

- Femoral triangle
- Popliteal fossa

Femoral Triangle

The femoral triangle is a hollow area in the anterior thigh providing relatively easy access to the femoral neurovascular bundle (Figure 6.1).

Boundaries

- Superior – inguinal ligament (attachments are ASIS and pubic tubercle)
- Lateral – sartorius
- Medial – adductor longus
- Floor – iliacus, pectineus, psoas muscles
- Roof – areolar tissue, fascia lata, subcutaneous tissue, skin

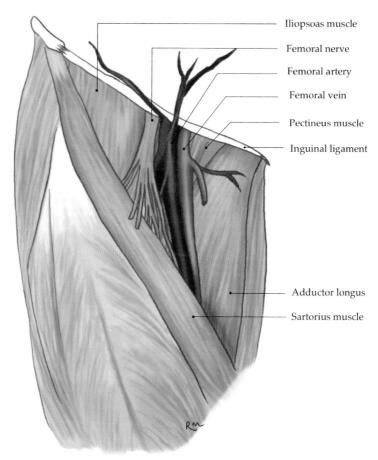

Iliopsoas muscle

Femoral nerve

Femoral artery

Femoral vein

Pectineus muscle

Inguinal ligament

Adductor longus

Sartorius muscle

Figure 6.1   Femoral triangle – boundaries and contents.

Contents (lateral to medial)

- Femoral nerve – invested in fascia iliaca
- Femoral branch of the genitofemoral nerve
- Femoral sheath – a prolongation of the transversalis fascia containing
  - Femoral artery
  - Femoral vein
  - Femoral canal – the medial component of the sheath containing lymphatics and possibly inguinal node (Cloquet's node). The femoral ring is the abdominal opening of the canal.

Why is the femoral triangle important to the anaesthetist?

It is an important anatomical landmark for anaesthetists to be able to access the neurovascular bundle.

- Femoral nerve: for femoral nerve block, 3-in-1 block, fascia iliaca block
- Femoral artery: for arterial cannulation (continuous BP, cardiac catheterisation, intra-aortic balloon pump)
- Femoral vein: for central venous catheters, vascaths, IVC filters

How do you locate the femoral artery on an actor? Where do the nerve and vein lie in relation to this?

The femoral artery is palpable at the mid-inguinal point, which is situated halfway between the pubic symphysis and the ASIS. The nerve lies lateral to the artery, and the femoral vein lies medial to the artery.

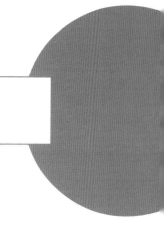

Popliteal Fossa

The popliteal fossa is a diamond-shaped area posterior to the knee joint. This is the site for popliteal nerve block for providing analgesia for procedures performed in the lower leg (Figure 6.2).

Boundaries

- Superomedial – semimembranosus
- Superolateral – biceps femoris
- Inferomedial – medial head of gastrocnemius
- Inferolateral – lateral head of gastrocnemius
- Floor – posterior capsule of the knee joint and posterior surface of the femur
- Roof – skin and popliteal fascia (continuous with the fascia lata of the leg)

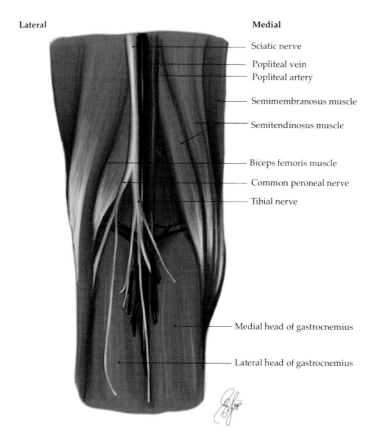

Figure 6.2 Popliteal fossa – boundaries and contents.

Contents (medial to lateral)

- Popliteal artery, vein and their genicular branches
- Popliteal lymph nodes
- Tibial nerve
- Common peroneal nerve: both nerves are branches of the sciatic nerve, which commonly divides around the fossa. Subject to anatomical variation this occurs approximately 5–10 cm above the popliteal skin crease.

Circulation

- Arterial supply
- Venous drainage

Arterial Supply of Lower Limb

The main blood supply to the lower limb is by the *femoral artery*, which is the continuation of the external iliac artery. The femoral artery continues as the popliteal artery in the lower leg (Table 6.1 and Figure 6.3).

See Femoral Triangle and Popliteal Fossa respectively for the relations of femoral artery and the popliteal artery.

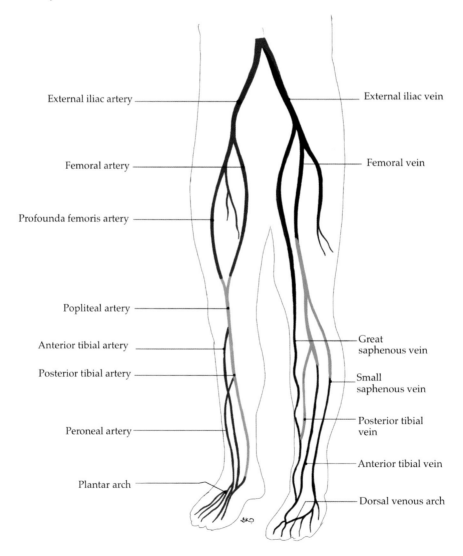

Figure 6.3   Arterial supply and venous drainage of the lower limb.

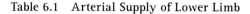

Table 6.1   Arterial Supply of Lower Limb

Thigh – femoral artery
Course: the external iliac artery continues as the femoral artery when it crosses the midpoint of inguinal ligament to enter the thigh. It treks down the anteromedial side of the thigh and passes through the adductor canal. At the junction of middle and lower one third of the thigh, it exits to the popliteal fossa through the opening in the adductor magnus and continues as the popliteal artery.
Branches and supply
<ul><li>*Profunda femoris*: largest branch of the femoral artery which supplies the hip joint, and most of the muscles in all compartments of the thigh</li><li>*Superficial and deep external pudendal arteries*: supplies the skin of perineum and lower abdomen</li><li>*Descending genicular artery*: supplies the upper and medial part of skin and some muscles of thigh and the knee joint</li><li>*Superficial epigastric artery and superficial circumflex iliac artery*: small branches which supply the skin, superficial fascia and superficial inguinal lymph nodes</li></ul>
Knee and lower leg – popliteal artery
Course: the popliteal artery passes through the popliteal fossa at the lower border of the popliteus muscle and terminates by branching into the anterior and posterior tibial arteries.
Branches and supply:
<ul><li>Anterior and posterior tibial arteries: they are the terminal branches of the popliteal artery and supply the muscles and bones of the lower leg</li><li>Genicular branches: there are five genicular branches that supply the knee joint and ligaments</li><li>Muscular and sural arteries: these supply the muscles of the lower leg</li></ul>
Ankle and foot – tarsal, malleolar, plantar and dorsalis pedis arteries
Course: dorsalis pedis and plantar branches are continuation of posterior and anterior tibial arteries, respectively, and these, along with their branches, supply the ankle and foot.

What are the causes of limb ischaemia?

Emboli rank first for being the culprit for acute limb ischaemia and most commonly arise from the heart, a proximal arterial aneurysm or atherosclerosis. Thrombosis may be induced by any of the three factors of Virchow's triad: static or turbulent blood flow, hypercoagulability and endothelial injury.

Other causes include vasculitis, trauma, compartment syndrome, fibrodysplasia and iatrogenic interventions (e.g. cannulation of vessels).

What are the features of an ischaemic limb?

- Acute: 6 Ps – pain, pallor, paraesthesia, paralysis, pulselessness, perishing cold
- Chronic: may be asymptomatic, intermittent claudication, ischaemic rest pain, ulceration and gangrene

What are the management options for an acutely ischaemic limb?

The management of a patient presenting with an acutely ischaemic limb begins with taking a thorough history and examination. Acute ischaemia caused by complete arterial blockage can cause irreversible damage in 6 hours.

History with particular mention to

- Onset of symptoms – sudden onset over the last few hours suggests an acute event whereas a slow onset over days/weeks suggests a more chronic problem
- Comorbidities – MI, AF, aneurysm would be suggestive of an embolism
- Use (or discontinuation) of anticoagulants

Examination

- Assess the viability of the limb (irreversible signs such as fixed staining, mottling, gangrene – surgical interest)
- Airway and targeted examination of other systems

Investigations

- FBC, clotting, creatine kinase, group and save, doppler, magnetic resonance angiography or computed tomographic angiography or intra-arterial angiography

General management

- ABC measures
- Analgesia

Specific management

- Immediate involvement of the vascular team
- Anticoagulation with heparin
- Surgical – embolectomy +/– fasciotomy, bypass procedures
- Endovascular – angioplasty, thrombectomy, local intra-arterial thrombolysis, etc.

Anaesthetic management

Patients are usually systemically ill, and the surgical procedure is often urgent, but a thorough anaesthetic and medical history and examination is carried out and system optimisation should be considered within the time available. Surgeons may choose to perform an embolectomy under local anaesthesia but given the high perioperative risks, anaesthetic presence is usually necessary. If more invasive surgery is planned, general anaesthesia is the preferred choice for various reasons (use of therapeutic doses of anticoagulant drug, non-fasted state, etc.)

Points to remember

- General measures of management of an acutely ill patient with the use of invasive monitoring, regular acid-base analysis, electrolyte corrections, fluid resuscitation and inotropic support.
- Reperfusion injury – hyperkalaemia, myocardial depression, arrhythmias, cardiac arrest, myoglobinaemia and acute renal failure can happen due to reperfusion of the ischaemic limb. In the case of muscle necrosis or irreversible ischaemia, these risks may be overwhelming and primary amputation may be indicated.

Venous Drainage of Lower Limb

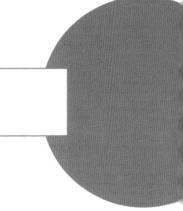

The venous drainage of the lower limb can be divided into two groups

- Deep venous system

  The deep veins accompany the arteries in the leg. The peroneal vein drains into the posterior tibial vein which, along with the anterior tibial vein, empties into the popliteal vein. The popliteal vein continues as the femoral vein and accepts the profunda femoris vein and becomes the external iliac vein.

- Superficial venous system

  The superficial veins form the dorsal venous arch which continue as the great saphenous vein on the medial side of the leg (drains into the femoral vein) and small saphenous vein laterally (drains into the popliteal vein).

What might be the indications for cannulating the femoral vein?
- Central venous access – which can be used to administer drugs/infusions
- Central venous pressure monitoring
- Dialysis catheters (vascaths)
- IVC filter insertion
- Port of access for interventional angiography (e.g. coronary angiogram)

What are the possible complications of femoral vein cannulation?
Immediate

- Arterial injury
- Haematoma
- Damage to the femoral nerve
- Bowel/bladder injury

Delayed

- Pseudoaneurysm
- Venous thrombosis
- Infection
- Septic arthritis (usually following the puncture of the hip capsule in infants)

What clinical features would make you suspect IVC thrombosis in a patient with a femoral vein catheter?

Features of local obstruction

- Lower limb pain and oedema
- Scrotal swelling

Features of clot migration

- Pulmonary embolism
- Budd Chiari syndrome – ascites, portal hypertension, collateral vein enlargement, hepatic fibrosis due to extension or migration of the thrombus to the hepatic veins
- Renal failure

Features of venous hypertension

- Bilateral lower-extremity oedema
- Varicose veins and non-healing venous ulcers
- Caput medusae (visibly dilated superficial abdominal veins from collateral drainage)

Bibliography

Darwood, R. Acute Limb Ischaemia. rcemlearning.co.uk.

Fraser, K., & Raju, I. (2014). Anaesthesia for lower limb revascularization surgery. *BJA Education, 15*(5), 225–230.

Gilroy, A. M., Voll, M. M., & Wesker, K. (2017). *Anatomy: An Essential Textbook.* New York, NY: Thieme Medical Publishers, Inc.

Nervous System

- Dermatomes and nerve distribution
- Lumbar plexus, femoral, saphenous and sciatic nerves
- Blocks
  - Lumbar plexus block
  - Femoral nerve block
  - 3-in-1 block
  - Fascia iliaca block
  - Adductor canal block
  - Sciatic nerve block
  - Popliteal nerve block
  - Ankle block

Dermatomes and Nerve Distribution

Figures 6.4 and 6.5 show the dermatomal and peripheral nerve distribution of the anterior and posterior parts of the lower limb.

- Thigh

  Cutaneous supply of the thigh from the groin to the knee is from the lumbar plexus. The femoral nerve is responsible for the anterolateral aspect of the skin of the thigh with an important branch being the lateral cutaneous nerve of the thigh. The obturator is responsible for the posteromedial aspect, with the posterior cutaneous nerve of the thigh being an important branch. Superiorly, iliohypogastric and subcostal nerves supply the skin directly over the anterior superior iliac spine (ASIS) and beneath the inguinal region.

- Knee

  Cutaneous innervation is derived from the lumbar plexus and the sacral plexus, more specifically, the femoral nerve and the sciatic nerve. The femoral nerve is responsible for the anteromedial aspect, whereas the sciatic nerve innervates the posterolateral aspect of the knee.

- Lower leg

  Like the knee, the femoral and sciatic nerves are responsible for the cutaneous innervation of the lower leg. The saphenous nerve (branch of the femoral nerve) supplies the medial aspect of the leg, including the medial malleolus. The sciatic nerve and its branches supply the rest of the leg and foot. This is covered in more detail under Ankle Block.

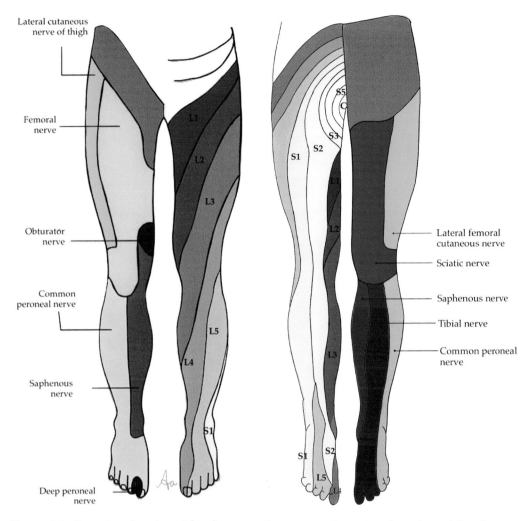

Figure 6.4 Dermatomal and peripheral nerve distribution of the anterior aspect of lower limb.

Figure 6.5 Dermatomal and peripheral nerve distribution of the posterior aspect of the lower limb.

The Lumbar Plexus

The lumbar plexus is a network of nerve fibres that provide motor and sensory innervation to the lower limb. They are formed of the anterior rami of the lumbar spinal nerves from L1–L4 with 50% of cases receiving contribution from T12. The plexus is found anterior to the transverse processes of lumbar vertebrae within the psoas major muscle compartment. These spinal nerves divide into cords and combine to form six major peripheral nerves (Table 6.2 and Figure 6.6).

Table 6.2 Summary of Lumbar Plexus

Lumbar plexus	
Origin	Anterior rami of L1–L4 and some contribution from T12
Course	Emerges from intervertebral foramina and lies within the psoas muscle, anterior to the transverse processes of the lumbar vertebrae
Supplies	Motor: all the muscles of the lower limb
	Sensory: innervation to inguinal/groin region, anterior thigh, medial aspect of leg
Six branches	Two nerves with one root, two nerves with two roots and two nerves with three roots
Indulgent	Iliohypogastric (L1)
Ian	Ilioinguinal (L1)
Got	Genitofemoral (L1–L2)
Leftovers	Lateral cutaneous nerve of the thigh (L2–L3)
On	Obturator (L2–L4)
Fridays	Femoral (L2–L4)
Blocks	Lumbar plexus block/psoas compartment block

L1 and, in 50% of cases, a branch of T12 splits into two divisions – upper and lower. Upper division gives rise to iliohypogastric and ilio-inguinal nerves. The lower division forms the genitofemoral nerve after joining with a branch from L2 anterior rami.

The rest of L2–L3 and some branches of L4 rami divide into two divisions – dorsal and ventral. Dorsal divisions of L2–L3 form the lateral cutaneous nerve of the thigh and that of L2–L4 form the femoral nerve. The ventral divisions of L2–L4 join to form the obturator nerve.

All nerves apart from the obturator emerge between the quadratus lumborum and the psoas muscles. The obturator nerve passes medially and travels under the iliac vessels to the lower limbs.

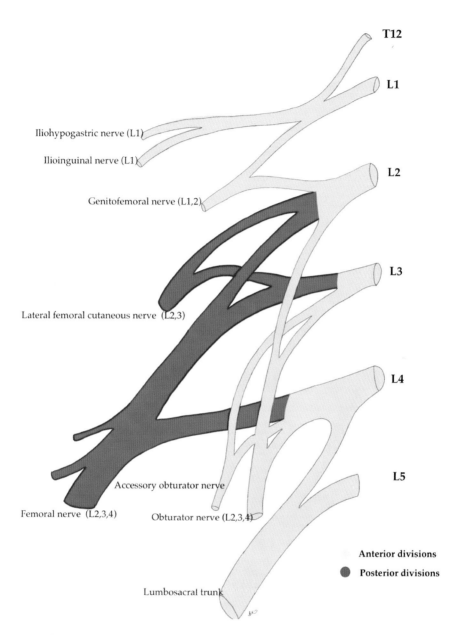

Figure 6.6   Lumbar plexus – origin and branches.

What do the branches of the lumbar plexus supply and what (if any) are their functions?

Table 6.3 Summary of Function of the Branches of the Lumbar Plexus

Nerve	Function
Iliohypogastric L1 ± T12	*Motor*: transversus abdominis and internal oblique *Sensory*: skin of posterolateral gluteal region
Ilioinguinal L1	*Motor*: transversus abdominis and internal oblique *Sensory*: skin of middle thigh and anterior scrotum (males) and mons pubis (females)
Genitofemoral L1–2	*Motor*: cremaster muscle *Sensory*: skin of anterior thigh and anterior scrotum (males) and mons pubis (females)
Lateral cutaneous N of thigh L2–3	*Motor*: none *Sensory*: anterior and posterior branches supply the skin of anterolateral and lateral aspect of mid thigh respectively
Obturator L2 –L4	*Motor*: obturator externus, adductor longus and brevis, gracilis, pectineus *Sensory*: skin of medial thigh
Femoral L2–L4	*Motor*: abductors – iliacus, sartorius, quadriceps femoris *Sensory*: skin of anterior and medial thigh

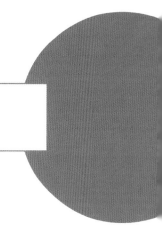

Femoral Nerve

The femoral nerve arises from primary rami of L2–L4 (dorsal divisions) within the lumbar plexus. It supplies

- Skin overlying medial aspect of anterior thigh and medial leg below the knee
- Pectineus, sartorius, quadriceps femoris muscles
- Femoral shaft, hip and knee joint

Course of the nerve

The nerve emerges from the lateral margin of the psoas muscle, passing inferiorly between the psoas and iliacus muscles and crosses beneath the inguinal ligament to enter the thigh. The nerve resides in the femoral triangle, lateral to the femoral artery and is invested in the fascia of iliacus muscle which separates it from the femoral sheath. It divides into its terminal branches at the base of the triangle.

Terminal branches

These stem from anterior and posterior divisions.

Anterior division

- Muscular branches which innervate sartorius and pectineus.
- Cutaneous branches which supply skin overlying medial aspect of anterolateral thigh – intermediate and medial cutaneous nerve of the thigh.

Posterior division

- Muscular branches which innervate quadriceps femoris.
- Saphenous nerve – largest cutaneous branch of the femoral nerve. This nerve arises in the femoral triangle and enters the adductor canal of Hunter. It crosses medially over the knee behind the sartorius, running down the medial border of the tibia immediately behind the great saphenous vein, crossing the vein in front of the medial malleolus. It is responsible for sensation of extensive cutaneous area over medial side of the leg (Figure 6.7 and Table 6.4).

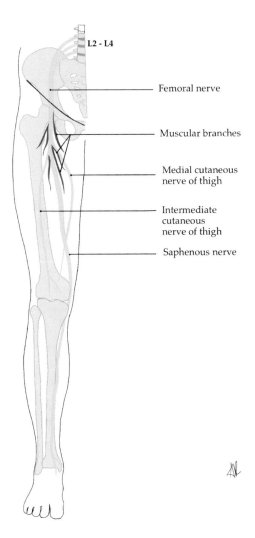

L2 - L4

Femoral nerve

Muscular branches

Medial cutaneous
nerve of thigh

Intermediate
cutaneous
nerve of thigh

Saphenous nerve

Figure 6.7   Femoral nerve – course.

Table 6.4   Summary of Femoral Nerve

Femoral nerve (L2–L4)	
Origin	Anterior rami of L2–L4 from lumbar plexus within the psoas muscle
Course	Crosses beneath the inguinal ligament and enters femoral triangle, dividing into its terminal branches at its base
Supplies	*Motor*: sartorius, pectineus, quadriceps femoris *Sensory*: femoral shaft, hip and knee joints, cutaneous supply of thigh and medial part of lower leg
Important branch	Saphenous nerve
Associated blocks	Femoral nerve, 3-in-1, fascia iliaca and adductor canal blocks Saphenous nerve can be blocked as part of ankle block

Sciatic Nerve

The sacral plexus is a collection of spinal nerves responsible for the innervation of the skin and muscles of the pelvis and leg. It is located anterior to the piriformis muscle on the surface of the posterior pelvic wall.

At each vertebral level, the paired spinal nerves exit the spinal cord through the intervertebral foramina and then divide into the anterior and posterior rami with the anterior rami of S1–S4 forming the basis of the sacral plexus. It also receives contributions from L4 and L5 with anatomical differences in how much the lumbar spinal nerves contribute to the plexus.

Shortly after exiting the spinal cord, the anterior rami of S1–S4 divide into cords, which subsequently combine together to from five peripheral nerves of sacral plexus

- Superior gluteal nerve (L4–L5, S1)
- Inferior gluteal nerve (L5, S1–S2)
- Sciatic nerve (L4–L5, S1–S3)
- Posterior femoral cutaneous nerve (S1–S3)
- Pudendal nerve (S2–S4)

These either leave the greater sciatic foramen to enter the gluteal region or remain in the pelvis to supply the pelvic muscles and organs.

Outline the course of sciatic nerve from the spinal cord. What does it supply?

The sciatic nerve is the largest peripheral nerve in the body. It arises from the sacral plexus from L4–L5, S1–S3 nerve roots and exits the pelvis posteriorly via the greater sciatic notch. It descends into the thigh between ischial tuberosity and greater trochanter and between two heads of biceps femoris. Commonly at the apex of the popliteal fossa, the sciatic nerve splits to give off its terminal branches – the common peroneal nerve and tibial nerve.

The sciatic nerve provides sensory innervation to most of the lower limb below the knee, apart from the skin overlying the medial side of knee, lower leg and ankle (supplied by the saphenous nerve). It supplies articular branches to the hip and knee joint as well as providing motor innervation to muscles of the thigh (semitendinosus, biceps femoris, semimembranosus and half of adductor magnus) and all muscles of the lower leg (posterior compartment as tibial nerve; anterior and lateral compartments as peroneal nerve) (Figure 6.8 and Table 6.5).

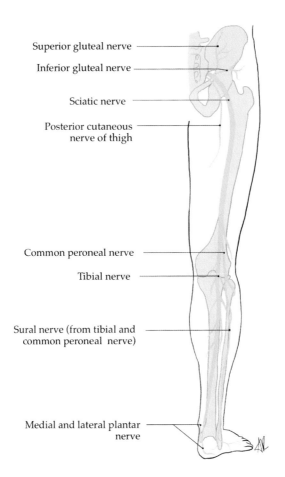

Superior gluteal nerve

Inferior gluteal nerve

Sciatic nerve

Posterior cutaneous
nerve of thigh

Common peroneal nerve

Tibial nerve

Sural nerve (from tibial and
common peroneal nerve)

Medial and lateral plantar
nerve

Figure 6.8   Sciatic nerve – course.

Table 6.5   Summary of Sciatic Nerve

Sciatic nerve (L4–S3)	
Origin	Anterior rami of L4–S3 from sacral plexus
Course	Leaves pelvis and enters gluteal region via greater sciatic foramen Separated from sacrum by piriformis muscle Exits posteriorly via sciatic notch and descends between two ischial tuberosities and greater trochanter between two heads of biceps femoris Terminates into common peroneal and tibial nerves at apex of the popliteal fossa
Supplies	*Motor*: sartorius, pectineus, quadriceps femoris *Sensory*: no direct sensory branches Supplies the skin of the lateral leg, heel and foot through its terminal branches
Important branches	Common peroneal nerve Tibial nerve
Associated blocks	Sciatic nerve block • Posterior approach – Raj and Labat's • Popliteal approach (also posterior) • Anterior approach – Beck's Terminal branches of the sciatic nerve are blocked as part of ankle block

Nerve Blocks

What is the sensory innervation of the hip?

Main sensory innervation to the hip joint and capsule are from femoral and obturator nerves, with the sciatic nerve contributing to the posterior aspect of the joint. All three of these nerves are involved in supplying the sensation of the femoral shaft.

The skin overlying the hip is supplied by the iliohypogastric nerve, lateral cutaneous nerve of the thigh, superior cluneal nerves (L1–L3) and occasionally lower thoracic cutaneous nerves.

What regional anaesthesia techniques can be used for analgesia following hip surgery?

- Central neuraxial techniques – spinal/epidural
- Lumbar plexus block (psoas compartment block)
- Femoral nerve block
- '3-in-1' block
- Fascia iliaca block

Lumbar plexus block

When would you consider a lumbar plexus block?

This block reliably blocks the femoral, obturator and lateral cutaneous nerve of the thigh and therefore can be used for

- Analgesia for fractured neck of femur (NOF)/fractured femoral shaft
- Intraoperative and postoperative analgesia for surgeries involving the groin, anterior thigh and/or knee but not generally used as a sole anaesthetic technique

How will you perform the lumbar plexus block (without ultrasound)?

- *General measures*

  Patient consented, IV access, AAGBI monitoring and 'stop before you block' after positioning patient and sterility ensured throughout
- *Patient position*

  Lateral decubitus position (hips and knees flexed), side to be blocked uppermost
- *Landmarks*

  Transverse process of L3 which lies 2–3 cm lateral to the dorsal midline
- *Needle insertion*

  Perpendicular to skin at transverse process L3

- *Needle direction*

  Needle directed cranially in order to penetrate psoas sheath and quadratus lumborum fascia

- *Depth*: 8–10 cm
- *Local anaesthetic volume*: 20–30 ml injected in 5 ml aliquots after negative aspiration
- *Technique*

  Mark the midline of the back along the spinous processes. Also mark the intercristal line – the line connecting the superior part of the iliac crests. A point approximately 3 cm lateral to the intersection of these two lines to be used as needle insertion point. Infiltrate the skin with local anaesthetic prior to needle entry, and nerve stimulation or loss of resistance technique using Touhy needle can be applied. Needle is inserted perpendicular to the skin until transverse process of L3 is encountered, aim cephalad and aim to 'walk off' the transverse process. It is advanced further until either quadriceps contraction is seen using nerve stimulator or until a change in resistance (less resistance) is felt if using a Touhy needle when fascia of psoas sheath is penetrated. A catheter may also be placed to allow top-ups or a continuous infusion (Table 6.6).

Table 6.6   Summary of Lumbar Plexus Block

Lumbar plexus block	
Indications	Intra/post op analgesia for hip, anterior thigh and knee surgery
Nerves blocked	Six branches of lumbar plexus
Volume of LA	20–30 ml
Patient position	Lateral, side to be blocked uppermost
Landmarks	<ul><li>Iliac crests (L4 level)</li><li>Spinous processes</li></ul>
Technique	3–4 cm lateral to lumbar spine at L3 Needle perpendicular and angled cephalad
End point for nerve stimulator	Patellar twitch (from quadriceps femoris contraction supplied by femoral nerve) at 0.5–1 mA
Limitations	Rarely dense enough block to use as sole anaesthetic procedure
Block-specific complications	Distribution of LA within psoas muscle causes systemic absorption of LA and risk of LA toxicity

What are the specific complications of a lumbar plexus block?

- Epidural spread due to the proximity of the lumbar plexus to the epidural space
- More local anaesthetic will be absorbed intravascularly given the excellent blood supply of the psoas muscle and therefore there is theoretically high risk of local anaesthetic toxicity
- Renal haematoma has been reported

Alternate question...

You are called to the Emergency Department to review a patient who has suffered a fractured NOF.

How should this patient's analgesia be managed?

In accordance with the NICE guideline on management of hip fractures (June 2011),

- Assessment of pain

    Pain assessment should be done immediately upon presentation, within 30 minutes of administering initial analgesia and hourly thereafter until settled in a ward environment. It should continue as part of routine nursing observations throughout admission. Pain should be well controlled so that the patient is able to tolerate movements necessary for investigations, nursing care and rehabilitation.

- Analgesia options

    Patients should be prescribed regular oral analgesics and offered analgesia on presentation, including those with cognitive impairment. Paracetamol regularly unless contraindicated and additional opioids if paracetamol alone does not provide sufficient preoperative pain relief. NSAIDs are not recommended. If further analgesia or opioid sparing technique is required, nerve blocks are the next option. Nerve blocks should not be used as substitute for timely surgical management.

    The following blocks can be considered.
    - Central neuraxial techniques – spinal/epidural
    - Lumbar plexus block (psoas compartment block)
    - Femoral nerve block
    - 3-in-1 block
    - Fascia iliaca block
- Surgical management

    Surgical fixation provides best analgesia and should be performed either on the day of or day after the injury.

    Of clinical interest, extracapsular fractures (requiring dynamic hip screw) are more painful than intracapsular fractures (requiring hemiarthroplasty/replacement) due to greater degree of periosteal damage.

Femoral nerve block

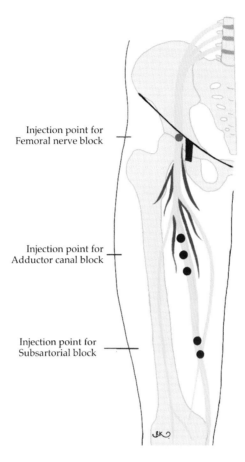

Injection point for
Femoral nerve block

Injection point for
Adductor canal block

Injection point for
Subsartorial block

Figure 6.9   Femoral nerve – level of blocks.

Can you tell me some of the other indications for femoral nerve block?

- Analgesia for femoral fracture
- Perioperative analgesia for knee surgery

How would you block the femoral nerve without ultrasound?

- *General measures*

  Patient consented, IV access, AAGBI monitoring and 'stop before you block' after positioning patient, sterility ensured throughout, ensure local anaesthetic drugs prepared and nerve stimulator available.
- *Patient position*: supine
- *Landmarks*: femoral artery below midpoint of inguinal ligament
- *Needle insertion*

  1 cm lateral to femoral arterial pulsation and 2 cm below inguinal ligament

- *Needle direction*: angled 45° to skin
- *LA volume*: <20 ml injected in 5 ml aliquots after negative aspiration
- *Technique*

    After identification of landmarks and needle insertion point, insert needle 45° to skin and advance until two 'pops' are felt as it penetrates fascia lata and iliopectineal facia.

What are the limitations of a femoral nerve block for hip surgery?

Due to the innervation of the hip, there is incomplete analgesia as the joint is also supplied by obturator and sciatic nerves, which are not blocked. Furthermore, site of incision of hip surgery will not be covered as cutaneous innervation is from superior cluneal nerves, lateral cutaneous nerve of thigh and iliohypogastric nerves. Therefore, it cannot be used as the sole anaesthetic technique and may be inadequate for analgesia on its own (Table 6.7).

Table 6.7   Summary of Femoral Nerve Block

Femoral nerve block	
Indications	Analgesia involving anterior thigh and knee Analgesia for femoral fracture
Nerves blocked	Femoral nerve
Volume of LA	<20 ml
Position	Supine
Landmarks	Femoral artery below midpoint of inguinal ligament
Technique with nerve stimulator	Needle 1 cm lateral to femoral artery and 2 cm below inguinal ligament Angle 45°; feel for two pops → fascia lata and iliopectineal fascia. Look for patellar twitch (from quadriceps femoris contraction, supplied by femoral nerve) at 0.5–1 mA. 10–20 ml injected after negative aspiration
Technique with ultrasound	Transducer is positioned transverse at the femoral crease to identify the femoral artery and nerve. The needle is inserted in-plane about 1 cm away from the lateral edge of transducer from lateral to medial direction to reach the femoral nerve between the two layers of the fascia iliaca. Local anaesthetic: 10–20 ml injected after haem-free aspirate and hydrolocation
Limitations	Incomplete analgesia for hip surgery as hip joint is also supplied by obturator and sciatic nerves. Site of incision of hip surgery is not covered as cutaneous innervation is from lateral cutaneous nerve of thigh, iliohypogastric and superior cluneal nerves. Mobility is limited due to motor block of quadriceps
Block-specific complications	Nil – general risks apply

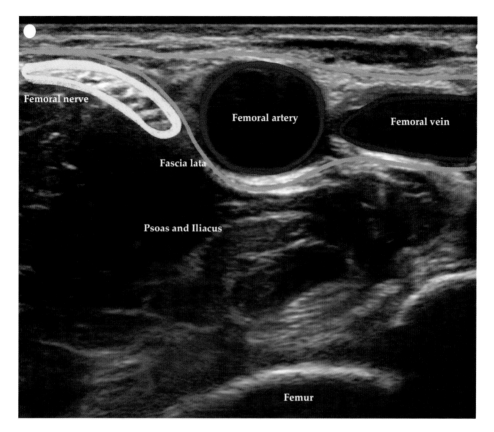

Figure 6.10   Ultrasound image of the right femoral nerve at the level of femoral triangle.

What are the differences between the femoral nerve block and the '3-in-1' block? Explain why the block may also fail to provide reliable analgesia for hip surgery.

The '3-in-1' block is essentially a femoral nerve block utilising a large volume (20–30 ml) with firm distal pressure on injection used to encourage cephalad spread of local anaesthetic in order to anaesthetise the lateral femoral cutaneous and obturator nerves. Apart from this difference, the approach and technique for both blocks are the same.

The major limitation to the 3-in-1 block is that the obturator nerve is rarely blocked and it is therefore unable to provide reliable analgesia for hip surgery (Table 6.8).

Table 6.8   Summary of 3-In-1 Block

3-in-1 block	
Indications	Intra/post op analgesia involving anterior thigh and knee Analgesia for femoral fracture
Nerves blocked	Femoral nerve Lateral cutaneous nerve of thigh Obturator (often missed)
Volume of LA	20–30 ml (more than femoral nerve)
Patient position	Supine
Landmarks	Same as femoral nerve block – femoral artery
Technique with nerve stimulator	Same as femoral nerve block but apply distal pressure on injection to cause cephalad spread of LA
Technique with ultrasound	Probe is placed transversely view the femoral artery distal to the inguinal ligament and then moved laterally to identify the nerve. From lateral to medial direction and with an in-plane approach, the needle is advanced and 20–30 ml of local anaesthetic injected after hydrolocation.
Limitations	Obturator rarely blocked Mobility limited due to motor block of quadriceps
Block-specific complications	Nil – general risks apply

What is the fascia iliaca compartment?

Fascia iliaca compartment is a potential space found within the boundaries as below.

- Anterior: skin, subcutaneous tissue, fascia lata and posterior surface of the fascia iliaca
- Posterior: anterior surface of iliacus muscle and psoas major muscle
- Medial: vertebral column and iliac crest
- Superior: continuous with space between quadratus lumborum muscle and its fascia

Describe the fascia iliaca block.

The fascial iliaca block attempts to block the femoral and obturator nerves using a different approach from the femoral and 3-in-1 blocks. The block infiltrates the fascia iliaca compartment which contains these nerves.

- *General measures*

  Patient consented, IV access, AAGBI monitoring and 'stop before you block' after positioning patient, sterility ensured throughout and ensure local anaesthetic drugs prepared
- *Patient position*: supine with affected limb abducted and externally rotated
- *Landmarks*

  1. Line joining ASIS and ipsilateral pubic tubercle

2. Mark a point dividing this line into medial two-thirds and lateral one third

3. Draw a point 1 cm caudal and distal from this point

- *Needle insertion and direction*: angled 60° to skin and advanced cranially

- *LA volume*: 20-30 ml injected in 5 ml aliquots after negative aspiration

- *Technique*

  Identify the landmarks and identify needle insertion point. Palpate the ipsilateral femoral pulse to ensure that the pulse is ideally 2 cm medial to needle insertion site. Clean the skin and infiltrate insertion site with 1% lignocaine. Insert short bevelled needle and once through the skin, angle 60° to skin and advance cranially, keeping needle in sagittal plane to avoid puncturing major vessels and peritoneal cavity. Advance until two 'pops' are felt as it penetrates the fascia lata and then the fascia iliaca. Reduce the needle angle and advance a further 1-2 mm. Inject local anaesthetic solution after haem-negative aspiration (Table 6.9).

Table 6.9 Summary of Fascia Iliaca Block

Fascia iliaca block	
Indications	Intra/post op analgesia involving anterior thigh and knee Perioperative analgesia for femoral fracture Analgesia for lower leg tourniquet pain in awake procedure
Nerves blocked	Femoral nerve Obturator (often missed)
Volume of LA	20–30 ml
Patient position	Supine
Landmarks	1. Line joining ASIS and ipsilateral pubic tubercle 2. Divide this line into thirds and identify a point 1/3 lateral and 2/3 medial on this line. 3. Draw a point 1 cm distal from this point and this is the needle insertion point.
Technique with nerve stimulator	Angle needle 60° to skin and advance cranially Advance until two 'pops' are felt as it penetrates the fascia lata and then the fascia iliaca. Reduce the needle angle and advance a further 1-2 mm. If used, patellar twitch is end point at 0.5–1 mA
Technique with ultrasound	Transducer positioned transversely below the inguinal ligament to identify the femoral artery, iliopsoas muscle, fascia iliaca and sartorius muscle. Needle is inserted in-line to reach the plane between the iliopsoas muscle and the fascia iliaca. For a successful block the local anaesthetic should spread medially towards the femoral nerve and laterally towards the iliac spine.
Limitations	Obturator not reliably blocked Not sole anaesthetic technique
Block-specific complications	Nil – general risks apply

Are there any contraindications to these blocks described?

When answering questions about contraindications to regional techniques, divide your answer into those common to all blocks and those specific to the block in question.

Common to all blocks

- Patient refusal
- Bleeding risk – anticoagulation/antiplatelet medications, bleeding disorders
- Local inflammation/infection over injection site
- Reported allergy to LA agents

Block specific
- Previous femoral bypass surgery

What is the adductor canal? When is adductor canal block used?

The adductor canal is a pyramidal-shaped tunnel running from the apex of the femoral triangle to the adductor hiatus. It runs anterolateral to the vastus medialis muscle and posteromedially to the adductor longus and magnus muscles. Important contents of this canal include the saphenous nerve, nerve to vastus medialis with femoral artery and vein.

The innervation of the knee comes from contributions from both the lumbar (femoral nerve) and sacral plexuses (sciatic nerve). By infiltrating the adductor canal with local anaesthetic only the medial aspect of the knee will be anaesthetised. Therefore, the adductor canal block can be used as part of a multimodal analgesic regime for knee surgery, which together will provide superior analgesia and enhance functional recovery after knee arthroplasty, while limiting the adverse effects of a single drug or procedure alone. Landmark or US guidance can be used to infiltrate a small amount (5–10 ml) of LA in the canal. Landmarks for this block are described in the table and can be difficult to identify, which is why US guidance is proving a popular technique.

Lateral   Anterior   Medial

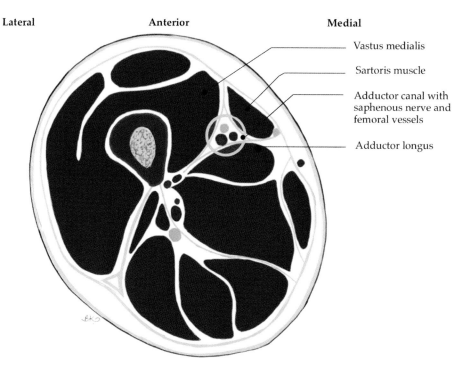

Vastus medialis

Sartoris muscle

Adductor canal with
saphenous nerve and
femoral vessels

Adductor longus

Figure 6.11   Adductor canal – relations.

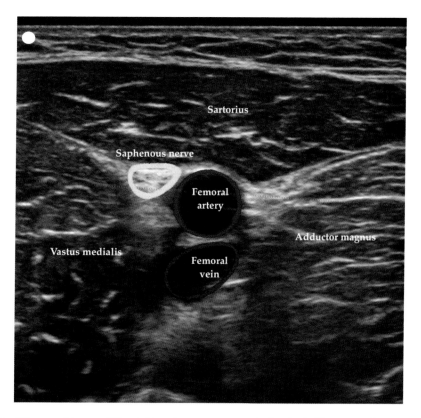

Figure 6.12   Ultrasound image of the right saphenous nerve at the level of adductor canal.

Table 6.10   Summary of Adductor Canal Block

Adductor canal block	
Indications	Saphenous vein grafting, multimodal analgesia for knee, medial foot and ankle surgery
Nerves blocked	Saphenous nerve (branch of femoral)
Volume of LA	5–10 ml
Patient position	Supine, knee of side to be blocked flexed and slightly rotated
Landmarks	Adductor canal in between sartorius and adductor longus muscle, at mid-thigh level Canal contains saphenous nerve, femoral artery and vein
Technique with ultrasound	With the patient supine, and the knee externally rotated and slightly flexed, the ultrasound probe is positioned axially at mid-thigh and femoral artery is visualised. The probe is then moved medially and distally to identify a point between the middle and distal third of the thigh where the artery lies deep to the sartorius and proximal to the adductor hiatus where the saphenous nerve is anterolateral to the artery. The needle is inserted in-plane from lateral to medial till the tip lies superficial to the artery. Local anesthetic: 10–15 ml after haem-free aspirate and hydrolocation
Limitations	Purely sensory block
Block-specific complications	Nil – general risks apply

Sciatic nerve block

What are the various approaches to blocking the sciatic nerve?

There are a variety of approaches to the sciatic nerve given its long course (Table 6.11; Figures 6.13, 6.14, 6.15 and 6.16).

Table 6.11   Summary of Sciatic Nerve Blocks

Sciatic nerve blocks		
Indications	Analgesia for knee surgery, lower limb surgery and foot	
Nerve blocked	Sciatic nerve	
Volume of LA	10–20 ml in 5 ml aliquots	
Position	Landmarks	Needle insertion/direction
Raj (posterior approach)		Needle inserted medial to midpoint of this line Perpendicular to skin ~6 cm depth
Supine Leg flexed 90° at hip and knee	Line from greater trochanter to ischial tuberosity	
Labat (posterior approach)		Needle inserted perpendicular to skin ~5–10 cm depth Nerve stimulation end point aim for gastrocnemius contraction at 0.5 mA – plantar flexion (tibial); dorsiflexion (peroneal)
Lateral, operative side up	Midpoint of line from greater trochanter to sacral hiatus	
Beck's (anterior approach)		Needle insertion at the intersection point which approximates inferior trochanteric position Insert until the needle hits femoral shaft. Then redirect medially to slide off and direct 5 cm into skin to catch the nerve in the lesser trochanter region.
Supine	Line 1: ASIS to pubic tubercle Line 2: parallel to line 1 but from greater trochanter Line 3: line drawn perpendicularly from the medial 2/3 of line 1 to intersect line 2	
Limitations	Beck's approach: 15% of sciatic nerves lie immediately posterior to femur and are therefore missed.	
Block-specific complications	Nil – general risks apply	

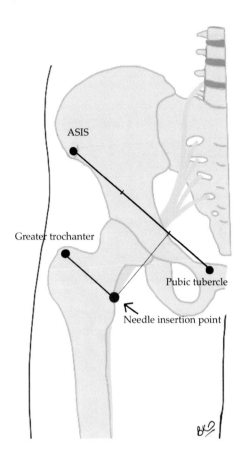

Figure 6.13   Sciatic nerve block – anterior approach.

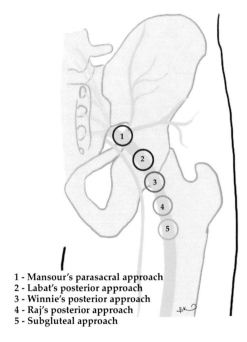

1 - Mansour's parasacral approach
2 - Labat's posterior approach
3 - Winnie's posterior approach
4 - Raj's posterior approach
5 - Subgluteal approach

Figure 6.14   Sciatic nerve block – posterior approaches.

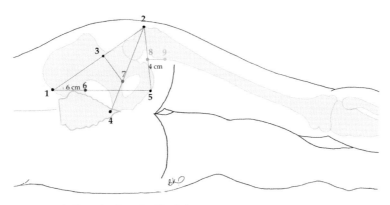

1 - Posterior Superior Iliac Spine
2 - Greater trochanter
3 - midpoint between 1 and 2
4 - Sacral hiatus
5 - Ischial tuberosity
6 - Injection point for Mansour's parasacral approach
7 - Injection point for Labat's transgluteal approach
8 - Injection point for Rāj's infragluteal approach
9 - Injection point for subgluteal approach

Figure 6.15   Sciatic nerve block – points of injection in different approaches.

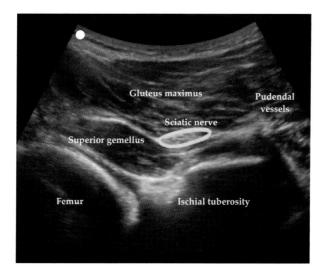

Figure 6.16   Ultrasound image of sciatic nerve at gluteal level.

What are the advantages and disadvantages of the posterior and anterior approaches to the sciatic nerve block?

The posterior approach described by Labat is the most popular and reliable technique but requires the patient to be turned into a lateral, almost semi prone position.

When patient positioning is difficult, e.g. due to trauma, the leg can be splinted in this position or another approach can be employed. The popular alternatives in this situation would be Beck's and Raj's approach with the patient supine, with Beck's approach easiest for patient positioning. There are disadvantages with Beck's approach compared with posterior approaches

- The needle crosses more tissue and muscle planes and is therefore more uncomfortable for the patient
- The block is more distal and therefore there is a higher chance of missing the posterior cutaneous nerve of the thigh meaning that if a procedure required a thigh tourniquet, it would not be well tolerated
- The sciatic nerve is blocked posteromedial to the lesser trochanter, and in 30% of the population the sciatic nerve is anterior to the lesser trochanter at this point
- The femoral vessels and femoral nerve lie anterior and medial to the femoral shaft and there is theoretical risk of injuring these structures

How would you perform the popliteal block?

The sciatic nerve consists of the tibial and common peroneal nerves enveloped by a common sheath (Vloka's sheath) and the nerves diverge 5–12 cm proximal to the popliteal fossa crease. In the popliteal fossa, the sciatic nerve components are lateral and superficial to the popliteal artery and vein (Table 6.12).

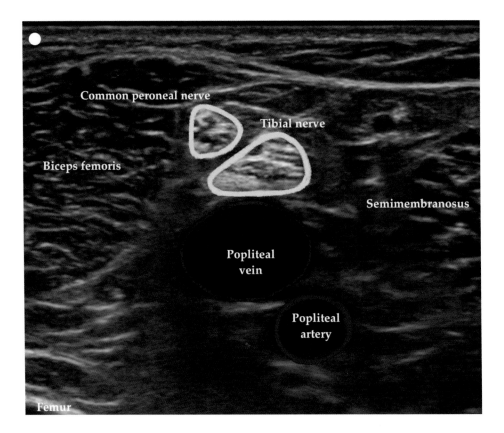

Figure 6.17   Ultrasound image of sciatic nerve at popliteal level.

Table 6.12 Summary of Popliteal Block

Popliteal block	
Indications	Foot and ankle surgery, lower limb angioplasty and stripping of short saphenous venous system
Nerves blocked	Components of the sciatic nerve
Volume of LA	20 ml
Patient position	Prone
Landmarks	Popliteal fossa crease, tendons of biceps femoris laterally, semitendinosus and semimembranosus medially
Technique with nerve stimulator	Patient in prone position, identify popliteal fossa crease, tendons of biceps femoris, semitendinosus and semimembranosus. The needle is inserted 7 cm above the popliteal fossa crease at the midpoint between the tendons. Nerve stimulator: 1.5 mA initially to 0.2–0.5 mA Endpoint: dorsiflexion and eversion of the foot if common peroneal nerve is stimulated, plantar flexion and inversion if tibial nerve is stimulated 20 ml of local anaesthetic is injected after negative aspiration
Technique with ultrasound	The popliteal vessels are identified with the transducer placed transversely in the popliteal crease. At this point, the tibial nerve is lateral and superficial to the popliteal vein and the common peroneal nerve more laterally. The probe is moved cranially to view the sciatic nerve before it divides, and this is usually 5–12 cm above the popliteal crease. An in-plane or out-of-plane approach can be used to target the nerve. Local anaesthetic: after haem-free aspirate, 20 ml is injected whilst observing the circumferential spread of the solution around the nerve.
Block-specific complications	Nil – general risks apply

How can the sciatic nerve be damaged in the perioperative setting?

Anaesthetic causes

- Direct damage from needle in regional techniques
- Drug toxicity from intraneural injections

Surgical causes

- Direct trauma to the nerve
- Retractor compression
- Stretch or compression due to positioning or traction
- Heat injury (cement)
- Compression from haematoma development

Medical causes
- IM buttock injections

Tell me about the cutaneous innervation to the ankle and foot.

Skin of the ankle and foot is supplied by five nerves

- Saphenous nerve (L2–L4)
- Tibial nerve (L4–L5, S1–S3)
- Superficial peroneal nerve (L4–L5, S1)
- Deep peroneal nerve (L4–L5, S1)
- Sural nerve (L5, S1–S2)

All are terminal branches of the sciatic nerve, except for the saphenous nerve which is a branch of the femoral nerve. These nerves originate from the lumbar plexus (femoral nerve) and the sacral plexus (sciatic nerve).

Branch of femoral nerve (L2–L4)

The femoral nerve originates from the anterior rami of L2–L4 nerves and the saphenous nerve is the largest cutaneous branch of the femoral nerve.

Saphenous nerve: arises from the base of the femoral triangle and descends the leg towards the ankle, remaining lateral to the femoral artery. It remains in the adductor canal in the thigh and emerges between the gracilis and sartorius muscles before descending down the medial border of the tibia, just behind the great saphenous vein. At the medial malleolus, the saphenous nerve crosses to be in front of the vein.

It has no motor function but supplies an extensive cutaneous area over the medial side of the foot and ankle, as well as the medial aspect of knee and leg.

Branches of sciatic nerve (L4–L5, S1–S3)

The sciatic nerve provides sensory innervation to most of the lower limb below the knee, apart from the skin overlying the medial side of knee, lower leg and ankle. At the apex of the popliteal fossa, the sciatic nerve splits to give off its terminal branches – the common peroneal nerve and tibial nerve.

The *tibial nerve* is the larger of the two branches and normally arises from the apex of the popliteal space and traverses the posterior aspect of the knee joint. It gives off branches to muscles in the superficial posterior compartment of the lower leg and here, it gives rise to the sural nerve. The tibial nerve continues its descent down the tibia alongside the posterior tibial vessels supplying the deeper muscles of the posterior leg. At the foot, the nerve passes posteroinferior to the medial malleolus through the tarsal tunnel and distal to this, the tibial nerve terminates by dividing into its sensory branches innervating the sole of the foot.

The *sural nerve* arises in the popliteal fossa between the two heads of the gastrocnemius, piercing its fascia halfway down the leg, and receives branches from the peroneal nerve before descending behind the lateral malleolus, running alongside the lateral side of the foot to the fifth toe. It is responsible for the innervation of the skin over the posterolateral part of the lower third of the calf, as well as the lateral side of the foot and of the fifth toe.

The *common peroneal nerve* descends from the apex of the popliteal fossa along the border of the biceps femoris. It wraps around the neck of the fibula and divides into its terminal branches (superficial and deep peroneal nerve).

The *superficial peroneal nerve* descends between the fibularis muscles and lateral side of the extensor digitorum longus. It gives rise to its motor branches before continuing down the leg with purely sensory fibres innervating the anterolateral aspect of the lower leg.

The *deep peroneal nerve* passes medially from the lateral compartment of the leg to the anterior compartment following the course of the anterior tibial artery. The two structures descend between the tibialis anterior muscle and the extensor digitorum longus and inferiorly between the tibialis anterior muscle and the extensor hallucis longus. The deep peroneal nerve crosses the ankle joint anterior to the distal tibia and lies deep to the extensor retinaculum before terminating in the dorsum of the foot into lateral and medial branches. It is responsible for innervation of the webbed space of the skin between the great and second toe.

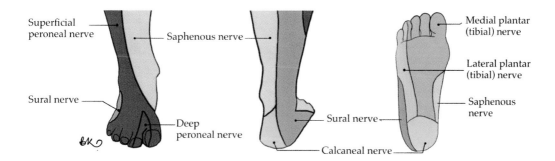

Figure 6.18   Peripheral nerve distribution of the leg and ankle.

You have a 78-year-old gentleman with a history of COPD for hallux valgus surgery on the orthopaedic list. **What are the options for regional block for this procedure?**

- Central neuraxial blockade
- Lumbar plexus block
- Popliteal fossa sciatic nerve block
- Digital block
- Surgical infiltration
- Ankle blank

What are the indications for ankle block?

Ankle block can be used as a sole anaesthetic technique for foot surgeries including bunionectomy, forefoot reconstruction, osteotomy, foreign body removal and amputation. It can also provide excellent postoperative analgesia for foot and ankle procedures. The block impairs ambulation to a lesser degree than the sciatic or popliteal blocks and this block may be preferable for outpatient forefoot surgery.

It can be used as analgesia for fracture, soft tissue injuries in the foot and for gout.

Furthermore, it can be used for diagnostic and therapeutic purposes with spastic equinovarus and sympathetically mediated pain. Depending on the type of the procedure, specific nerves could be blocked rather than all of the five nerves.

Using landmark technique, describe how you would perform an ankle block. What volume of local anaesthetic is commonly injected for each nerve?

Ankle blocks can be performed under ultrasound guidance, but the nerves are blocked more proximally due to the difficulty in obtaining a good view with bony prominences and it can be difficult to see exact margins of smaller nerves.

- *General measures*

  Patient consented, IV access, AAGBI monitoring and 'stop before you block' after positioning patient, sterility ensured throughout, ensure local anaesthetic drugs prepared and nerve stimulator available (tibial nerve is the only nerve which can be located with aid of nerve stimulation).

- *Patient position*: supine
- *Landmarks*

  See table below for landmarks for these nerves. Always start with the tibial nerve as it is the largest nerve and takes longest to block (up to 20 minutes).

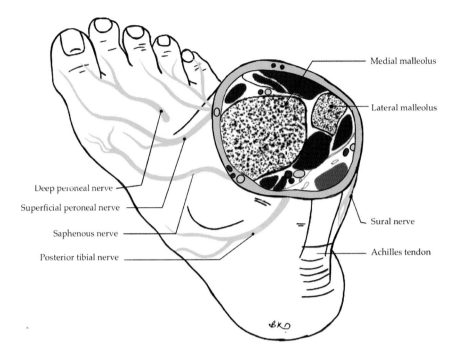

Figure 6.19   Ankle block – position of individual nerves.

Table 6.13   **Summary of Ankle Block**

Nerve and volume	Supply	Landmarks and technique
Tibial 5 ml	Sole of the foot	Landmark: medial malleolus, Achilles tendon, posterior tibial artery Technique: needle insertion halfway between medial malleolus and tip of calcaneum. Insert needle behind the pulsation of posterior tibial artery. Nerve stimulation end point: plantar flexion of toes
Saphenous 5 ml	Medial aspect of foot down to great toe	Landmark: medial malleolus, great saphenous vein Technique: inject immediately above medial malleolus or palpate great saphenous vein and introduce needle posterior to it
Sural 2-3 ml	Lateral aspect of foot	Landmark: lateral malleolus, Achilles tendon Technique: needle inserted halfway between lateral malleolus and Achilles tendon towards lateral malleolus
Superficial peroneal 5 ml	Dorsum of foot	Landmark: lateral and medial malleolus Technique: subcutaneous injection along intermalleolar line to raise a subcutaneous wheal
Deep peroneal 2-3 ml	1st web space	Landmark: extensor hallucis longus, dorsalis pedis Technique: seek nerve lateral to dorsalis pedis

What are the consequences to a patient following inadvertent wrong-sided peripheral nerve block?

- May lead to wrong site surgery
- Increased risk of local anaesthetic toxicity (if another block is required)
- Exposing patient to unnecessary block and risks associated with the block
- Delayed hospital discharge
- Reduced mobility or dexterity

What measures can be taken to prevent a wrong-sided block?

The RCOA have introduced the 'stop before you block' process on top of the routine WHO checklist. During the procedure, they recommend that following the routine WHO sign in immediately prior to the needle insertion, the correct site is confirmed again. The anaesthetist and the assistant must check

- Surgical site marking
- Side of the block on consent

When are the factors that may increase wrong-sided peripheral nerve block?

The 'stop before you block' campaign has highlighted some circumstances where particular vigilance is required.

- When there has been a distraction in the anaesthetic room, e.g. extra personnel, discussion of other cases, etc.
- There is a time delay in WHO sign in and performance of the block
- After turning the patient – block site will be on a different side relative to the anaesthetist
- When the person performing the block does not routinely perform regional anaesthesia

Other clinical application questions...

1. Local anaesthetic toxicity

Bibliography

Al-Haddad, M. F., & Coventry, D. M. (2003). Major nerve blocks of the lower limb. *BJA CEPD Reviews*, *3*(4), 102–105.

Bricker, S. (2017). *The Anaesthesia Science Viva Book.* Cambridge University Press, Cambridge, UK.

Ellis, H., & Mahadevan, V. (2018). *Clinical Anatomy: Applied Anatomy for Students and Junior Doctors.* Wiley-Blackwell.

Ftouh, S., Morga, A., & Swift, C. (2011). Management of hip fracture in adults: Summary of NICE guidance. *BMJ, 342*, d3304.

Kopka, A., & Serpell, M. G. (2005). Distal nerve blocks of the lower limb. *Continuing Education in Anaesthesia, Critical Care & Pain, 5*(5), 166–170.

Maxwell, L., & White, S. (2013). Anaesthetic management of patients with hip fractures: An update. *Continuing Education in Anaesthesia, Critical Care & Pain, 13*(5), 179–183.

Nysora.com. (2019). [Online] Retrieved 9 August 2019 from www.nysora.com/files/2013/pdf/. (v12p24-27) sciaticanteriorapproach.pdf.

O'Donnell, R., & Dolan, J. (2018). Anaesthesia and analgesia for knee joint arthroplasty. *BJA Education*, *18*(1), 8–15.

Prout, J., Jones, T., & Martin, D. (Eds.). (2014). *Advanced Training in Anaesthesia*. Oxford: OUP.

RCOA.ac.uk. (2019) [Online] Retrieved 9 August 2019 from www.rcoa.ac.uk/sites/default/files/CSQ-PS-sby b-supporting.pdf.

Teachmeanatomy.info. (2019). *The Femoral Triangle - Borders - Contents - TeachMeAnatomy* [Online]. Retrieved 9 August 2019 from https://teachmeanatomy.info/lower-limb/areas/femoral-triangle/.

Teachmeanatomy.info. (2019). *The Lumbar Plexus - Spinal Nerves - Branches - TeachMeAnatomy* [Online]. Retrieved 9 August 2019 from https://teachmeanatomy.info/lower-limb/nerves/lumbar-plexus/.

Teachmeanatomy.info. (2019). *The Sacral Plexus - Spinal Nerves - Branches - TeachMeAnatomy* [Online]. Retrieved 9 August 2019 from https://teachmeanatomy.info/lower-limb/nerves/sacral-plexus/.

MISCELLANEOUS

7

- Nerve – structure and damage
- Pain pathway
- Nerve stimulators and ultrasound in regional anaesthesia
- AAGBI guidelines for regional anaesthesia in patients taking anticoagulants and antiplatelets
- Autonomic nervous system
- Labour analgesia
- Placenta
- Fetal circulation
- Bone circulation
- Anatomical differences between paediatric and adult airway

Anatomy of the Nerve

Peripheral nerves are formed of axons of neurons with cell bodies that reside in the central nervous system.

Endoneurium surrounds the axon from its origin in the spinal cord to where it synapses. The endoneurium also surrounds the myelin sheath and Schwann cells in some peripheral nerves.

Perineurium is a connective tissue layer that surrounds the axons which are arranged in fascicles by axon diameter with the largest being most proximal.

Epineurium surrounds the perineurium which acts as a selective barrier producing endoneurial fluid that surrounds the axons.

The blood supply to nerves is formed from the anastomosis of a plexus of vessels in the epineural space and the intrinsic circulation of the endoneurium (Figures 7.1, 7.2 and 7.3).

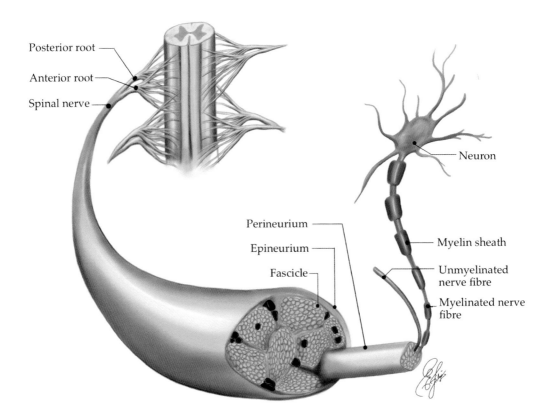

Figure 7.1 Nerve structure.

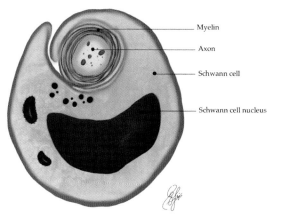

Figure 7.2   Cross section of myelinated nerve.

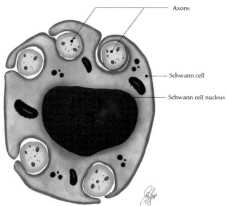

Figure 7.3   Cross section of unmyelinated nerve.

What are the causes of perioperative peripheral nerve damage?

The main causes of perioperative nerve damage are listed below.

- Direct nerve damage (trauma) – e.g. surgery, regional anaesthesia
- Drug toxicity – local anaesthetic agents produce cytotoxic axonal damage especially with intraneural injection
- Stretch and compression – e.g. poor padding, extreme positioning of limbs, tourniquet use
- Double crush syndrome – explains that patients with pre-existing peripheral neuropathy are at increased risk of peripheral nerve damage. Nerves which have experienced a compressive lesion or previous insult renders them less tolerant to compression at the same or at another location.
- Ischaemia – this is the final common pathway of nerve injury, e.g. prolonged immobility, tourniquet use, haematoma and local anaesthetic agents

What are the risk factors of perioperative peripheral nerve damage?

Patient risk factors

- Pre-existing peripheral neuropathies, e.g. rheumatoid arthritis, diabetes
- Pre-existing vascular disease, e.g. severe peripheral vascular disease, diabetes mellitus, smoking, hypertension
- Advancing age
- Male sex
- Extremes of body habitus
- Anatomical abnormalities, e.g. thoracic outlet syndrome

Anaesthetic risk factors

- General anaesthesia and neuraxial blocks are associated with higher incidence of peripheral nerve damage compared to sedation
- Perioperative hypotension, hypoxia, hypothermia, electrolyte disturbances

Surgical risk factors

- Neurosurgery, cardiac surgery, GI and orthopaedic surgery are associated with higher chance of nerve damage
- Prolonged surgery
- Improper patient positioning and extremes of positioning
- Use of tourniquets and other direct surgical mechanical compression/stretch to the nerve
- Use of compressive dressing/casts
- Haematoma/abscess formation

What are the different types of nerve damage that can occur and what are their prognoses?

Damage to a peripheral nerve may manifest as a sensory and/or motor deficit. Seddon and Sunderland are two different classifications of peripheral nerve damage that are commonly used and classify nerve damage according to the damage seen histologically (Figure 7.4).

These different types of nerve damage may be distinguished using electromyography (EMG). Prognosis is dependent upon the amount of damage to the nerve with full recovery seen in months in those cases with little damage and absence of complete recovery in nerves with more damage (Table 7.1).

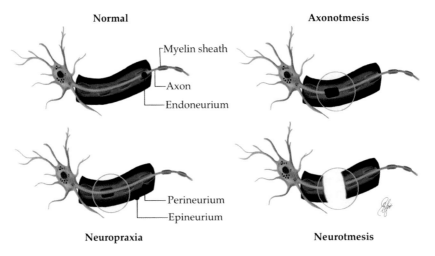

Figure 7.4   Types of nerve damage. A – undamaged nerve; B – neuropraxia; C – axonotmesis; D – neurotmesis.

Table 7.1   Seddon's and Sunderland's Classifications of Nerve Damage and Their
Characteristics

Seddon	Sunderland	Pathophysiology	EMG findings	Prognosis
Neuropraxia (compression)	*Type 1*	Local myelin damage only. Nerve is intact.	Normal or decreased	Recovery within months
Axonotmesis (crush)	*Type 2*	Axon structure and flow disrupted with Wallerian degeneration. Endo-, peri- epineurium still intact.	May be normal in acute phase. Abnormal activity after 10–14 days	Recovery within months
	Type 3	Type 2 + endoneurial injury		Poor once endoneurium is breached. Surgery may be required; recovery is dependent on nerve regeneration.
	Type 4	Type 3 + perineural injury (Epineurium still intact)		
Neurotmesis (transection)	*Type 5*	Disruption of all three layers	Abnormal activity – fibrillation and positive sharp waves	Surgery required; prognosis is guarded.

Which peripheral nerves are most commonly injured perioperatively?

Upper limb

- Ulnar nerve (C7–T1) – most common perioperative peripheral nerve injury (incidence 0.037%) due to the proximity of the nerve to medial condyle. Damage is caused by direct pressure on ulnar groove and prolonged forearm flexion.
- Brachial plexus injury (C5–T1) – due to the superficial positioning of the plexus and its course through limited space between clavicle and first rib. Damage is caused by compression, stretching or direct injury from regional technique.
- Radial nerve (C5–T1) – due to course of radial nerve along spiral groove of humerus. Damage is caused commonly by compression of non-invasive blood pressure cuffs, tourniquets and incorrectly positioned arm boards.
- Median nerve (C5–T1) – due to direct nerve damage from regional techniques or compression in carpal tunnel
- Axillary (C5–C6) and musculocutaneous nerves (C5–C7) – result from shoulder surgery or dislocations

Lower limb

- Sciatic nerve (L4–S3) – due to the long course of the sciatic nerve, there are multiple points where it can be injured. Damage is caused by surgical positioning in lithotomy, frog leg and sitting positions (hyperflexion of hip, extension of leg).

- Femoral nerve (L2–L4) – often compressed at pelvic brim by retractors used in abdominal or pelvic surgery. Damage is usually caused by surgical positioning (lithotomy) and ischaemic damage seen during aortic cross clamp.

- Superficial peroneal nerve (L4–S2) – often compressed at the fibular head. Direct injury during knee surgery and surgical positioning (lateral and lithotomy) also brings about the damage.

How do we prevent peripheral nerve damage in the perioperative period?

The American Society of Anesthesiologists (ASA) formulated advice for prevention of peripheral nerve damage but this is based on empiric knowledge and consensus opinion as there is currently little evidence to substantiate this advice.

- A thorough history and examination of the patient to identify any predisposing conditions as well as a thorough knowledge of anatomy and risks posed by positioning of patient perioperatively is crucial.

- Utmost care with positioning of patient in theatre

  ○ Brachial plexus: arm abduction limited to <90° in supine position

  ○ Median and ulnar nerves: padding and flexion of elbow limited to ≤90°

  ○ Femoral and sciatic nerves: adequate padding in lithotomy and lateral positioning and hip flexion ≤120°

- Early postoperative assessment of the patient may lead to early recognition of peripheral nerve damage. Currently, no nerve monitoring technique has been shown to successfully prevent peripheral nerve damage intraoperatively.

Bibliography

Lalkhen, A. G., & Bhatia, K. (2011). Perioperative peripheral nerve injuries. *Continuing Education in Anaesthesia, Critical Care & Pain, 12*(1), 38–42.

Marhofer, P. (2010). *Ultrasound Guidance in Regional Anaesthesia: Principles and Practical Implementation.* Oxford: OUP.

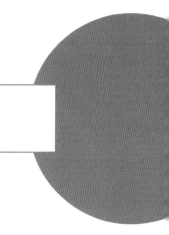

Pain Pathway

Can you explain how pain sensation is transmitted from the periphery to the brain?

- *Nociceptors*

  Nociceptors are free, unmyelinated nerve endings of primary afferent (or first order) neurons and are responsible for sensing the initial nociceptive stimuli (mechanical, thermal and chemical). These stimuli include histamine, leukotrienes, potassium, bradykinin and prostaglandins which indicate tissue damage. Nociceptors can be unimodal (responding to only one stimulus) or polymodal (responding to multiple stimuli) and initiate an action potential which is carried up the first order neuron.

- *First order neuron/primary afferents*

  First order neurons relay action potentials from peripheral nociceptors to the spinal cord. There are two different types of first order neurons which carry pain sensation centrally

  - Type Aδ fibres – respond to mechanical and thermal stimuli and have large (2–5 μm) myelinated axons with higher conduction velocities (12–30 m/s). They are responsible for carrying sharp and well localised sensations of pain.

  - Type C fibres – respond to thermal, mechanical and chemical stimuli. These have smaller (0.4–1 μm) unmyelinated axons with slower conduction velocities (0.5–2 m/s) and produce a pain of dull, poorly localised character which is felt often after pain mediated by Aδ.

  These first order neurons have their cell bodies in the dorsal root ganglion and synapse with interneurons or second order neurons in the laminae of Rexed I and IV (Aδ fibres) or the laminae II and III of substantia gelatinosa (C fibres).

- *Second order neuron*

  Secondary afferents continue transmission of nociceptive signal to the brain and decussate near the level of entry of the primary afferent and ascend in the lateral spinothalamic tract. These afferents synapse in the thalamus with third order neurons. Second order neurones also give off projections (e.g. to peri-aqueductal gray, locus coeruleus) to areas of the brain involved in pain modulation.

- *Third order neuron*

  These neurones are responsible for relaying nociceptive signals to somatosensory areas in cortex which are then interpreted as pain.

What can you tell me about modulation of pain impulses?

This area is of great research interest and debate. To summarise, there are three best known theories.

- *The gate theory*

  Inhibitory interneurons 'gate' transmission between first and second order neurones in the substantia gelatinosa. These interneurons can be activated by afferents carrying different sensory stimulation, e.g. light touch from Aβ fibres, and from descending neurons from higher centres. Once activated, the interneurons have an inhibitory effect on the transmission between the first and second order neurons of the pain pathway.

- *Descending inhibitory pathways*

  Neurons from the higher centres project to the dorsal horn of the spinal cord and influence the ascending second order neurons. Periaqueductal gray is believed to be the main control for descending inhibition but it also receives inputs from hypothalamus, thalamus and cortex. Other significant inhibitory pathways include locus coeruleus and raphe nuclei. Serotonin and noradrenaline are thought to be the main neurotransmitters of these descending pathways.

- *Endogenous opioid system*

  Centrally located opioid receptors in the periaqueductal gray, ventral medulla and spinal cord bind to endogenous opioids (enkephalins, endorphins) causing a reduction in transmission of nociceptive signals.

What is 'wind-up'?

This describes the central sensitisation to repeated nociceptive transmission and is an important concept in chronic pain conditions. NMDA (*N*-methyl-D-aspartate) receptors normally have a tightly bound magnesium plug which inactivates the receptor in acute pain. With continuous stimulation, there is prolonged depolarisation of neurons at the dorsal horn causing a huge influx of calcium ions displacing the magnesium plug, thus allowing glutamate to bind. This augments neuronal response to peripheral nociceptive signal, i.e. there is an increased number of action potentials propagated for a given peripheral stimulus. This is an example of neuroplasticity following continuous nociceptive transmission which demonstrates the physiological differences between acute and chronic pain.

Which neurotransmitters are involved in nociceptive transmission?

There are numerous neurotransmitters with more being implied in pain transmission and modulation with ongoing research in this field.

Periphery

- Excitatory neurotransmitters at the periphery include serotonin, substance P, leukotrienes and bradykinins

Dorsal horn

- Glutamate are excitatory at AMPA (α-amino-3-hydroxy-5-methyl-4-isoxazole propionic acid) receptors as well as NMDA receptors in wind up phenomenon
- Substance P is excitatory at natural killer (NK) cell receptors

Spinal cord and higher centres

- Glutamate is the most important excitatory and GABA (gamma-aminobutyric acid) is the main inhibitory neurotransmitter

- Endogenous opioids (enkephalins, endorphins and dynorphins) have an inhibitory effect on receptors in periaqueductal gray
- Serotonin and noradrenaline are important neurotransmitters of the descending inhibitory pathways which modulates ascending nociceptive signals

Where do analgesic drugs act in these pathways?

- NSAIDs – cyclo-oxygenase inhibitors which reduce inflammation and the production of endogenous algogens (i.e. reduce stimulation of nociceptors)
- Opioids – ligands for G-protein coupled opioid receptors in the CNS (esp. the periaqueductal gray and substantia gelatinosa) and in the periphery
- Ketamine – non-competitive antagonist of the NMDA calcium channel pore, may have some effect on opioid receptors
- Gabapentin – exact mechanism unknown. Inhibits voltage dependent calcium channels in CNS and may stimulate production and release of GABA
- Tricyclic antidepressants – prevent reuptake of noradrenaline and 5-hydroxy tryptamine thereby increasing modification of nociceptive signals by descending pathways
- Local anaesthetics – block sodium influx into neurons and prevent propagation of action potential
- Clonidine – agonist of pre- and postsynaptic $\alpha2$ receptors
- Capsaicin – depletes neurones of substance P

Bibliography

Singh, V. (2014). *Textbook of Clinical Neuroanatomy.* Elsevier Health Sciences.

Nerve Stimulators for Regional Anaesthesia

There are two types of nerve stimulators commonly used in anaesthesia

1. For localisation of nerves during regional nerve blocks
2. Monitoring of neuromuscular blockade

We will be focusing on the first type in this chapter.

What is the physiological basis of nerve stimulation?

Ultimate aim of nerve stimulation is to cause depolarisation of motor nerve in order to cause muscle contraction (twitch) visible to the eye.

The electrical energy delivered by a nerve stimulator should be sufficient to cause increase in membrane potential so as to exceed the threshold potential leading to depolarisation and propagation of an action potential.

The stimulus applied must be strong enough and long enough in duration to produce an action potential and therefore, the current amplitude and the duration of the stimulus can be adjusted. The energy delivered to the nerve per stimulus can be quantified by multiplying the current amplitude and the duration of the stimulus. The other variables that can be controlled in nerve stimulation are frequency of the stimulus, polarity of the electrode and proximity of the electrode to the nerve.

What is meant by rheobase and chronaxie?

The current required to initiate an action potential in a certain nerve is known as the *rheobase*.

Chronaxie is the duration a current must be applied to the nerve to initiate an impulse when the current level is twice the rheobase. The term is often used to describe excitability of different tissues and nerves and below is a table of the chronaxie time for different nerves (Table 7.2).

Table 7.2   Chronaxie Times for Different Nerve Types

	Nerves	Chronaxie time (msec)
Unmyelinated	C	0.40
Myelinated	Aδ	0.17
Myelinated	Aα	0.05–0.10

Describe the components of a nerve stimulator.

The following components are incorporated in a nerve stimulator

- Power supply
- Constant current generator

- Oscillator – to interrupt the constant current generator and influence the frequency and duration of stimulus. This can be controlled and adjusted.
- User interface of display and controls – to adjust the amplitude and frequency of stimulation
- Complete electrical circuit using a positive anode (a standard ECG electrode) and a negative cathode (needle used for block)

What are the ideal electrical characteristics of a nerve stimulator?

- Constant current generator
- Monophasic (rectangular) output pulse, i.e. current flows in one direction only. Shape of current output is rectangular but provides no proven benefit over other shapes
- Ability to vary pulse duration: short pulse duration (0.1 msec) to ensure only motor neurons are stimulated, thereby sparing sensory neurons
- Lead should be marked to avoid confusion of cathode and anode ends
- Stimulation frequency: affects the speed of nerve localisation, normally 1–2 Hz
- Accuracy: actual current generation is close to the current dialed on display
- Alarms for circuit disconnection, low battery and high impedance

What are the characteristics of a nerve stimulator needle?

They are normally short bevelled, hollow needles with Luer lock connection at the connector end. The whole shaft of the needle is insulated apart from the tip.

They come in different sizes (20–25G) and lengths (25–150 mm) with some having depth markings on the shaft of the needle. Different procedures will require different lengths of nerve stimulator needle depending on the depth of the structure to be targeted (see Table 7.3).

Table 7.3 Needle Lengths Required for Various Regional Anaesthetic Techniques

Needle length	Regional techniques
25 mm	Interscalene block
50 mm	Cervical plexus, supraclavicular, axillary and femoral nerve block
100 mm	Infraclavicular, paravertebral, lumbar plexus and sciatic nerve block
150 mm	Anterior sciatic approach

How would you use a nerve stimulator for an axillary nerve block?

General preparation

- Informed consent, AAGBI monitoring, IV access, presence of trained assistant and emergency resuscitation equipment including intralipid
- WHO checklist and Stop Before You Block
- Ultrasound guidance available if required

- Functioning nerve stimulator (checked prior to starting) and appropriate needle for axillary nerve block (50 mm insulated 23–25G needle)
- Local anaesthetic solution prepared correctly and drawn up in sterile syringe
- Aseptic technique and sterile conditions employed throughout procedure

Use of nerve stimulator

- Ensure correct placement of electrodes – positive anode attached to ECG dot on patient and negative cathode attached to needle to complete the circuit
- Local anaesthetic syringe should be attached to the flexible tubing of the needle and both the needle and tubing are flushed with the local anaesthetic solution
- Nerve stimulator should be checked prior to use – the machine may have a flashing light and/or audible beep to indicate that there is a complete electrical circuit and is thus ready to use
- Initial stimulation should be set: 1–2 mA current, 0.1 msec duration and 2 Hz frequency.
  - Large current amplitude is required initially in order to locate target nerve
  - Duration of 50–100 msec is used as there is less stimulation of sensory fibres as motor fibres have a shorter chronaxie
- Point of needle entry is located by identifying anatomical landmarks, in this case, anterior to the axillary artery at the level of pectoralis major muscle insertion. Needle direction roughly 30–45° aiming cranially.
- Nerve stimulation should begin as soon as the needle is inserted under the skin and desired muscle twitch (stimulation end point) should be observed for as the needle is advanced slowly. Stimulation end point should correspond to the motor component of the target nerve; therefore, in the case of axillary nerve block
  - Median nerve: flexion of lateral digits
  - Ulnar nerve: flexion of fifth digit and adduction of thumb
  - Radial nerve: thumb abduction/extension of wrist
- Once end point is visualised, current amplitude is decreased until muscle contraction disappears and the current on the nerve stimulator is noted. This is to check the distance from the needle tip to the nerve and that it is not too close to risk an intraneural injection, but close enough for a successful nerve block. Acceptable current amplitude for the muscle twitch to disappear is between 0.2–0.5 mA. 0.5 mA has been traditionally thought to indicate that the needle is 1–2 mm from the nerve but recent ultrasound studies have demonstrated huge variations and therefore this estimate is inaccurate
- Inject the local anaesthetic solution once the needle is in the correct position aspirating every 3–5 ml to prevent intravascular injection

What would happen if the positive electrode were attached to the needle?

Less energy is required to stimulate the nerve that is next to the cathode rather than the anode. Therefore, the current required to produce depolarisation at a constant distance would be increased and thus increasing the risk of intraneural injection.

Bibliography

Aston, D., Rivers, A., & Dharmadasa, A. (2013). *Equipment in Anaesthesia and Critical Care: A Complete Guide for the FRCA*. Royal College of General Practitioners: London, UK.

McGrath, C. D., & Hunter, J. M. (2006). Monitoring of neuromuscular block. *Continuing Education in Anaesthesia, Critical Care & Pain*, *6*(1), 7–12.

Prout, J., Jones, T., & Martin, D. (Eds.) (2014). *Advanced Training in Anaesthesia*. Oxford: OUP.

Ultrasound for Regional Anaesthesia

Ultrasound is the use of high frequency sound waves (>20 kHz wavelength) to image soft tissues.

Soft tissue image is formed from an ultrasound probe which acts as a transducer to transmit and receive ultrasound via piezoelectric effect. The probe is made from piezoelectric crystals which have the ability to change shape and vibrate when voltage is applied thus producing sound waves, and vice versa. Ultrasound which is generated is transmitted to the patient, propagated into the tissues and is either reflected or scattered at tissue interfaces.

The reflected portion is picked up by the probe and these sound waves distort the piezoelectric material, creating electrical charge which is then amplified and used to generate an image on a monitor.

Time taken for the reflection gives the depth of tissue from the surface, i.e. distance travelled by the sound waves. The amount reflected is tissue dependent and can be referred to as the *echogenicity* of the tissue.

Highly reflective (*hyperechoic*) tissue appears white, e.g. bone; poorly reflective (*hypoechoic*) appears grey, e.g. fat; no reflection (*anechoic*) appears black, e.g. blood/air. This can also be described in terms of *tissue acoustic impedance*, i.e. the ability of sound to propagate through tissue which is greater with increasing density of the tissue (bone has high acoustic impedance). The relative changes of acoustic impedance at the interface between two tissue boundaries are picked up by the transducer to generate a two-dimensional (2-D) image.

What equipment is needed for medical ultrasound imaging?

The pieces of equipment needed for ultrasound imaging are

- An imaging system
- A transducer probe
- Conductive medium for the ultrasound to pass from the probe to the tissue with minimal attenuation. This is normally in gel form.

What types of transducers are available?

There are three types of transducers used for 2-D ultrasound imaging for regional anaesthesia.

Linear array probes: piezoelectric crystals arranged in a long line and are typically used to produce images with best axial resolution, and therefore have poor penetration of tissue. They produce a rectangular field of view and frequencies of 6–13 MHz are used with these probes.

Curved array probes: crystals arranged along a curved surface and produce lower resolution images that have better penetration and allow visualisation of deeper structures. They typically produce a diverging field of view and frequencies of 2–5 MHz are used.

Phased array probes: these probes consist of multiple active piezoelectric elements (compared to the linear and curved probes which contain a single element to generate and receive ultrasound

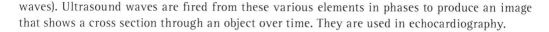

waves). Ultrasound waves are fired from these various elements in phases to produce an image that shows a cross section through an object over time. They are used in echocardiography.

Tell me about 'resolution' of an image. What are the other adjustments to the image that can be made using controls on an ultrasound machine?

Axial resolution describes the ability to separate two points when these points are in the path-line of the beam. The higher the frequency of ultrasound (and therefore shorter the wavelength), the more likely it is to distinguish these points as separate entities. However, attenuation of sound at these wavelengths is greatest and therefore depth of tissue that can be visualised is limited. To get a picture of deeper structures, resolution will be sacrificed.

The *focus* of the image can be adjusted, which concentrates the beam of ultrasound produced to the region of interest to be narrow and thus improves the lateral resolution.

The brightness of the overall image or *gain* can be changed by amplifying or attenuating the overall received signal to obtain an optimal image.

Time-gain compensation (TGC) – allows for differential amplification of signals from different depths. Signals that are received from structures that lie deep are attenuated more than signals that are received from similar structures that are more superficial; this is to compensate for using TGC. It allows for equal amplitudes from all depths to be displayed.

Tell me about the different modes used in ultrasound study.

Modern scanners that are in use come in various modes.

- *A-mode (Amplitude)* is rarely used alone

  This is the simplest of ultrasound modes and allows depth of tissue structures to be noted from single ultrasound wave emitted

- *B-mode (Brightness)* is the most common mode

  Linear array of ultrasound waves are emitted and provides a cross-sectional 2-D image of the body. Different echogenicity of tissue can be seen

- *M-mode (Motion)*

  It is a specialised B-mode used in medical imaging where the soft tissue imaged is repeatedly bombarded with one particular ultrasound line (the 'm-line'). In other words, the mechanism of image generation is to ensonify the tissue with the 'm-line' of ultrasound. It generates a time motion display of ultrasound wave and due to its high sampling rate and high time resolution, rapid movement of structures can be seen

- *C-mode (Colour)*

  In *C-mode*, the direction of blood is estimated and encoded as a colour image which is superimposed on B-mode

- *D-mode (Doppler)*

  It utilises the doppler effect whereby soundwaves change in frequency when reflected off a moving object, e.g. blood. There are various forms

  - *Continuous wave (CW)*: image formed is a result of velocities of all objects that ultrasound beam has encountered. It is displayed as a velocity against time in a graph or produces a corresponding audible sound of flow, e.g. of arterial blood. Used in transoesophageal cardiac output monitoring

○ *Pulsed wave (PW)*: similar to CW but doppler information sampled from only a small volume and presented on a velocity against time graph. It alternates transmission and reception of ultrasound in a similar way to M-mode.

○ *Colour*: velocity information presented as colour on a 2-D image

○ *Duplex PW*: doppler information presented simultaneously in 2-D form

Other modalities that are increasingly used include 3-D (which takes several contiguous B-mode slices and stacks them together), contrast imaging and elastography.

How may physical factors influence the image quality of an ultrasound device?

Factors to do with tissue/structure of soft tissue

- Similarities in acoustic impedance of tissue can make them difficult to distinguish due to the lack of contrast resolution between two materials.

Factors to do with interaction of ultrasound with tissues

- *Attenuation*: echo energy reflected from deeper structures will be weaker compared to superficial structures of similar composition as more energy is scattered and absorbed. TGC is used to overcome this.

- *Refraction*: much like light energy, when ultrasound waves travel through different mediums, a change in its velocity can alter its direction and cause it to bend. Refraction of ultrasound beams can produce artefacts whereby returning signals are incorrectly located.

- *Diffraction*: weakening of power intensity of the ultrasound beam from its source. This can be adjusted by adjusting the focus of the beam.

- *Scattering*: most of the ultrasound beam will be lost (scattered) if it is directed perpendicular to an object. The energy is lost to surrounding structures and will alter the echo image generated. Regions of increased scatter are hyperechoic compared to adjacent tissues, the reverse is true for hypoechoic appearances.

- *Speckle*: describes the grainy appearance of images on ultrasound. This is a form of visual artefact due to scattering waves returning at different velocities and depends on the nature of the tissue and its depth.

- *Acoustic enhancement*: this occurs where a fluid-filled cyst acts as a lens focusing the beam on deeper structures and therefore, distorting the image produced.

- *Reverberation*: multiple reflections occur resulting in overlapping images.

Factors to do with use of ultrasound probe

- Frequency of sound waves used
- Type of probe used
- *Anisotropy*: small changes in angle of the transducer held in relation to the organ can dramatically reduce the amount of beam reflected to transducer and thus the echogenicity of the object will vary.

What do nerves look like in ultrasonography?

The correct description of appearance of peripheral nerves in ultrasonography is based on echogenicity of the nerve and its form or shape. Nerve structures appear hypoechoic (due to large percentage of neuronal structures) with a hyperechoic surrounding (due to increased percentage

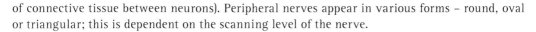

of connective tissue between neurons). Peripheral nerves appear in various forms – round, oval or triangular; this is dependent on the scanning level of the nerve.

In regional anaesthesia, nerves are normally visualised in a transverse view, with the longitudinal view being of little clinical importance.

Which two needling techniques are commonly used in ultrasound guided nerve blocks and what are the advantages and disadvantages of each?

One of the main advantages of using ultrasound to guide procedures is that the needle used can be visualised and thus the procedure is no longer a blind one. Adequate visualisation of needles is mandatory for safe and effective blocks. There are two main techniques of doing this

- *Out-of-plane technique*

  Needle insertion is along the short axis of the ultrasound probe, i.e. perpendicular to transducer. Only the needle tip can be seen, and it will appear as a hyperechoic dot (white dot) on the monitor as it crosses the beam. Depending on the depth of the structure to be targeted, the angle of the needle needs to be adjusted with flat angles for superficial structures and steeper angles for deeper structures. Steeper angles are associated with better visibility of the tip compared to flat angles.

- *In-plane technique*

  Needle insertion is along the long axis of the probe, i.e. parallel to ultrasound beams. In this technique, the entire needle should be visualised longitudinal to the scanning head. This technique necessitates that the needle is located inside a 1 mm longitudinal area; slight deviations to this will cause the needle to disappear from the ultrasound window. The ultrasound appearance of the needle is significantly better at shallow angles of insertion. Historically, this has been the preferred technique used in regional anaesthesia but there have been adaptations to block technique in recent years to meet anatomical requirements (Table 7.4).

Table 7.4   Advantages and Disadvantages of In-Plane and Out-Of-Plane Techniques

Out-of-plane technique	In-plane technique
Advantages 1. Shorter distance between the needle to target structure and this may limit patient discomfort and make reaching deeper structures easier. 2. Catheter placement may be easier in this plane.	Advantages 1. Able to visualise tip and shaft of needle throughout procedure making puncture of vasculature less likely. 2. Insertion of angle relative to probe is fairly superficial making it useful for superficial nerve blocks.
Disadvantages 1. Accurate identification of tip is challenging – it may be difficult to differentiate between the shaft and the tip.	Disadvantages 1. Needle may need to travel further through tissue to get to target site and this will be painful for the patient and may cause additional tissue damage. 2. May be technically difficult requiring excellent hand-eye coordination and experience. 3. Advancing the needle using this technique produces reverberation artefacts.

What is the optimal approach to a nerve?

The aim of ultrasound guided nerve blocks in regional anaesthesia is to get the tip of the needle as close to the epineurium as possible, i.e. extraepineural needle tip position which will give a safe and effective block.

How would you tell if an intraneural injection has been given?

The anaesthetist may feel a 'pop' sensation as the needle goes through the fascial layer into the nerve. Additionally, in a conscious patient, they may describe paraesthesia or dysaesthesia.

If using ultrasound guidance, the injection that has been given forms black hypoechoic shadow in the nerve with some of the solution leaking out to form a small black ring around the nerve.

Bibliography

Aston, D., Rivers, A., & Dharmadasa, A. (2013). *Equipment in Anaesthesia and Critical Care: A Complete Guide for the FRCA*. Royal College of General Practitioners: London, UK.

Marhofer, P. (2010). *Ultrasound Guidance in Regional Anaesthesia: Principles and Practical Implementation*. Oxford: OUP.

Regional Anaesthesia in Patients Taking Anticoagulants and Antiplatelets

This is the summary of recommendations related to drugs used to modify coagulation and platelet function (Table 7.5).

Bibliography

www.aagbi.org/sites/default/files/rapac_2013_web.pdf AAGBI guidance Nov 2013

Table 7.5 AAGBI Guidelines for Regional Anaesthesia in Patients Taking Anticoagulants and Antiplatelets

Drug		When to stop (before central neuraxial block or catheter removal)	Administration of drug while catheter in place	When to recommence (after block or catheter removal)
Anticoagulation (oral)				
Coumarins	Warfarin	INR ≤ 1.5	Not recommended	After removal
Factor Xa inhibitor	Rivaroxaban (prophylaxis)	18 h	Not recommended	6 h
	Rivaroxaban (treatment)	48 h	Not recommended	6 h
	Apixaban (prophylaxis)	24–48 h	Not recommended	6 h
Thrombin inhibitor	Dabigatran prophylaxis or treatment		Not recommended	6 h
	(CrCl >80 ml.min^{-1})	48 h		
	(CrCl 50–80 ml.min^{-1})	72 h		
	(CrCl 30–50 ml.min^{-1})	96 h		
Anticoagulation (intravenous IV/subcutaneous SC)				
Heparins	UFH IV (treatment)	2–4 h or APTTR normal	Caution[1]	4 h
	UFH SC (prophylaxis)	2–4 h or APTTR normal	Caution[2]	1 h
	LMWH SC (prophylaxis)	12 h	Caution	4 h
	LMWH SC (treatment)	24 h	Not recommended	4 h[3]
Heparin alternatives (Factor Xa inhibitor)	Fondaparinux (prophylaxis)	26–42 h (consider anti-Xa levels)	Not recommended	6–12 h
	Fondaparinux (treatment)	Avoid (consider anti-Xa levels)	Not recommended	12 h

(*Continued*)

Table 7.5 (Continued)   AAGBI Guidelines for Regional Anaesthesia in Patients Taking Anticoagulants and Antiplatelets

	Drug	When to stop (before central neuraxial block or catheter removal)	Administration of drug while catheter in place	When to recommence (after block or catheter removal)
Antiplatelets				
COX inhibitors	NSAIDS	Nil	Yes	Nil
	Aspirin	Nil	Yes	Nil
PDE inhibitors	Dipyridamole	Nil	Yes	Nil
ADP receptor inhibitors	Clopidogrel	7 days	Not recommended	6 h
	Prasugrel	7 days	Not recommended	6 h
GP2a3b inhibitors	Tirofiban	5 days	Not recommended	6 h

Notes to table

[1] *Common for IV heparin to be given following spinal block or epidural catheter insertion – follow local guidelines.*
[2] *LMWH commonly given in prophylactic doses twice daily after surgery, but many clinicians recommend only one dose in first 24 h following block or catheter placement.*
[3] *Consider increasing this to 24 h if block is traumatic.*

Autonomic Nervous System

The autonomic nervous system is the unconscious nervous system that deals with a series of involuntary functions controlling a number of actions within organs in the body. It is separated into the sympathetic and the parasympathetic nervous systems which can be mostly seen to have complementary effects on each other. These can be identified broadly as the 'fight or flight' response or the 'rest and digest' response, respectively.

Basic anatomy

- There is an afferent and an efferent limb along with a connecting pathway
- Afferent: the afferent limb conveys data from the peripheries to the central nervous system, the receptors being located in various thoracic and abdominal organs, e.g. vagal nerve afferents which have baroreceptors in the aortic arch
- Reflex arc pathway: these are transmitted via the dorsal root ganglion or to the brain stem via the cranial nerves. The reflex arc is predominantly completed within the organ involved except some complicated reflexes which will involve the higher centres such as the brain stem and hypothalamus
- The efferent limb consists of myelinated preganglionic fibres which then synapse with unmyelinated postganglionic fibres. The synapses most often occur at ganglia, a cluster of nerve cell bodies

Sympathetic nervous system

The sympathetic nervous system consists of a chain of fused ganglia that lie adjacent to the spinal cord bilaterally.

The preganglionic fibres have cell bodies in the lateral horn of the spinal cord between the first thoracic to the second lumbar vertebrae (thoraco-lumbar outflow). These fibres travel in the primary ventral rami of a mixed spinal nerve via the white rami communicantes. They then synapse in the sympathetic chain to the postganglionic unmyelinated fibres via the grey rami communicantes to join the spinal or visceral nerve to the effector organ.

The sympathetic chain itself can be subdivided into four sections depending upon which parts it supplies

- Cervical part (superior, middle and inferior) supplies the head, neck and thorax
- Thoracic part – supplies the cardiac, pulmonary and thoracic plexus
- Lumbar part – supplies part of the coeliac plexus
- Pelvic part – supplies the sacrum

Parasympathetic nervous system

The parasympathetic nervous system consists of preganglionic fibres originating from the brain stem of the motor nuclei of cranial nerves III, VII, IX and X and from the ventral rami of sacral nerves two, three and four (cranio-sacral outflow).

The longer preganglionic fibres synapse at the ganglia and shorter postganglionic fibres synapse to the effector organ. (In the sympathetic nervous system the preganglionic fibres tend to be short and postganglionic long; the parasympathetic nervous system has long preganglionic fibres and short postganglionic part as the ganglia tend to be relatively close to the effector organ).

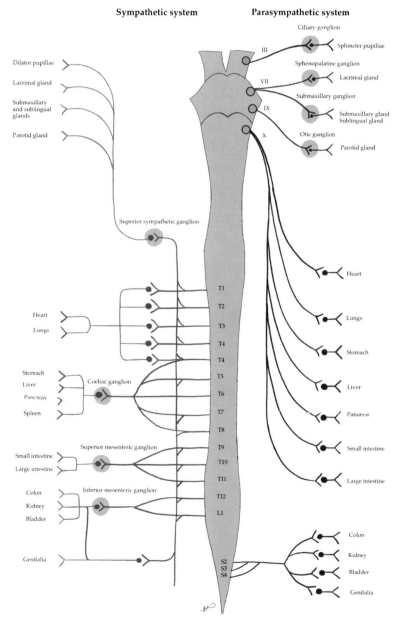

Figure 7.5   Autonomic nervous system – an overview.

Table 7.6   Comparison of Sympathetic and Parasympathetic Nervous System

Characteristics	Sympathetic system	Parasympathetic system
Origin	Thoraco-lumbar outflow Lateral horns of spinal cord segments T1–L3	Cranio-sacral outflow Brain stem nuclei of cranial nerves 3, 7, 9, 10 and Spinal cord segments S2–S4
Preganglionic fibres	Short with extensive branching	Long with minimal branching
Ganglia location	Prevertebral and paravertebral	At effector organ
Postganglionic fibres	Long	Short
Rami communicantes	White and grey rami communicantes	Absent
Neurotransmitters	Preganglionic – acetylcholine Postganglionic – norepinephrine (except sweat glands)	Preganglionic – acetylcholine Postganglionic – acetylcholine
Receptor types	Preganglionic – nicotinic Postganglionic – α1, α2, β1, β2	Preganglionic – nicotinic Postganglionic – muscarinic
Function	Prepares body for activity 'Fight and flight'	Conserves energy 'Rest and digest'

What are the differences between the white and grey rami communicantes?

The ramus communicans is a communicating branch that connects two other nerves. With respect to the sympathetic nervous system, it is the branch that transmits signals between the spinal nerves and the sympathetic trunk. There are two types of rami communicantes – white and grey.

- The white rami communicantes appear white as they have more myelinated fibres than the grey. These only exist in the intermedio-lateral column, T1 to L2, and contain preganglionic fibres **from** the spinal cord **to** the paravertebral ganglia.
- The grey rami exist at every level throughout the spinal cord and contain postganglionic fibres, they connect **from** the sympathetic trunk **to** the spinal nerves.

There are exceptions to this with some preganglionic fibres ascending or descending to other levels before they synapse.

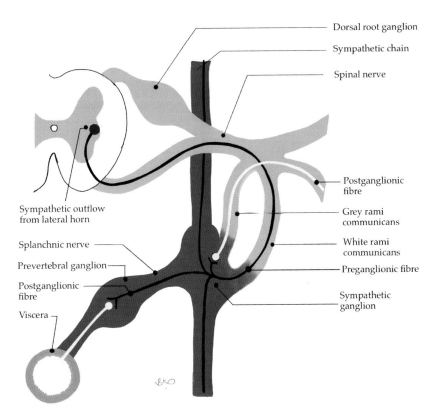

Dorsal root ganglion

Sympathetic chain

Spinal nerve

Postganglionic fibre

Grey rami communicans

White rami communicans

Preganglionic fibre

Sympathetic ganglion

Sympathetic outflow from lateral horn

Splanchnic nerve

Prevertebral ganglion

Postganglionic fibre

Viscera

Figure 7.6   Rami communicantes.

What are the main neurotransmitters at autonomic synapses?

- **Preganglionic** fibres are **cholinergic fibres** and acetylcholine is the neurotransmitter
- Postganglionic fibres
  - **Sympathetic** postganglionic fibres are **adrenergic fibres** and mainly release noradrenaline. Exception: acetylcholine is the neurotransmitter at piloerector muscles of hair, sweat glands and the occasional blood vessel
  - **Parasympathetic** postganglionic fibres are **cholinergic fibres** releasing acetylcholine (Table 7.7)

Table 7.7   Clinical Effects of Sympathetic and Parasympathetic Stimulation on Effector Organs

Organ	Sympathetic stimulation		Parasympathetic stimulation	
	Receptor	Effect	Receptor	Effect
Heart	β1, β2 α1, β1, β2	↑ Heart rate ↑ Contractility ↑ Conduction velocity	M2	↓ Heart rate ↓ Contractility ↓ Conduction velocity
Lung	α1 β2	Bronchoconstriction Bronchodilatation	M1, M3	Bronchoconstriction ↑ Bronchial secretions
GI tract	α1, α2, β2 α1, α2	↓ Motility Sphincter contraction	M2, M3	↑ Motility and tone Sphincter relaxation
Bladder	β2 α1	Detrusor relaxation Sphincter contraction	M	Detrusor contraction Sphincter relaxation
Kidney	β1	↑ Renin secretion		

Uterus	α1
	β2
		Contraction of pregnant
		    uterus
		Relaxation of pregnant
		    and non-pregnant
		    uterus		

Eyes	α1	Pupillary dilatation	M	Pupillary constriction
Liver	α1, β2	↑ Glycogenolysis ↑ Lipolysis	M	Glycogen synthesis
Adipose	α1, β1, β3	↑ Lipolysis		
Arteries	β1 β2 α1, α2	Coronary vasodilatation Vasodilatation Vasoconstriction	M	Vasodilatation
Veins	β2 α1, α2	Vasodilatation Vasoconstriction		
Platelets	α2	↑ Platelet aggregation		
Salivary glands	α1	Viscous secretions		Watery secretions

M – muscarinic receptors

What are the causes of autonomic dysfunction?

Primary	Acquired
Familial dysautonomia	Diabetes mellitus
Multisystem atrophy	Chronic alcoholism
Amyloidosis	Drug/toxin induced (e.g. amiodarone, chemotherapy drugs)
Fabry disease	Infections (e.g. Lyme's disease, tetanus, HIV, botulism)
Porphyria	Autoimmune: Guillain-Barré, SLE, Lambert-Eaton myasthenic syndrome
	Vitamin B12 deficiency
	Paraneoplastic syndromes

How would someone with autonomic neuropathy present?

Symptoms

- Cardiovascular: dizziness, fainting, painless myocardial infarction
- Gastrointestinal: gustatory sweating, constipation, nocturnal diarrhoea, reflux, nausea, vomiting
- Genito urinary: nocturia, urgency, incontinence, impotence
- Miscellaneous: lack of sweating, cold peripheries

Signs

Resting tachycardia, fixed heart rate and lack of heart rate variability, episodic hypertension, postural hypotension, decreased pupil size, absent or delayed light reflex and dependent oedema

How will this be investigated?

- Lying and standing blood pressures (greater than 20 mmHg suggests autonomic dysfunction)
- Valsalva manoeuvre (with lack of heart rate variability, blood pressure will consistently fall as the compensatory mechanisms are lost)
- ECG changes (prolonged QTc interval)
- Cold pressor test (placing a hand in a mixture of 50/50 ice and water for one minute: normal response is an increase of approximately 20 mmHg in systolic pressure, this is blunted or absent in those with autonomic dysfunction)
- Tilt table test
- Investigations of underlying cause (e.g. nerve biopsy)
- Power spectral analysis of biological variables, i.e. R-R interval or BP variables

How would you manage these patients during an anaesthetic?

Preoperative

- Full investigations to the nature and extent of autonomic dysfunction
- Premedication with a H2 antagonist/proton pump inhibitor and a prokinetic such as metoclopramide to reduce the risk of gastric aspiration
- Ensure adequate hydration

Intraoperative

- Consider invasive monitoring preinduction. CM5 ECG lead configuration for monitoring of ischaemia may be considered in those at risk.
- Rapid sequence induction if there is a risk of gastric aspiration. Be aware of a reduced pressor response to tracheal intubation.
- Neuraxial blockade is a controversial subject; it should be decided on an individual basis. Significant hypotension can be seen.
- Positive pressure ventilation may be poorly tolerated if the patient is hypovolaemic.
- Significant hypotension may occur when position of patient is changed suddenly (due to lack of compensatory mechanisms). Hence any position changes need to be slow and/ or staged.
- Atropine and directly acting vasopressors should be available for cardiovascular instability (such as the alpha 1 agonist, phenylephrine).
- Ensure adequate temperature monitoring and control.

Postoperative

- If significant autonomic dysfunction is present, then a high dependency care with full monitoring is considered. These patients may be at risk of haemodynamic instability and also silent ischaemia.

What is autonomic hyperreflexia?

Autonomic hyperreflexia develops in individuals with a spinal cord injury above the T6 vertebral level. It is a medical emergency with complications resulting from severe and sustained peripheral hypertension.

Stimulus caused by bladder distension, urinary tract infection, bowel impaction and various surgical procedures trigger this condition.

A stimulus below the level of injury causes a peripheral sympathetic response through the spinal nerves resulting in vasoconstriction below the level of injury. The central nervous system, not being able to detect the stimuli below the cord due to lack of continuity, detects only sympathetic response and then sends inhibitory response down the spinal cord. This reaches only until the level of injury and does not cause a desired response in the sympathetic fibres below the injury, leaving the hypertension unchecked.

Above the level of injury: predominant unopposed parasympathetic response leading to flushing and sweating, pupillary constriction and nasal congestion and bradycardia

Below the level of injury: sympathetic overactivity giving a pale, cool skin

Why T6?

The level depicts the autonomic supply to the biggest reservoir of blood, the splanchnic circulation. The greater splanchnic nerve arises at T5–T9, and any lesions above T6 allow the strong uninhibited sympathetic tone to constrict the splanchnic bed causing systemic hypertension. Lesions below T6 results in a good parasympathetic inhibitory control and prevents hypertension.

What is the physiological explanation for this response?

Not fully known. One theory is that the peripheral alpha-adrenergic receptors associated with the blood vessels become hyper-responsive below the level of spinal cord injury due to the low resting catecholamine levels. These 'orphaned' receptors have a decreased threshold to react to adrenergic stimuli with an increased responsiveness.

It has also been postulated that the loss of descending inhibition is responsible for this mechanism.

How would you tailor your anaesthetic for this patient and minimise risk of hyperreflexia?

Seek senior help

Use of regional anaesthesia +/– sedation

- Difficult positioning
- Prepare vasopressors

General anaesthesia

- Prepare vasopressors and atropine (excessive hypotension on induction)
- May need RSI because of reflux – avoid suxamethonium (increase in K+!)
- Possible difficult intubation due to positioning
- Adequate anaesthesia and remifentanil to reduce stimulus

Others

- Careful temperature control due to altered temperature regulation
- Arterial line in severe cases
- Ensure bladder is not distended

How will you treat severe hypertension associated with dysreflexia?

- Short-acting antihypertensives, such as nifedipine or nitrates
- Remifentanil or other short-acting opioids
- Deepening of anaesthesia

Autonomic Supply of Eye

The eye receives supply from both the parasympathetic and the sympathetic fibres (Figure 7.7).

- Parasympathetic supply

  The preganglionic fibres originate in the Edinger-Westphal nucleus in the brain stem and then pass in the third cranial nerve to the ciliary ganglion. The postganglionic fibres then enter the eye via the short ciliary nerve and innervate the ciliary muscles.

  Activation of the parasympathetic pathway constricts the pupil (miosis).

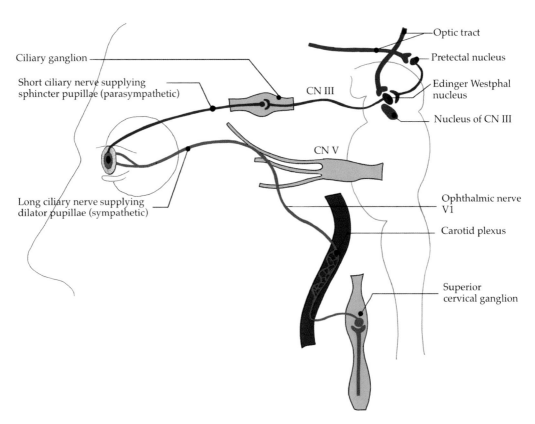

Figure 7.7   Autonomic supply – eye.

- Sympathetic supply

  This originates in the hypothalamus, passing through the midbrain (uncrossed) and lateral medulla and emerges from T1 (close proximity to the lung apex) and passes to the superior cervical ganglion via the dorsal roots. The superior cervical ganglion is located deep to the carotid sheath at the level of the second and third cervical vertebrae. From there, the fibres synapse and project cranially and innervate the eye either via the short ciliary nerve, long ciliary nerve or directly into the orbit. These will then innervate the radial fibres of the iris.

  Activation of the sympathetic pathway dilates the pupil (mydriasis).

The autonomic nervous system is also involved in the increased production ($\beta2$) and reduced production ($\alpha2$) of aqueous humour and enhanced drainage of aqueous humour via the canal of Schlemm and the trabecular network (muscarinic effect).

Can you describe the pupillary light reflex?

The pupillary light reflex constricts the pupil in response to light, through the innervation of the iris sphincter muscle. This is the result of the neuroanatomical pathways described below. Pupillary light reflex is used to assess the brain stem function. Abnormal pupillary light reflex can be found in optic nerve and oculomotor nerve damage, brain stem lesions and in use of medications such as barbiturates.

Light is shone into the eye which enters the pupil and stimulates the retina.

Afferent limb: retinal ganglion cells transmit the light signal to the optic nerve and the action potential travels along the axon. The optic nerve enters the optic chiasma where the nasal retinal fibres cross to contralateral optic tract and the temporal retinal fibres stay in the ipsilateral optic tract.

Centre: fibres from the optic tracts project and synapse in the pretectal nuclei in the dorsal midbrain. The pretectal nuclei project fibres to the Edinger-Westphal nuclei bilaterally (therefore responsible for the direct and consensual response to light) via the posterior commissure.

Efferent limb: the Edinger-Westphal nucleus projects preganglionic parasympathetic fibres, which travel along the oculomotor nerve and then synapse with the ciliary ganglion, which sends postganglionic parasympathetic fibres (short ciliary nerves) to innervate the sphincter muscle of the pupils resulting in pupillary constriction.

When can there be an abnormal response to the light reflex?

Table 7.8   Abnormal Pupillary Responses

Bilateral abnormal pupillary response	Unilateral abnormal pupillary response
Mid-brain lesions (mid-position pupils)	Isolated cranial nerve III lesion
Pontine lesions (pinpoint pupils)	Horner's syndrome
Argyll-Robertson pupil (large fixed pupils, still able to accommodate)	Holmes-Adie pupil – dilated pupil that reacts slowly to light
Brain stem death	Brain stem herniation due to the stretching of cranial nerve III

What is Horner's syndrome?

A group of signs caused by the unilateral interruption to the ascending sympathetic supply to the eye and face and is characterised by miosis, anhydrosis, partial ptosis, pseudoenophthalmos, bloodshot conjunctiva and loss of ciliospinal reflex.

Causes of Horner's syndrome can originate anywhere along the sympathetic path.

- Central and cervical spinal cord
  - Massive cerebrovascular accident
  - Brain neoplasm
  - Syringomyelia
  - Cord tumours

- Along the sympathetic chain in the neck
  - Carotid artery dissection
  - Postsurgical, i.e. thyroid or laryngeal surgery
  - Cervical lymphadenopathy

- T1 root
  - Pancoast tumour
  - Brachial plexus trauma
  - Cervical rib

- Sympathectomy and nerve blocks

What is oculo-cardiac reflex?

This occurs during ophthalmic procedures especially seen in children and in squint surgery. It is parasympathetically activated causing profound bradycardia and even sinus arrest due to traction on the extraocular muscles or compression of the globe. The afferent pathway is via the trigeminal nerve and the efferent pathway is via the vagus nerve.

This condition is treated by removal of initial stimulus, anticholinergics, deepening of anaesthesia and very rarely CPR may be warranted. Local anesthetics used prior to the procedure may reduce this phenomenon.

Autonomic Supply of Heart

The heart has sympathetic and parasympathetic control with modulator centres within the medulla which regulate the outputs (Figure 7.8).

Centre: the nucleus tractus solitarius (NTS) in the medulla is the major regulator of autonomic nerve outflow to the heart and blood vessels. The hypothalamus and higher centres modify the activity of the medullary centres and are particularly important in stimulating cardiovascular responses to emotion and stress. Neural connections from the NTS modulate sympathetic neuronal activity in the upper ventrolateral medulla, and the activity of parasympathetic neurons located in the dorsal vagal nucleus and nucleus ambiguus. Stimulation of the NTS reciprocally activates vagal neurons and inhibits sympathetic neurons.

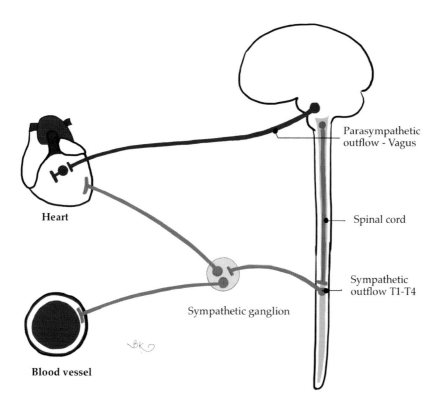

Figure 7.8   Autonomic supply of the heart.

- The sympathetic nerves exit the medulla and travel down the spinal cord where they synapse with the sympathetic ganglia. The fibres within the sympathetic chain originate from the superior, middle and inferior cervical ganglia, along with T1 to T4. Longer postganglionic efferent fibres from the ganglia travel to the heart and vessels.
- The parasympathetic nerves in the form of vagus nerves (cranial nerve X) exit the medulla as long preganglionic efferent fibres that synapses with short postganglionic fibres within the heart or vasculature.

Heart: the autonomic supply to the heart is via the superficial and deep cardiac plexus formed by branches from the sympathetic and parasympathetic efferents. Sympathetic efferent nerves are present throughout the atria, ventricles and conducting system including the sinoatrial (SA) and atrioventricular (AV) nodes.

The parasympathetic nervous system innervates the SA and AV nodes, atrial muscle and sparsely innervates the ventricles.

What are the effects of sympathetic and parasympathetic stimulation on the heart?

Table 7.9   Effects of Sympathetic and Parasympathetic Stimulation on the Heart

Sympathetic stimulation	Parasympathetic stimulation
Increased heart rate	Reduction in heart rate
Increased inotropy (contractility)	Reduction in contractility
Increased dromotropy (conduction velocity)	Reduction in conduction velocity
Increased lusitropy (rate of relaxation)	

What autonomic effects are seen in a transplanted heart?

Loss of sympathetic effects

- Increased refractory time with an increased tendency for first degree heart block and potential need for pacemaker insertion
- Loss of normal response to hypovolemia or hypotension (i.e. no increased tachycardia or increased contractility). The denervated heart is said to be preload dependent.
- Blunted response to exercise

Loss of parasympathetic effects

- Loss of parasympathetic innervation with resultant higher resting heart rate (in the region of 90 to 110 bpm)
- Absent vagal reflexes (such as those with laryngoscopy, carotid massage and the Valsalva manoeuvre)

Effects on drug action

- Absent response of the heart to drugs that work by blocking the parasympathetic supply, i.e. glycopyrronium and atropine. Drugs that have a direct effect on the heart should be used instead (isoprenaline, glucagon, adrenaline and noradrenaline).
- Increased effect of certain drugs such as adrenaline and noradrenaline as there will be no reflex reaction of a reduced heart rate when the blood pressure increases

Sympathetic Blocks

a. Stellate ganglion block
b. Coeliac plexus block
c. Lumbar sympathectomy

What are the indications and contraindications for a sympathetic block?

Indications (the specific indications and contraindications are explained in detail with respective blocks)

- Neuropathic pain
  - Acute herpes zoster
  - Carcinomatous neuropathy
  - Complex regional pain syndrome (CRPS) types I and II

- Vascular insufficiency
  - Acute: post-traumatic vasospasm, arterial or venous occlusion, frostbite and inadvertent intra-arterial injection of irritants
  - Chronic: Raynaud's syndrome and atherosclerosis

- Visceral pain
  - Malignancy
  - Chronic non-cancer related pain syndromes (e.g. refractory angina)
  - Perioperative pain

- Other
  - Hyperhidrosis

General contraindications

- Patient refusal
- Coagulopathy/ongoing anticoagulation
- Abnormal anatomy
- Local infection
- Local neoplasm

Discuss the different type of drugs used for sympathetic blocks.

Local anaesthetics: 1% lignocaine for diagnostic blocks and 0.25–0.5% bupivacaine for therapeutic blocks

Neurolytics

- Phenol: 2–3% phenol causes selective sensory block; 6% phenol destroys both motor and sensory fibres. They are temporary due to nerve fibre regeneration and phenol is shorter acting and produces a less profound effect compared to alcohol.
- Alcohol: 50–100% alcohol produces neurolysis but has a higher incidence of neuritis.

Stellate ganglion block

The stellate ganglion is formed by the fusion of the inferior cervical and the first thoracic sympathetic ganglion bilaterally and is present in 80% of the population. It consists of sympathetic innervation for the head, neck, heart and upper limbs. The ganglion lies anterior to the neck of the first rib and extends to the inferior aspect of the transverse process of C7 and is located posteromedial to the vertebral artery close to the dome of pleura (Figure 7.9).

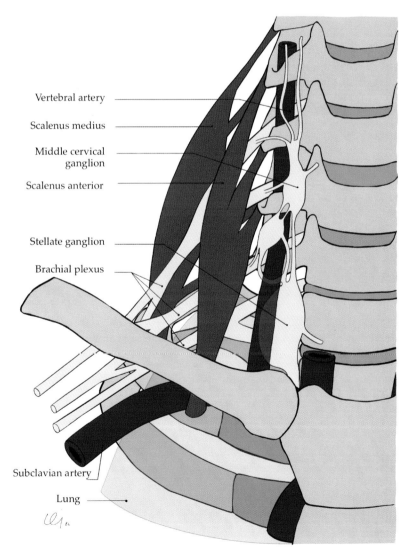

Vertebral artery
Scalenus medius
Middle cervical ganglion
Scalenus anterior
Stellate ganglion
Brachial plexus
Subclavian artery
Lung

Figure 7.9   Stellate ganglion – position and relations.

The important relations are as follows

- Anterior
  - Subcutaneous tissue and sternocleidomastoid muscle
  - Subclavian artery and carotid sheath

- Posterior
  - Transverse process of C7
  - Vertebral artery
  - Sheath of the brachial plexus

- Inferior
  - Pleural dome of the lung

- Lateral
  - Superior intercostal artery and vein
  - Ventral ramus of first thoracic nerve

- Medial
  - Vertebral column (at C7 body)
  - Thoracic duct
  - Oesophagus

What are the specific indications and contraindications for this block?

Specific indications

- Pain syndromes
  - Complex regional pain syndrome 1 & 2
  - Refractory angina
  - Phantom limb syndrome
  - Herpes zoster affecting the appropriate dermatomes

- Vascular insufficiency
  - Raynaud's syndrome
  - Embolic phenomena (e.g. inadvertent intra-arterial injection of thiopentone)
  - Frostbite

- Other
  - Hyperhidrosis

Specific contraindications

- Contralateral phrenic nerve palsy
- Glaucoma
- Recent myocardial infarction

How would you perform the procedure using the landmark technique?

General measures

- Informed consent discussed and signed
- IV access, trained assistant, access to emergency equipment and drugs
- Appropriate AAGBI monitoring attached
- Sedation if appropriate
- Asepsis
- Local anaesthetic dose within the toxic limit

Procedure

- Position: supine with neck partially extended and head turned slightly to the opposite side
- Landmarks: sternocleidomastoid muscle, carotid sheath are identified and pulled away laterally (correlating with C6). This block can be performed with the use of ultrasound guidance, CT guidance and fluoroscopy.
- Needle type: 22G spinal needle, 9 cm long
- Needle entry point: 2–3 cm above and 2 cm lateral to the suprasternal notch – between trachea and the carotid sheath, at the level of cricoid cartilage and Chassaignac's tubercle (C6)
- Technique: the needle is directed medially and inferiorly to hit the C6 body. Then the needle is withdrawn by 2 mm.
- Confirmation: under fluoroscopic guidance, contrast is injected which if seen to be spreading both caudally and cranially will confirm the position.
- Drug: 10–15 ml of the appropriate agent should then be injected with frequent aspirations. The drug used is determined by the clinician's preference and local hospital policies.

What are the possible complications?

General

- Haematoma
- Neuralgia
- Local infection over injection site
- Local anaesthetic toxicity
- Allergy to local anaesthetics

Specific

- Horner's syndrome (indicates a successful block)
- Hoarse voice (recurrent laryngeal nerve palsy)
- Post sympathectomy neuralgia

- Unilateral phrenic nerve palsy
- Vertebral artery and intrathecal or epidural injection
- Damage to adjacent structures
  - Pneumothorax
  - Oesophageal perforation
  - Brachial plexus injury
  - Chylothorax

Coeliac plexus block

The coeliac plexus is the largest sympathetic plexus located in the upper abdomen at the origin of the coeliac trunk from the abdominal aorta (T12/L1 level). It is made of the right and the left ganglia: the right ganglion lies posterior to the inferior vena cava and the left lies posterior to the origin of the splenic artery (Figure 7.10).

The plexus provides autonomic nerve supply to the upper abdominal organs (pancreas, spleen, liver, stomach, kidney and the bowel up to the splenic flexure).

Sympathetic innervation of the coeliac plexus begins from the anterolateral horn of the spinal cord at the level of T5 to T12. Each coeliac ganglion receives preganglionic sympathetic fibres from the greater (T5–T9), lesser splanchnic nerves (T10–T11) and the least splanchnic nerve (T12) and the postganglionic sympathetic nerves leave the ganglion in periarterial plexuses. It also contains the preganglionic parasympathetic fibres from the vagal trunks (passes through but does not connect here).

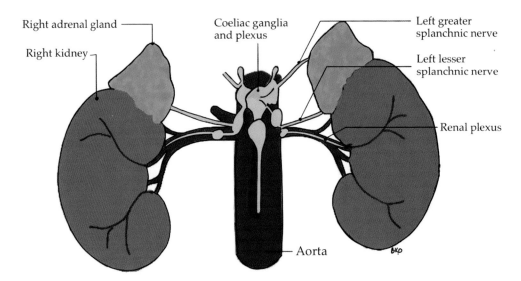

Figure 7.10   Coeliac plexus – position and relations.

What are the specific indications and contraindications for this block?

Specific indications

- Intractable visceral pain
  - Malignant and benign tumours of the abdominal organs. Common indication is to treat pain associated with pancreatic cancer.
- Chronic pancreatitis (controversial)

Specific contraindications

- Dangerous in the presence of a large aortic aneurysm

How would you perform the procedure?

General measures: as before

Intravenous fluid is started prior to the block in an attempt to minimise hypotension.

- Procedure
- Position: prone
- Landmarks: with x-ray guidance, identify the tip of 12th rib. Done with two needle approach on each side
- Needle type: 22G, 15 cm long
- Needle entry point: below the tip of the 12th rib
- Technique: aimed medially to make contact with the body of the L1 and then redirected so that it is in front of the vertebra in the vicinity of the coeliac plexus, avoiding the major blood vessels
- Confirmation: under fluoroscopic guidance, contrast is injected to confirm the position
- Drug: 10 ml of the appropriate agent should then be injected with frequent aspirations (as per clinician's preference and local hospital policies). Local anaesthetics and steroids are used for patients with benign pathology whereas neurolytic agents are reserved for cancer-related pain

What are the specific complications?

Common

- Orthostatic hypotension (even after a unilateral block)
- Diarrhoea

Uncommon
- Retroperitoneal haematoma (due to aortic or vena cava puncture)
- Paraplegia (damage of the artery of Adamkiewicz)
- Bowel, pancreas or other visceral injury
- Diaphragmatic injury
- Pneumothorax
- Sexual dysfunction

Lumbar sympathectomy

The lumbar sympathetic chain is situated along the anterolateral fascial plane of L1 to L4 vertebrae. It is separated from the somatic nerves by the psoas muscle and corresponding fascia.

It continues superiorly with the thoracic sympathetic chain at the diaphragm and inferiorly it passes behind the common iliac vessels over the sacral ala and is continuous with the sacral sympathetic chain. The right lumbar sympathetic chain lies posterior to inferior vena cava and the left lies posterolateral to the aortic lymph nodes.

What are the indications for this block?

Specific indications

- Pain syndromes
  - Intractable cancer pain
  - Rectal tenesmus secondary to malignancy
  - Intractable back pain
  - Phantom limb pain

- Vascular insufficiency
  - Peripheral arteriosclerosis and claudication pain

How would you perform the procedure?

General measures: as before

Procedure

- Position: prone
- Landmarks: using an image intensifier, the L3 spinous process is located
- Needle type: 20G, 15 cm long
- Needle entry point: 10 cm lateral to the midpoint of L3/L4
- Technique: needle aimed at the anterolateral edge of L3 to contact the vertebral body and then the needle is 'walked off', therefore avoiding the great vessels
- Confirmation: under fluoroscopic guidance, contrast should be injected with adequate caudal and cranial spread ideally covering L1 to L3
- Drug: 10–20 ml of local anaesthetic should be injected (depending on local policies and clinician's preference)

What are the specific complications?

- Post sympathectomy neuralgia
- Intrathecal or epidural injection
- Intravascular injection
- Damage to the renal pelvis
- Perforation of intervertebral disc
- Ejaculation disorders

Bibliography

Assadi, R., Motabar, A., & Lange, R. A. Heart nerve anatomy [Internet]. New York, NY: WebMD; c2016. Retrieved 28 June 2016.

Kawashima, T. (2005). The autonomic nervous system of the human heart with special reference to its origin, course, and peripheral distribution. *Anatomy & Embryology, 209*(6), 425–438.

Klabunde, R. (2011). *Cardiovascular Physiology Concepts.* Lippincott Williams & Wilkins: Philadelphia, PA.

Menon, R., & Swanepoel, A. (2010). Sympathetic blocks. *Continuing Education in Anaesthesia, Critical Care & Pain, 10*(3), 88–92.

Labour Analgesia

Labour is an active process and is characterised by regular painful uterine contractions which increase in frequency and intensity with progressive cervical dilatation (Table 7.10).

Table 7.10 Stages of Labour

1st Stage	From establishment of labour to full cervical dilatation
2nd Stage	Full cervical dilatation to delivery of baby
3rd Stage	Delivery of baby to delivery of placenta

The pain pathways during the first and second stages of labour are explained below (Figures 7.11 and 7.12).

First stage

- Latent phase – onset of regular uterine contraction to cervical dilatation of 5 cm
- Active phase – latent phase to full cervical dilatation

The first stage of labour involves stretching and dilatation of the cervix and uterine contractions – *visceral pain (diffuse and poorly localised)*.

Visceral pain pathway

- C pain fibres from the uterus and cervix coalesce at the paracervical region and pass through the uterine, cervical and hypogastric plexuses to reach the main sympathetic chain. They then reach the spinal cord through the paravertebral sympathetic fibres (T10–L1) and via spinothalamic tracts to higher centres. The poor localisation is due to the cross over and extensive anterior and posterior extensions of some nerve fibres at the level of dorsal horn. Because of the involvement of T10–L1, the pain is referred to these dermatomal levels and a dull pain is felt in the lower abdomen, sacrum and back.
- Displacement of other intra-abdominal structure by the gravid uterus can cause pain transmitted by the coeliac plexus.
- Chemical mediators involved are bradykinin, leukotrienes, prostaglandins, serotonin, substance P and lactic acid.

Hence it is easy to understand how pain relief during the first stage of labour can be accomplished by lumbar epidural, paracervical and paravertebral blocks.

The upper dermatomal level needed for adequate analgesia is about T10.

Second stage

- Spans from full cervical dilation to delivery of baby
- The second stage of labour deals with perineal distension and hence *somatic pathways (sharp and well localised)* are involved (along with visceral pain due to uterine contraction)

Somatic pain pathway

- Myelinated Aδ fibres carry somatic pain via the pudendal nerves (S2/3/4), genitofemoral nerve (L1/2), ilioinguinal nerve (L1) and posterior cutaneous nerve of the thigh (S2/3)
- Impulses from the bladder, urethra and rectum are transmitted along S2/3/4 and those from the periuterine tissues and lumbosacral area (due to fetal malposition) are transmitted via the lumbosacral plexus L5–S1
- All impulses are conducted to the brain via the spinothalamic tract

Somatic pain is easily localised, sharp in character and radiates to adjacent dermatomes and again can be controlled by lumbar epidural analgesia. Table 7.11 summarises the types of pain.

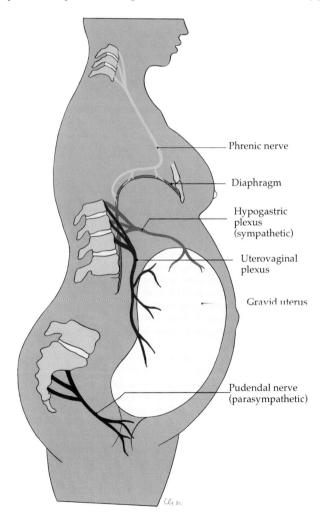

Figure 7.11   Pain pathways in pregnancy.

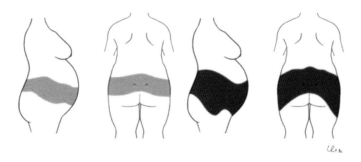

First stage of labour

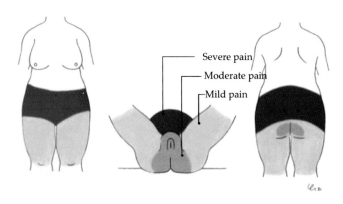

Early second stage of labour

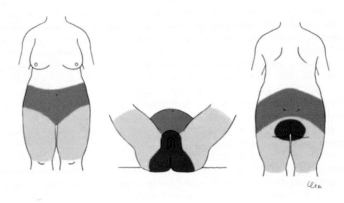

Late second stage of labour

Figure 7.12   Pain during labour. A – first stage; B – early second stage; C – late second stage.

Table 7.11 Summary of Visceral and Somatic Pain

Visceral pain	Somatic pain
Occurs in early first stage and second stage	Occurs in late first stage and second stage
Due to dilatation of cervix and lower uterine segment	Due to stretching and distension of pelvic floor, perineum and vagina
Transmitted via small unmyelinated C fibres	Transmitted via fine myelinated A delta fibres
Pain is dull and diffuse with poor localisation	Pain is sharp and localised

Why do you need a higher dermatomal level for caesarean section, compared to labour analgesia?

When considering using regional anaesthesia for surgery, it is important to remember that the skin, muscles, bones and all organs in one area have a different nerve supply. This is because spinal segmental innervation for dermatomes and myotomes and organ innervation do not coincide.

Definition of an adequate block height for caesarean section is when T6 is 'either blocked, or expected to be blocked to touch before surgery has reached the peritoneal cavity'.

In the classic Pfannenstiel incision, the skin innervation is T12/L1 and uterine innervation is T10, but peritoneal innervation can go as high as T4. During the procedure after closing the uterus the para colic gutters are cleaned and there is peritoneal irritation needing block levels for caesarean section to be as high as T4.

As alluded to before, effective analgesia from labour pain needs block only up to T10 but for caesarean section the block level needs to be up to T4.

Why do you observe bradycardia during regional anaesthesia for caesarean section?

Reported incidence of bradycardia during caesarean section under spinal anaesthesia is 2.9%.

The most probable reasons are noted below.

- Classic reason is a high spinal block – sensory block higher than T4 due to the blocking of the sympathetic cardio accelerator fibres to the heart (T1–T4). This can cause severe bradycardia which if not treated can lead to asystole.
- Reflex bradycardia due to the use of vasopressors (phenylephrine) to maintain the feto-placental circulation
- Reflex cardiovascular depression due to decrease in venous return, known as Bezold–Jarisch reflex or neurocardiogenic syncope
- Severe reflex bradycardia has been supported in case studies during the time of placental expulsion and traction
- Manipulation of the abdominal viscera, peritoneum or traction of the visceral ligaments, uterine exteriorisation and inversion
- Patient with pre-existing cardiac disease such as sick-sinus syndrome can also have bradycardia

How may pain following caesarean section be managed?

Good quality analgesia post caesarean section using a multimodal approach leads to better bonding with baby, motivation and faster recovery.

Principles of intraoperative analgesia during caesarean section under general anaesthesia

- Avoid systemic opioids until delivery of the baby and cord clamping (exceptional circumstances in hypertensive disorders of pregnancy)
- Simple analgesia
  - Paracetamol intravenously
  - NSAIDS, if not contraindicated
- Morphine intravenously or equivalent
- Regional blocks
  - Transversus abdominis plane (TAP) block
  - Bilateral ilio-inguinal/ilio-hypogastric (II/IH) nerve block
- Antiemetics to prevent postoperative nausea and vomiting which can worsen pain

Postoperative analgesia

Regular simple analgesics: paracetamol and NSAIDS.

Codeine phosphate is usually avoided in breast feeding mothers for fear of neonatal respiratory depression and seizures. DF118 is a suitable alternative.

Opioids: oral morphine or morphine patient-controlled analgesia as per hospital protocol

Do regional blocks play a role in providing analgesia in the postoperative period?

Regional nerve blocks such as TAP and bilateral II/IH nerve blocks are excellent modes of pain relief as they are opioid sparing.

Meta-analysis and systemic reviews support the use of TAP block for analgesia after caesarean section by showing significant improvement in postoperative analgesia in women who did not receive intrathecal opioids and little benefit in those who received them. In those patients who received TAP blocks, pain scores and opioid consumption are lower for up to 24 hours.

Bibliography

Eisenach, J. Anatomy of pain fibres important in the first stage of labour. Neurophysiology of labour pain. esahq.org.

Labor, S., & Maguire, S. (2008). The pain of labour. *Reviews in Pain, 2*(2), 15–19.

Ousley, R., Egan, C., Dowling, K., & Cyna, A. M. (2012). Assessment of block height for satisfactory spinal anaesthesia for caesarean section. *Anaesthesia, 67*(12), 1356–1363.

Russell, I. F. (2004). A comparison of cold, pinprick and touch for assessing the level of spinal block at caesarean section. *International Journal of Obstetric Anesthesia, 13*(3), 146–152.

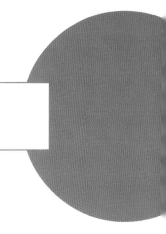

Placenta

The placenta is a disc-shaped organ measuring 20 cm in diameter and weighs around 500 g. The maternal surface is made up of 20–40 cotyledons separated by grooves giving it a nodular appearance. The fetal surface is smoother and houses the umbilical cord.

The placenta is a feto-maternal organ with the fetal and maternal parts held together by the anchoring villi (Figure 7.13).

The *fetal portion* is known as the villous chorion and is made up of the chorionic plate (consisting of the amnion, the extraembryonic mesenchyme, the cytotrophoblast and the syncytiotrophoblast) with its placental villi and the intervillous spaces.

The *maternal portion* is otherwise called the decidua basalis (specialised endometrium) with uterine vessels and glands.

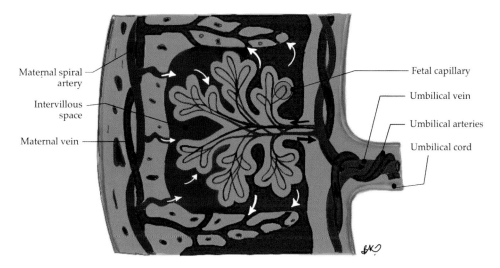

Figure 7.13   Structure of placenta.

Explain in detail the source of blood in the placenta.

Maternal component

- Uterine artery, arising from the anterior division of internal iliac artery
- Ovarian artery, a direct branch of the aorta
- Vaginal vessels, from the anterior division of internal iliac artery

All these vessels anastomose extensively which explains why ligation of the smaller vessels does not control uterine haemorrhage and that aortic clamping might be necessary. Maternal blood circulates freely within the intervillous space. The mean pressure at the arterial side is 70 mmHg, 10 mmHg in the intervillous space and less than 10 mmHg in the venous side of the maternal circulation.

Fetal component

- Two umbilical arteries which arise from the internal iliac arteries of the fetus
- One umbilical vein draining into the fetal inferior vena cava

It is a closed vascular system with an average pressure of 30 mmHg which is higher than the intervillous pressure preventing the collapse of the villous vessels.

What are the functions of the placenta?

Transfer: of gases, nutrients, water, electrolytes, amino acids, free fatty acids, glucose and many other compounds that take part in fetal development. It also acts as a means of removing wastes such as carbon dioxide, urea, uric acid, creatine, creatinine and bilirubin.

Endocrine function: the placenta produces various hormones such as

- Beta human chorionic gonadotropin – stimulates the corpus luteum to produce progesterone
- Human placental lactogen – decreases maternal insulin sensitivity and increases glucose levels. It helps in the development of maternal breasts and synthesis of fetal pulmonary surfactant.
- Oestrogen and progesterone – promote uterine growth and development of breasts

Synthetic function: the placenta plays a role in the production of glycogen, cholesterol and fatty acids.

Immune function: immunoglobulins are transferred from mother to the fetus through the placenta by pinocytosis, thus improving the immunity of the fetus. It also acts as a barrier to some microorganisms.

Metabolic function: phase 1 and 2 reactions occur in the placenta to varied extents depending on placental development, length of gestation and maternal health.

What is the role of placenta in the transfer of gases and drugs?

All gases are transferred through the same principles that govern the laws of gas exchange in the lung.

Oxygen

Oxygen is transferred by simple diffusion and relies on the partial pressure gradient (materno-fetal PaO_2 gradient is ~4 kPa) between the fetal and maternal blood at the villi and the intervillous spaces.

Bohr and double Bohr effect: the tendency of the oxygen dissociation curve (ODC) to shift in response to carbon dioxide is called the Bohr effect.

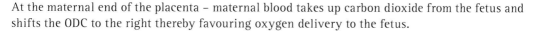

At the maternal end of the placenta – maternal blood takes up carbon dioxide from the fetus and shifts the ODC to the right thereby favouring oxygen delivery to the fetus.

At the fetal end of placenta – fetus becomes alkalotic by giving up carbon dioxide shifting the oxygen dissociation curve to the left, which aids in oxygen uptake.

Carbon dioxide

Similarly, this is exchanged by simple diffusion depending on the feto-maternal partial pressure gradient of carbon dioxide which is ~1.8 kPa.

Haldane and Double Haldane effect: the increased capacity of deoxygenated blood to take up more carbon dioxide is called the Haldane effect.

When maternal blood delivers oxygen to the fetus and becomes deoxygenated, it binds avidly to carbon dioxide and transfers it out. Conversely, at the fetal end, absorption of oxygen makes it less attractive to carbon dioxide.

Carbon monoxide (CO)

Mother: CO has 250 times more affinity to adult Hb than oxygen. So, it binds avidly to Hb and decreases O_2 binding and delivery. Hence although the PaO_2 is normal, Hb saturation is low and the ODC shifts to the left.

Fetus: CO readily crosses placenta and binds to fetal Hb, which has greater affinity to CO compared to adult Hb, so it binds even more fiercely!

As the fetus already lives in an oxygen-deprived environment, this depletes it further and causes fetal distress and death.

Drug transfer

The different methods by which the drugs cross the placenta are

- Simple/passive diffusion, e.g. gases, small molecules

  It is dependent on concentration gradient and does not use energy
- Facilitated diffusion, e.g. glucose, some antibiotics

  Also dependent on concentration gradient, but uses a carrier substance to transfer without using energy
- Active transport, e.g. most drugs

  Energy is utilised primarily from ATP and works against the concentration and electro-chemical gradients. The transporter proteins are usually positioned on the cell membrane
- Pinocytosis, e.g. immunoglobulins

  Drugs are engulfed by invagination of membrane on one side and released on the other after traversing along the body of the cell

Three drug types are identified depending on their readiness to transfer and the resultant feto-maternal concentrations (F/M) (Table 7.12).

Table 7.12   Drug Types with Respect to Placental Transfer

Type 1 drugs	Complete transfer (e.g. thiopentone)
	Good transfer across the membrane and F/M = 1
Type 2 drugs	Exceeding transfer (e.g. ketamine)
	The drugs readily cross the barrier and F/M >1
Type 3 drugs	Incomplete transfer (e.g. suxamethonium)
	Little or no transfer and F/M <1

What are the factors that affect drug transfer?

Table 7.13   Factors Affecting Placental Drug Transfer

Drug characteristics
Size (drugs with molecular weight <500 Da cross the placenta, and most drugs with MW >1000 Da do not cross the placenta)
Lipid solubility
Protein binding
Concentration gradient
pKa (along with pH of the maternal and fetal blood)
Membrane characteristics
Diffusion capacity
Diffusion distance – thickness of the membrane
Surface area
Presence of transporters
Miscellaneous
Utero placental blood flow
pH of maternal and fetal blood
Metabolism
Presence of disease states – diabetes, preeclampsia

Laws of diffusion

Henry's law: gas transfer into solution is proportional to the partial pressure of the gas.

Graham's law: rate of transfer of a substance is directly related to solubility and inversely proportional to the square root of molecular weight.

Fick's law: the rate of transfer is directly proportional to the partial pressure or concentration gradient.

Hence,

$$\text{Rate of diffusion} \left(Q\right) \text{per unit time} \left(t\right) = K \times \frac{SA \times \left(Cm - Cf\right)}{T}$$

SA – surface area

T – thickness

Cm–Cf – materno-fetal concentration gradient

K – diffusion constant, which depends on molecular weight, protein binding, lipid solubility and degree of ionisation

How and to what extent do the commonly used anaesthetic drugs cross the placenta?

The use of any drug in the first trimester of pregnancy should be avoided unless it is positively justified because most drugs have some side effects that could affect the development of the fetus.

Intravenous anaesthetic agents

All agents undergo placental transfer with some drugs achieving greater F/M concentrations owing to their lipid solubility.

Thiopentone, for example, is highly lipid soluble and at normal maternal pH 60% is available as unionised portion. Hence it crosses the placenta rapidly in both directions attaining F/M <1. Ketamine reaches the fetus and the F/M becomes greater than 1 even with standard induction doses probably attributed to its least protein binding property.

All drugs cause neonatal depression and reduce APGARs to varying extents.

Inhalational agents

The anaesthetic gases including nitrous oxide are smaller molecules and highly lipid soluble and hence cross by simple diffusion. Longer induction to delivery interval causes lower APGARs.

Opioids

Being lipid soluble, opioids easily pass in both directions across the placenta.

Pethidine: F/M increases and becomes greater than 1 within 2–3 hours of injection. As pethidine is not metabolised in the placenta and if feto-maternal transfer fails to occur, fetal concentration increases several folds and causes neonatal depression.

Morphine: despite being hydrophilic, F/M of morphine reaches closer to 1 which is attributed to less protein binding.

Fentanyl, alfentanil and sufentanil: these drugs are lipophilic and easily cross the placenta. Sufentanil in particular has a higher CNS uptake and hence has a lower systemic absorption.

Remifentanil: it crosses the placenta rapidly and is metabolised by the fetus. Owing to reduced fetal side effects, it is the preferred choice for use in patient-controlled analgesia in labour wards.

Local anaesthetics

Fetal toxicity with local anaesthetic agents during maternal epidural analgesia should not occur in the absence of direct intravascular injection, severe maternal hepatic disease or fetal acidosis.

Maternal pH ~7.38–7.42

Fetal pH ~7.32–7.38

Local anaesthetics are weakly basic drugs that are principally bound to alpha-1-acid glycoprotein and their placental transfer depends on pKa, maternal and fetal pH, degree of protein binding, type of the drug, dosage and timing of doses and uterine blood flow.

The greater protein binding of bupivacaine and ropivacaine, compared with that of lidocaine, likely accounts for their lower fetal blood levels. Also, the esters are metabolised rapidly to have minimal effects on the fetus as very little remains in the maternal circulation to cross the placenta. Amide local anaesthetics are more likely to cross the placenta.

'Ion-trapping'

The unionised portion of the local anaesthetics from maternal blood crosses the placenta and in the presence of fetal acidosis, the ionised/unionised fraction increases and the ionised form gets accumulated or 'trapped' in the fetus to exhibit side effects. This becomes relevant when larger amounts are used for epidural anaesthesia or other nerve blocks around the time of delivery.

Muscle relaxants

Non-depolarising muscle relaxants: they are quaternary ammonium compounds which are poorly lipid soluble, exist in ionised form and hence do not cross placenta readily. Although detectable in fetal blood (F/M @ 0.1) when used in high doses, they rarely affect neonatal muscle tone.

Depolarising muscle relaxants: more than 300 mgs of suxamethonium is required to cross the placenta and can exhibit effects only in the presence of maternal and fetal pseudocholinesterase deficiency.

Anticholinesterases and anticholinergics

Neostigmine is a quaternary amine, available as smaller molecules but in ionised form and hence limited transfer occurs. Atropine being a tertiary amine and lipid soluble crosses the placenta easily, whilst glycopyrrolate, a quaternary ammonium compound is fully ionised at normal pH and does not cross. When neostigmine-glycopyrrolate is given as a reversal agent, neostigmine crosses the placenta to a greater extent leading to bradycardia which can be prevented by giving neostigmine-atropine combination.

Antibiotics

Most antibiotics are lipid soluble and readily cross the placenta to varying F/M concentrations.

Vasopressors

Ephedrine and phenylephrine are the two most commonly used drugs and they cross the placenta. Studies have shown that ephedrine causes fetal acidosis which is not the case with phenylephrine.

Antihypertensives

All classes of drugs cross the placenta to varying extents with F/M around 0.2–1.

Some drugs cause fetal anomalies and should be avoided during organogenesis.

Beta blockers: may decrease uteroplacental blood flow, cause growth restriction and may be associated with neonatal hypoglycemia at higher doses. Labetalol is the only beta blocker licensed for use during pregnancy and breast feeding.

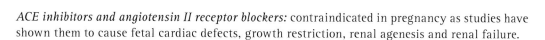

ACE inhibitors and angiotensin II receptor blockers: contraindicated in pregnancy as studies have shown them to cause fetal cardiac defects, growth restriction, renal agenesis and renal failure.

Calcium channel blockers: nifedipine is safe to use and does not cause any fetal side effects but may inhibit labour and have synergistic action with magnesium sulphate.

Hydralazine: its use has proven safety and efficacy with few documented adverse events.

Anticoagulants

Warfarin is contraindicated in pregnancy as it crosses placenta and causes fetal loss and congenital anomalies. Heparin (no transfer) and LMWH (little transfer) are safe to use.

How would you compare placenta and lung with respect to gas exchange?

Table 7.14   Comparison Between Lung and Placenta with Respect to Gas Exchange

	Placenta	Lung
Surface area	16 m^2	50 m^2
Thickness (diffusion distance)	3.5 microns	0.5 microns

It is obvious that the gas exchange is insufficient in the placenta compared to the lung. This is overcome by

- Increased maternal blood supply
- Increased placental blood supply
- Increased fetal Hb concentration (fetal Hb: 170–180 g/L and adult Hb: 120–140 g/L)
- Increased affinity of fetal Hb to oxygen (P50 of fetal Hb is 2.9 kPa and adult Hb is 3.5 kPa)
- Double Bohr effect

Bibliography

Lagan, G., & McClure, H. A. (2004). Review of local anaesthetic agents. *Current Anaesthesia & Critical Care, 15*(4–5), 247–254.

Principles and Practice of Pharmacology for Anaesthetists: Calvey and Williams Pharmacology for Anaesthesia and Intensive Care. Peck, Hill and Williams

Tuckley, J. M. (1994). Pharmacology of local anaesthetic agents. *Update in Anaesthesia, 4,* 19–24. Retrieved from www.world-anaesthesia.org.

Fetal Circulation

The placenta is the organ of gas exchange in fetuses. A specialised type of shunt-dependent fetal circulation forms with arterial and venous connections to ensure

- Adequate oxygen delivery despite low partial pressure of oxygen (maternal venous blood is the source of oxygenated blood to the fetus!)
- Blood with highest amount of oxygen is delivered to vital organs – heart and brain

This is achieved by important cardiopulmonary adaptations which are listed below (Figure 7.14).

- Distinctive quality of fetal haemoglobin (HbF) – *higher affinity and higher capacity*
  - Fetal Hb is made of two α and two γ globin chains. The absence of β chains (present in adult Hb, HbA) makes it less sensitive to 2,3– diphosphoglycerate (2,3–DPG) and reduces the P50 to 2.9 kPa (P50 of HbA is 3.5 kPa). A lower P50 shifts the oxygen dissociation curve to the left promoting increased uptake of oxygen in the placenta.
  - Normal concentration of fetal Hb is 150–180 g/L (adult Hb 130–140 g/L) at birth which increases the capacity to bind to oxygen.
- Presence of extra- and intracardiac shunts (discussed in detail later)
  - Ductus venosus (ensures oxygen enriched blood is directed to vital organs)
  - Foramen ovale (ensures oxygen-enriched blood is directed to vital organs)
  - Ductus arteriosus (shunts blood away from the lungs to the lower body)

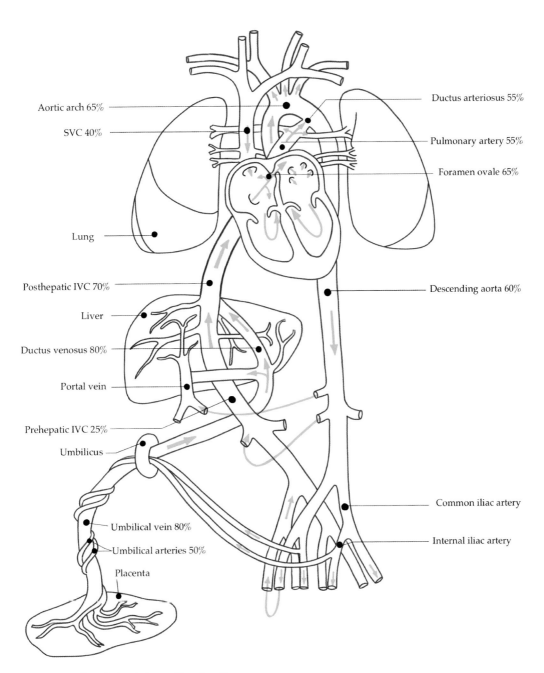

Aortic arch 65%
SVC 40%
Lung
Posthepatic IVC 70%
Liver
Ductus venosus 80%
Portal vein
Prehepatic IVC 25%
Umbilicus
Umbilical vein 80%
Umbilical arteries 50%
Placenta

Ductus arteriosus 55%
Pulmonary artery 55%
Foramen ovale 65%
Descending aorta 60%
Common iliac artery
Internal iliac artery

Figure 7.14   Foetal circulation with saturations.

Let's start with the placenta!

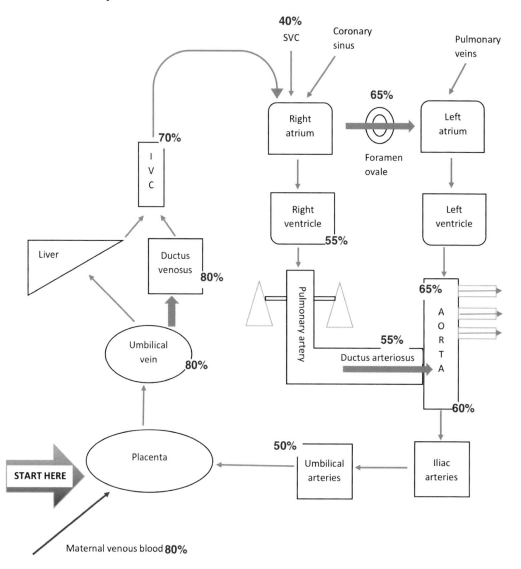

Figure 7.15   Schematic diagram of foetal circulation.

The maternal venous blood in the placenta is the source of oxygen and nutrients to the fetus. The umbilical cord contains one umbilical vein and two umbilical arteries.

Umbilical vein: carries oxygenated blood from the placenta (PO$_2$ ~4.7 kPa; oxygen saturation ~80%). Fifty percent of blood from the umbilical vein enters the liver and mixes with the hepatic sinusoids with the rest shunted to the ductus venosus.

Liver: the blood that enters hepatic sinusoids reaches the IVC at a later time via hepatic veins, containing less oxygenated blood due to mixing with the portal venous system.

Ductus venosus: connects umbilical vein to the inferior vena cava (IVC) at its inlet to the right atrium. Through a process of flow dynamics called 'preferential streaming', the ductus venosus blood enters the right atrium at the posterior aspect of the IVC bypassing the hepatic route. At the right atrial inlet, the eustachian valve directs the posterior stream to the second shunt called the foramen ovale to the left atrium.

Foramen ovale: a flap-like opening in the interatrial septum connecting the right and left atrial cavities. It is assumed that the ductus venosus blood enters with a higher pressure, which is sufficient enough to push open the flap of the foramen ovale. From the left atrium, the blood (PO_2 ~3.6 kPa; oxygen saturation ~65%) enters the left ventricle and the aorta and supplies the three proximal branches of the aorta (brachiocephalic, left common carotid and left subclavian arteries). This shunt plays a major role in delivering the oxygen-enriched blood to the heart, brain and upper part of the body.

Right atrium: (PO_2 ~2.7 kPa; oxygen saturation ~55%) is now left with the remaining blood from the IVC, venous drainage from the upper part of the body (SVC) and the heart (coronary sinus). This then enters the right ventricle and the pulmonary artery.

Ductus arteriosus: a wide muscular vessel that shunts blood from the pulmonary artery (PO_2 ~2.7 kPa; oxygen saturation ~55%) to the aorta bypassing the lung. The fetal lung is solid and filled with fluid resulting in a high pulmonary vascular resistance (PVR). This diverts the flow from the pulmonary artery to the ductus arteriosus such that only 12% of the right ventricular output enters the lungs. The remaining 88% of the blood enters the aorta after the origin of the three proximal branches and mainly supplies the lower part of the body.

Distal aorta: blood entering the distal aorta (oxygen saturation ~60%) originates from the left and right sided circulations and supplies the abdomen and lower part of the fetal body. The aorta branches into common iliac arteries, then to external and internal iliac arteries.

Umbilical arteries: branches from the anterior division of the internal iliac artery (two umbilical arteries in total) carrying deoxygenated blood (PO_2 ~2.3 kPa; oxygen saturation ~50%). They enter the placenta for oxygen and nutrient uptake.

Table 7.15   Values of Oxygen Saturation and PO_2 at Various Points in the Fetal Circulation (Different Articles Give Different Values, Use This as a Rough Guide)

Structure	Hb Sats	PO_2
Umbilical vein and ductus venosus	80%	4.7 kPa
Hepatic vein	25%	
Pre hepatic IVC	35%	
Post hepatic IVC	70%	
SVC	40%	
Right atrium	55%	
Right ventricle, pulmonary artery and ductus arteriosus	55%	2.7
Left atrium, left ventricle and proximal aorta	65%	3.6
Distal aorta	60%	
Umbilical arteries	50%	2.3 kPa

What are the main differences between the fetal and adult circulations?

Table 7.16   Differences Between Fetal and Adult Circulation

	Fetal circulation	Adult circulation

Circulation	In series
	Mixed blood in the right and left
	  side of the circulation
		In parallel
		Deoxygenated in the right and
		  oxygenated blood in the left

Oxygen supply	Placenta	Lung
Shunts	3 (DV, DA, FO)	0 (ignore the true shunts – bronchial veins and venae cordis minimae)
Cardiac output	Combined ventricular output (CVO) Left – 33% and Right – 66%	Combined cardiac output (CCO)
Right ventricle	Larger and thicker	Smaller
Left ventricle	Smaller	Larger and thicker
PVR	Higher than SVR	10-fold lower than SVR
SVR	Low	High

What happens to all these adaptations at birth?

This is a transition stage where the placenta is replaced by the lung as the organ of oxygenation. The cardiopulmonary adaptations will become obsolete from birth to a few days.

Thermal and tactile stimuli after birth and the initial breaths cause a lot of changes to the fetal circulation followed by clamping of the cord that hastens the changes.

- Initial breaths or gasps
  - This expands the lungs and increases the PAO_2, which obliterates the pulmonary vasoconstriction and decreases PVR
  - The resultant increase in PaO_2, to above 6.6 kPa, reduces prostaglandin E_2 levels (remember: PGE_2 is produced during hypoxia)
  - Decreased PGE_2 due to increased oxygen tension promotes the closure of the ductus arteriosus and venosus by contraction of specialised smooth muscle in their walls
- Clamping of the umbilical cord
  - Increase in SVR due to occlusion of umbilical arteries
  - Decreased flow to the ductus venosus due to clamping of umbilical vein
  - This results in decreased blood flow and hence decreased pressures in the right atrium and along with increased SVR and increased volume load from the pulmonary veins in the left atrium, the left and right pressures revert and the right to left shunt at the foramen ovale stops
  - Heart rate slows as a result of baroreceptor response to increase SVR

- Maintenance of normoxia, normocarbia, normothermia, normal pH in the baby
  - The change is transitional for a few days and can revert back to the original fetal circulation if there is acidosis and hypoxia in the neonate, hence it is important to maintain normal O_2, CO_2, pH and temperature in the newborn

When and by what mechanism do the shunts close after birth?

Foramen ovale

When: physiological and functional closure at birth. It takes months or even years for a complete closure with 25% of individuals having a patent foramen ovale.

How: due to decreased flow from the right atrium and increased pressure in the left atrium.

Ductus venosus

When: physiological closure at birth and complete obliteration in 2–5 days. It is replaced with a fibrous remnant, the ligamentum venosum, in a few months.

How: cold and decreased PGE_2 causes vasoconstriction that is hastened by clamping of the umbilical cord decreasing the blood flow.

Ductus arteriosus

When: closes almost immediately following birth. The physiological closure is complete in 1–4 days. Complete obliteration into a fibrous remnant, the ligamentum arteriosum, occurs in the months following birth.

How: lung expansion leads to increased bradykinin and decreased PGE_2 levels which cause contraction of the muscular wall of the ductus arteriosus and subsequent closure of the vessel.

What are the remnants of these shunts in the adult?

Table 7.17   Fetal Structures Persisting as Remnants in the Adult

Fetal structure	Adult remnant
Foramen ovale	Fossa ovalis
Ductus venosus	Ligamentum venosum
Ductus arteriosus	Ligamentum arteriosum
Umbilical arteries	Medial umbilical ligaments and superior vesicular artery
Umbilical vein	Ligamentum teres hepatis

What are the different types of congenital heart diseases?

This can be classified as in Table 7.18.

Table 7.18   Classification of Congenital Heart Diseases

Cyanotic	Rare. Due to abnormal blood flow from the right to the left side of the circulation resulting in poor oxygenation
Structural	Tetralogy of Fallot – discussed below Hypoplastic left heart disease – underdevelopment of all structures on the left side of the heart including the mitral and aortic valves and aorta
Valvular	Tricuspid atresia Pulmonary atresia Ebstein's anomaly – presence of abnormal tricuspid valve leaflets leading to tricuspid regurgitation
Vascular	Transposition of the great vessels – the positions of the aorta and pulmonary artery are reversed. Total anomalous pulmonary venous return – all four pulmonary veins drain into systemic veins or the right atrium.
Mixed	Truncus arteriosus – VSD with a single great vessel (truncus) carrying both systemic and pulmonary blood
Acyanotic	**Common**
Structural	ASD – atrial septal defect VSD – ventricular septal defect AVSD – atrioventricular septal defect PDA – patent ductus arteriosus
Valvular	Aortic stenosis Pulmonary stenosis
Vascular	Coarctation of aorta – narrowing of the aorta usually distal to left subclavian branch

An 11-month-old baby with Tetralogy of Fallot is booked for washout and suture of a dog bite wound by plastic surgeons.

What is Tetralogy of Fallot?

Tetralogy of Fallot (TOF) is the commonest cyanotic heart disease, accounting for 3.5% of all cases of congenital heart disease. The cause is unknown, but there is associated chromosomal abnormality in 25% of patients (microdeletion at 11q position on chromosome 22). It can also be associated with Di George syndrome, hypospadias, skeletal anomalies and a submucous cleft palate.

TOF consists of four anatomical components

- Ventricular septal defect
- An abnormally positioned aortic valve above (overriding) the ventricular septum
- Right ventricular outflow tract (RVOT) obstruction
- Right ventricular myocardial hypertrophy

What might be the symptoms and signs of TOF?

History

- Failure to thrive
- Dyspnoea and decreased exercise tolerance
- Hypercyanotic episodes: cyanosis after an episode of crying is a sign of acute reduction in pulmonary blood flow associated with sudden increase in the dynamic obstruction to the right ventricular outflow tract. This occurs due to muscular spasm at the sub-pulmonary infundibulum secondary to elevated levels of endogenous adrenaline and may be relieved in the knee-chest or squatting position

Examination

- Central cyanosis: suggests a saturation of less than 85% and is not improved by breathing 100% oxygen
- Clubbing, seen from 3–6 months of age
- Long harsh ejection systolic murmur with or without a thrill, best heard over the pulmonary area and the left sternal border. A thrill may be felt along the left sternal border
- Polycythaemia and its complications

Chest radiograph classically reveals a 'boot-shaped' heart with right ventricular hypertrophy and reduced pulmonary markings.

What do you mean by duct-dependent circulation?

Congenital cardiac lesions that are compatible with life only if the ductus arteriosus remains open are called 'duct-dependent'. In the right-sided lesions, there is no or limited blood flow to the lungs and the children present with cyanosis and hypoxia. In left-sided lesions, there is limited blood flow to the aorta, hence the whole of the body (Table 7.19).

Table 7.19 Examples of Duct-Dependent Circulation

Heart disease with duct-dependent pulmonary circulation
Pulmonary atresia/stenosis
Tetralogy of Fallot with pulmonary atresia
Tricuspid atresia
Ebstein's anomaly
Heart disease with duct-dependent systemic circulation
Coarctation of the aorta
Hypoplastic left ventricle
Hypoplastic aortic arch
Heart disease with duct-dependent mixed circulation
Transposition of the great arteries

For example,

In *pulmonary atresia* (duct-dependent pulmonary circulation), the lung receives blood solely from the aorta via the ductus arteriosus.

In *critical coarctation of the aorta* (duct-dependent systemic circulation), blood supply to the lower half of the body mainly comes from the pulmonary artery through the ductus arteriosus. The blood in the pulmonary artery is deoxygenated, so the oxygen saturation in the feet ('post-ductal') will be lower than the oxygen saturation in the right hand ('pre-ductal').

Continued survival of these babies requires infusion of prostaglandin E_1 or E_2 to keep the duct open until urgent cardiac surgery can be performed.

What are the intraoperative goals when you anaesthetise a child with TOF for non-cardiac surgery?

(Key points: pre- and post-ductal saturation monitoring and keeping ductus arteriosus patent)

- Appropriate centre carrying out paediatric and cardiothoracic surgery
- Invasive monitoring including pre- and post-ductal saturations
- Avoid hypothermia, hypoglycaemia and hypovolemia
- Avoid duct closure by
  - preventing hypoxia
  - avoiding rises in SVR and surges in blood pressure
  - avoiding NSAIDS
  - prostaglandin administration

What does the medical and surgical management of TOF involve?

Medical treatment: hypercyanotic spells can be treated with propranolol to reduce the spasm of the sub-pulmonary infundibulum.

If right ventricular outflow obstruction is severe, then a palliative shunt may be required, or corrective surgery expedited.

Surgical management

Palliative shunt: this is usually with a modified Blalock–Taussig shunt, directing blood from the subclavian artery to the pulmonary artery, allowing blood to flow to the lungs to receive oxygen, thus functioning like a patent ductus arteriosus.

Corrective surgery: complete repair consists of two main steps – closure of the VSD with a patch and reconstruction of the right ventricular outflow tract on cardiopulmonary bypass. It is ideally performed in the first year of life, usually at 4–6 months of age. It is important to manage a hypercyanotic spell to reduce infundibular spasm, improve oxygenation and increase cardiac output.

Cyanosis intraoperatively is treated with

- Supplementary oxygen
- Intravenous fluid boluses

- Deepen anaesthesia and/or fentanyl bolus
- Phenylephrine boluses or noradrenaline infusion to increase SVR
- Esmolol infusion to reduce infundibular spasm

Bibliography

Hepburn, L., & Kelleher, A. A. (2009). Grown-up congenital heart disease. *Anaesthesia & Intensive Care Medicine, 10*(9), 451–456.

Murphy, P. J. (2005). The fetal circulation. *Continuing Education in Anaesthesia, Critical Care & Pain, 5*(4), 107–112.

Walker, I. (2004). anaesthesia for non-cardiac surgery in children with congenital heart disease. Special Edition, 46.

Bone Circulation

How do you assess for dehydration in a child? What do you do if intravenous access fails?

Alternative opening question

What is the anatomy of the interosseous (IO) space? (Opening question specifically framed this way to see candidates' response to an unexpected enquiry.)

Anatomy of the interosseous (IO) space (Figure 7.16)

The epiphysis of long bones is the typical insertion site for IO access. The three main layers are

1. Periosteum – the outermost layer that surrounds the bone.
2. Cortical bone – the middle layer, which is heavily mineralised and contains a network of blood vessels. The Haversian canals are vertical channels for blood vessels and nerves found on the outermost region of cortical bone and are connected by horizontal Volkmann canals. Concentric layers (lamellae) containing osteophytes surround the Haversian canals and interconnections between the channels and osteophytes are called canaliculi.
3. Cancellous bone – the innermost layer and consists of multiple trabeculae in a lattice-like structure. The space between the trabeculae contains blood vessels and bone marrow. With correct placement, the tip of the IO needle lies within the cancellous bone.

How do you assess for dehydration in a child?

Assessment of dehydration in a child depends on their age and degree of dehydration. A structured approach would include history, examination and investigations.

- History is key to elicit reduced oral intake and sources of excessive fluid loss such as diarrhoea and vomiting
- Examination would include skin turgor, sunken eyes/fontanelles, evidence of tachycardia and hypotension (a late sign), reduced urine output and with a reduction in consciousness (a very late sign)
- Investigations may reveal hypernatraemia, a raised urea and haematocrit

How would you define failed intravenous access? What do you do in such a case?

The definition of failed IV access refers to either two to three attempts at cannulation or greater than 90 seconds to establish IV access. In this situation, IO should be attempted (Resus Council, 2015).

What are the layers encountered whilst performing an IO access?

Layers punctured from outside to inside would include

1. Skin
2. Subcutaneous tissue
3. Periosteum
4. Cortical bone
5. Cancellous bone

Can you explain in detail the blood supply of the medullary cavity?

The medullary cavity is the central cavity that contains bone marrow. Within long bones, it is usually located in the diaphysis (long bone shaft).

The arterial supply is from the *nutrient arteries* that enter the diaphysis, through a specific foramen. Within the medullary cavity the nutrient arteries divide into ascending and descending branches, which further subdivide into epiphyseal and metaphyseal arteries. Together they supply a capillary bed in all three layers of the bone, which allows nutrients to be delivered.

In the cortical bone this is via the Haversian canals and Volkmann canals. The *Haversian canals* contain blood vessels in the centre of the osteon, and the *Volkmann canals* are perpendicular to allow blood vessels to reach between different osteons in cortical bone. Since the IO needle tip sits in the cancellous bone most of the drugs injected bypass the Haversian and Volkmann canals.

The venous drainage from the sinusoids is into a central venous sinus that runs the length of the diaphysis and leaves the bone via the nutrient vein into the systemic venous system.

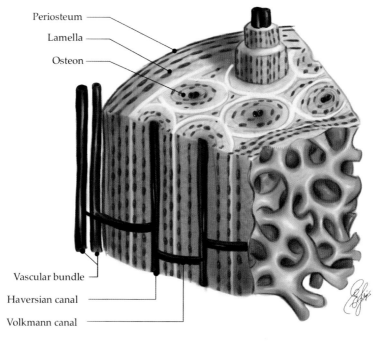

Figure 7.16   Bone circulation.

Tell me about the intraosseous needle. What does it look like?

There are several different types of IO needles and devices available. These can be classified into three subtypes

1. Manual trocar – needles are screwed into the medullary canal
2. Spring-loaded devices – to reduce the force required to penetrate the medullary canal
3. Drill-based devices – battery powered drill (e.g. EZ-IO™ drill)

The EZ-IO™ drill is commonly used in the UK and taught on both adult and paediatric resuscitation courses.

Each needle set has a catheter with a Luer lock system, stylet and a safety cap. They are all 15G, made from stainless steel and are available in various sizes with 10 mm markings on the needle.

- 15 mm (pink) for 3–39 kgs/paediatrics
- 25 mm (blue) for >39 kgs/adults
- 45 mm (yellow) for >40 kgs in adults (presence of excessive tissue or for humeral access)

What are the indications for IO access?

In any adult or paediatric patient who is shocked, where peripheral IV access is difficult or impossible. This is defined as greater than 90 seconds or two to three attempts at cannulation of peripheral vein. Given the speed, success rate and availability of IO devices, emergency central venous access is less frequently attempted outside specialist settings, for example ICU or theatres.

What are the contraindications for its use?

Absolute

- Bone trauma including fractures and previous IO attempts (within 48 hours) in the target bone
- Infection overlying insertion point
- Patient refusal
- Lack of skilled operator

Relative

- Prosthesis in target limb – interference with injectables and risk of infection
- Bone disease – osteomyelitis, osteoporosis, osteogenesis imperfecta
- Difficulty assessing landmarks
- Coagulopathy

What are the sites of insertion for IO access?

- Proximal humerus
  - 1 cm above the greater tubercle
  - The patient's palm should be kept on their abdomen with the elbow adducted

- Greatest flow rates up to 5 L/min and quickest time for medications entering the systemic circulation
- Proximal tibia
  - Two finger breadths below the patella and 1–2 cm medial to the tibial tuberosity in adults
- Distal tibia
  - 3 cm proximal to the most prominent aspect of the medial malleolus
- Femoral
  - Anterolateral surface, 3 cm above lateral condyle
- Iliac crest
- Sternum

What is the point of insertion on proximal tibia?

2 cm below patella and 2 cm medial to the tibial tuberosity. It is performed on the medial side due to the proximity of the common peroneal nerve wrapping around the head of the fibula on the lateral aspect risking nerve injury. The medial side of the proximal tibia is also an easier landmark to palpate.

How do you confirm position?

- Aspiration of bone marrow (not always obtained)
- Secure position – it should feel 'fixed'
- During insertion the cortical bone provides a high degree of resistance, but once the softer cancellous bone is reached, there should be a 'give' or loss of resistance
- No evidence of subcutaneous swelling or pain on injection
- X-ray confirmation if necessary

How are drugs and fluid given? What drugs can be given?

Once position is confirmed, secure the IO needle with the supplied dressing. Connect a three-way tap and pressured fluid bag. Fluid boluses will need to be given under pressure, and medication with a 20 ml flush.

All resuscitation drugs and fluids can be given via IO.

There are no drugs contraindicated via the IO route, with the greatest research carried out on the pharmacokinetics of resuscitation drugs. Certain medication may not reach the same peak plasma concentrations as IV administration (e.g. ceftriaxone, vancomycin, phenytoin). Drugs with significant side effects if extravasated, such as amiodarone, need to be carefully considered when taking this route.

What problems can occur on injecting some drugs?

- Pain – 1 or 2% lignocaine can be injected before drugs
- Problems with extravasation – e.g. amiodarone
- Decreased peak plasma concentrations with certain drugs as above
- Infection (osteomyelitis)

- Compartment syndrome
- Embolisation
- Dislodgement
- Skin necrosis

Once you have performed IO access, how long can you leave it in for?

Up to 48 hours and until an alternative, more permanent access is established. IO needles require the same care and assessment as intravenous devices and may need to be removed before 48 hours if necessary.

How will you diagnose compartment syndrome?

Compartment syndrome is a clinical diagnosis. It should be suspected in patients presenting with pain that is disproportionally high in the affected limb. As the intracompartment pressure increases, further neurovascular compromise occurs which is a late sign. Normal pressure is between 0–10 mmHg and ischaemia can occur at >30 mmHg. If compartment syndrome is suspected, stop using the IO device and measure the compartment pressure. This is a time-critical emergency as irreversible neurovascular injury can occur 4–8 hours after the onset of symptoms.

Treatment is usually surgical with fasciotomies to relieve compartment syndrome.

Bibliography

Bradburn, S., Gill, S., & Doane, M. (2015). Understanding and establishing intraosseous access. *World Federation of Societies of Anaesthesiologists*, 1–8.

EZ-IO – www.teleflex.com/vascular-access

Soar, J., Nolan, J. P., Böttiger, B. W., Perkins, G. D., Lott, C., Carli, P et al. (2015). European resuscitation council guidelines for resuscitation 2015: section 3. Adult advanced life support. *Resuscitation, 95*, 100–147.

Anatomical Differences between Paediatric and Adult Airway

'A child is not a small adult, but you are still an anaesthetist.'

Anonymous

There are significant differences between the adult and paediatric airways. As an airway management specialist, it is important to have knowledge of the anatomical, physiological and pathological features related to the airway, as well as knowledge of the various tools and methods that have been developed for this purpose (Table 7.20).

Table 7.20   Anatomical Differences Between the Paediatric and Adult Airways

Paediatric Anatomy	Airway management
Large head and a prominent occiput	Shoulder roll (support placed under the shoulder) to enable neutral position and prevent airway obstruction
Short neck and prominent occiput	Poor laryngoscopy views
Short trachea	Appropriately sized endotracheal tubes
Omega-shaped epiglottis	Use of straight blade laryngoscope (Miller) which lifts epiglottis directly out of view
Obligate nasal breathers, large tongue, large adenoids and tonsils – all these factors reduce upper airway space and predispose to difficult mask ventilation and rapid desaturation	Vigilance and awareness of rapidity of desaturation. Reduce periods of circuit disconnection and avoid hypoxic gas mixtures.
Location of cricoid cartilage • C4 at birth • C5 by age 6 • C6 in adults MRI and bronchoscopic views have found the glottic opening to be smaller than the cricoid. But the indistensibility of the cricoid makes it narrow functionally. Elliptical shape of cricoid ring – largest in the antero-posterior diameter	Cricoid cartilage is functionally the narrowest part of the paediatric airway which may mean that an endotracheal tube that passes easily though the vocal cords may not be small enough to pass through the cricoid ring. The elliptical cricoid ring affects the seal of cuffed and uncuffed endotracheal tubes and may guide selection of tracheal tubes.
Larynx is higher in the neck than in adults	In some positions, the mandible may lie in line with the upper glottic structures.
Highly compressible/compliant airway structures	The compliant cartilaginous tracheal rings can predispose to dynamic obstruction with negative pressure ventilation, especially with partial airway obstruction. There is a risk of breaching the posterior tracheal wall during needle cricothyroidotomy. Experts therefore suggest that direct approach to surgical cricothyroidotomy is likely to be ideal.

Bibliography

Harless, J., Ramaiah, R., & Bhananker, S. M. (2014). Pediatric airway management. *International journal of critical illness and injury science, 4*(1), 65–70. doi:10.4103/2229-5151.12801

Index

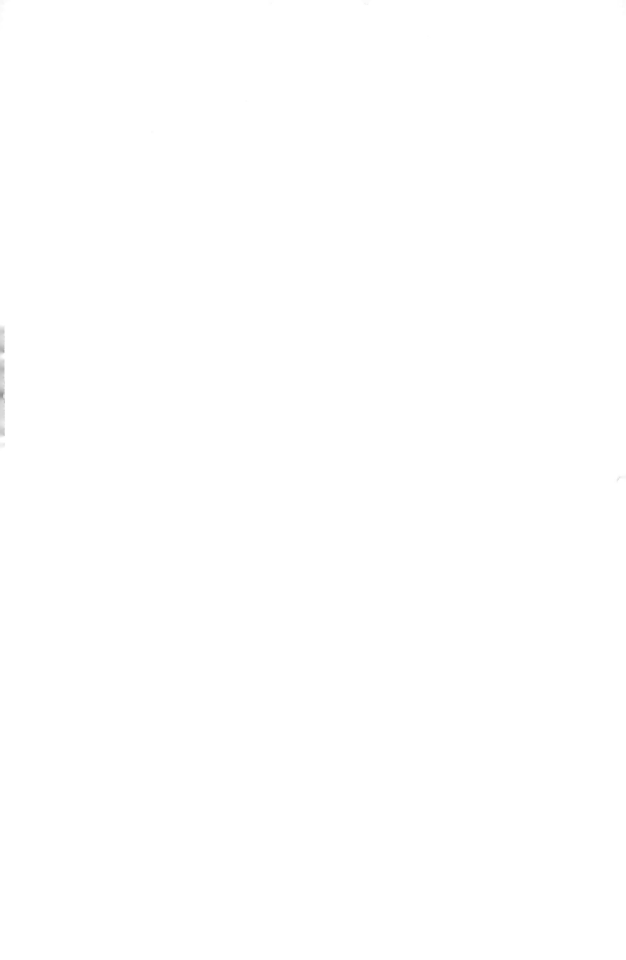